YOU

Having a Baby

The Owner's Manual to a Happy and Healthy Pregnancy

MICHAEL F. ROIZEN, MD
AND MEHMET C. OZ, MD

with Ted Spiker, Craig Wynett, Lisa Oz, Linda G. Kahn,
and Margaret L. McKenzie, MD

Illustrations by Gary Hallgren

Free Press

NEW YORK   LONDON   TORONTO   SYDNEY

Free Press
A Division of Simon & Schuster, Inc.
1230 Avenue of the Americas
New York, NY 10020

First Free Press trade paperback edition December 2010

FREE PRESS and colophon are trademarks of Simon & Schuster, Inc.

For information about special discounts for bulk purchases,
please contact Simon & Schuster Special Sales at
1-866-506-1949 or business@simonandschuster.com

The Simon & Schuster Speakers Bureau can bring authors to your live event.
For more information or to book an event contact the Simon & Schuster Speakers Bureau
at 1-866-248-3049 or visit our website at www.simonspeakers.com.

Designed by Ruth Lee-Mui

Manufactured in the United States of America

3   5   7   9   10   8   6   4   2

The Library of Congress cataloged the hardcover edition as follows:

Roizen, Michael F.
You : having a baby : the owner's manual to a happy and healthy pregnancy /
by Michael F. Roizen, and Mehmet C. Oz ; with Ted Spiker . . . [et al.] ;
illustrations by Gary Hallgren.
p.   cm.
1. Pregnancy—Popular works.   2. Childbirth—Popular works.
I. Oz, Mehmet, 1960–   II. Title.
RG525.R665   2009
618.2—dc22   2009024107

ISBN 978-1-4165-7236-7
ISBN 978-1-4165-7237-4 (pbk)
ISBN 978-1-4165-7240-4 (ebook)

NOTE TO READERS

This publication contains the opinions and ideas of its authors. It is intended to provide helpful and informative material on the subjects addressed in the publication. It is sold with the understanding that the authors and publisher are not engaged in rendering medical, health, or any kind of personal professional services in the book. The reader should consult his or her medical, health, or other competent professional before adopting any of the suggestions in this book or drawing inferences from it.

In addition, this book sometimes recommends particular products, websites, or other reference materials. Drs. Oz and Roizen are not affiliated in any way with such products or material or the entities sponsoring them with the exception of the Real Age website and doctoroz.com, and an algal DHA product (for which Dr. Roizen heads the scientific advisory board). In all instances, bear in mind that there are many products, websites, and reference materials other than those recommended here that may be useful to you.

The authors and publisher specifically disclaim all responsibility for any liability, loss, or risk, personal or otherwise, which is incurred as a consequence, directly or indirectly, of the use and application of any of the contents of this book.

To mothers, who bring life into the world, and their babies, who are the future

CONTENTS

Appendixes

Hey, You! Having a Baby?

Stand at the edge of the Grand Canyon, and your body rockets into sensory overload. Your eyes widen, your jaw drops, and your neurons spit out more adjectives than a novice novelist. Majestic, awe inspiring, glorious, astonishing, so my-oh-my beautiful that you want to fall to your knees and bow to the deity that created this masterpiece.

Then you freak out.

That, in essence, is pregnancy: On one hand, it's the most breathtaking thing you've ever experienced. On the other, it's a *looooong* way to the bottom of the canyon, just as it is a *looooong* way from conception to birth—so you can't help but have some anxiety about taking a wrong step along the way. There's no doubt that pregnancy evokes a similar diversity of emotional and physiological responses as do such natural wonders: laughing, crying, screaming, dry mouth, dry skin, dry heaves (and that's just the first day). What we're here to do is help you manage both extremes of the emotional spectrum, so you can appreciate such a miraculous process and conquer the anxiety and tension through a very powerful weapon: knowledge.

Whether this is your first pregnancy or your fourth, or you're trying so hard that you're spending more time on your bed than a throw pillow, you probably think you know a thing or two about being pregnant. Either you've gone through it before or you've had friends, sisters, and sixteen trillion baby bloggers to give you the inside-the-womb scoop.

However, we'd ask that you hold on one diaper-changing minute. We're here to bust myths, challenge your brain, and prepare your body for the greatest journey that any human can ever take—from the moment two cells become one to the second that your little squirt makes its first appearance outside the comforting shell of your belly.

To whet your appetite, we'd bet a case of Gerber bananas that you didn't know things like:

- The whole notion of nature versus nurture is as wrong as a three-legged crib. That's because a cutting-edge field called epigenetics has shown us that you have control over how the genes of your baby will express themselves.
- What happens during these 280 days on the inside actually teaches your child about how his body should act on the outside. He's actually forecasting his future—and that teaches him how healthy or unhealthy he will be years down the road.
- While most people assume that a mom's biological cocoon supports the child unconditionally, the truth is that your body is actually engaged in a very delicate dance to balance the often competing needs of mom and child.
- There's a biological reason why your areolas are dark, why your feet swell, and why one minute you gag at the thought of eating a cracker and the next minute you can't wait to get your hands on a salsa-smothered cantaloupe.

The good news is that we're here to help by teaching you crazy-cool things about your body and giving you the tools to maximize your experience and get the result you want: a healthy and happy baby.

Now, if you're like most women, we're guessing that you've already spent a lot of time thinking about what's in store. You've probably spent all-nighters scouring pregnancy websites and parked yourself in cushy bookstore chairs with thigh-high stacks of mom-to-be manuals. Maybe you haven't been this nervous since your sixth-grade oral report on rain forests, or maybe you haven't been this obsessed with something since McDreamy made his prime-time debut a few years back. You're probably poring over baby names, wondering why you crave pretzels dipped in marinara sauce, and debating about whether the nursery walls should have the hue of sunshine, cotton candy, or pomegranate juice.

Nope, there's nothing quite like this internal conflict that is pregnancy. One moment, you're thrilled, elated, and impatient for your baby's first smile, babble, and soothe-your-soul hug. The next, you feel anxious about a million unknowns—about what's going on inside your belly, about whether your little one is growing properly, about how you're going to function on zippo sleep. Since this happens to just about everyone, it must, in fact, be strangely ideal. The truth is that vigilance has great benefits. You're supposed to pay close attention. Our goal is to ensure that you focus on the right clues.

As you struggle to maintain your equilibrium, we want you to relax and take time to enjoy the beauty of the process. The most important thing to keep in mind is that most pregnancies turn out absolutely fine. *Absolutely fine.* Women's bodies are designed to carry children safely and efficiently. That doesn't mean everything will be smooth sailing on this journey, but it does mean that the odds are greatly in your favor. If you can learn how to maximize your chances that nature runs the course it's supposed to, you will increase those odds even further. This book will help show you how.

Introducing Your New Dance Partner

So let's start by rethinking our perception about conception (and beyond). Back in sex-ed class, most of us were taught a pretty simple recipe for how pregnancy works:

Ingredients
1 egg, mature
100 million sperm, very, very excited

Instructions
Preheat oven. Mix ingredients romantically. Cook bun for forty weeks. Sprinkle with love and serve to the world.

The bun-in-the-oven image has served us well over the years, underscoring the belief that mom is protector and baby is protected, that mom is cook and baby is concoction, that mom is in control and baby is not. But there's a fundamental problem with this analogy when it comes to the true biology of pregnancy (besides the fact that nobody bakes buns anymore): Baby has a heck of a lot more say about the whole process than a cinnamon raisin roll does.

In fact, pregnancy is more like dancing than cooking. You and your baby have a dynamic, choreographed relationship—one in which you lead and the baby follows. Your subtle movements and directions help show your baby how to grow and develop. After all, it takes two to tango, or in pregnancy terms, it's uter-*us,* not uter-*I.*

But your baby isn't always the most cooperative partner. Sometimes he'll want to take the lead, sometimes he'll send you signals about which way he wants you to move, sometimes he'll improvise, sometimes he'll do flips, and sometimes he'll step on your feet and get everything all tangled up. Part of the reason he'll act this way is that your body has a certain amount of biological ambivalence about this little cellular critter; after all, only half his genes are yours. Your relationship with him isn't exactly hostile, but it's not always warm and fuzzy either. Even at this young age, he's going to try to assert himself, and your body may try to resist. There are evolutionary reasons for this, which we'll discuss in the pages to come, but you can also think of these initial rebellious acts as practice for the years ahead.

Pregnancy can be as elegant as a waltz, as high-energy as a salsa, and as scattered as a twist (with a whole lot of shouting). Our main goal in *YOU: Having a Baby* is to teach you about this ingenious biological dance—a dance in which you have the ability and the artistry to guide your baby not only to a healthy delivery, but to a lifetime of good health as well.

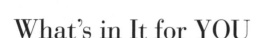

What's in It for YOU

While many pregnancy books tell you *what* to do, we aim to add a deeper level of meaning in true *YOU* style and explain *why*. After all, when you truly understand the *why*, the *what* is much easier to adopt. Instead of giving you a week-by-week or hiccup-by-hiccup guide to pregnancy, we're going to take a more holistic approach, focusing on how your mental and physical health affect your baby, and how—at the same time—pregnancy affects *your* mind and body. Of course, we'll provide plenty of our signature YOU Tips and YOU Tools to help you make the best choices for a safe and healthy pregnancy, but we're going to take you there a little bit differently than other pregnancy guides may. Here's what you can expect★ from us:

We want you to understand at the base level how epigenetics works and why it's important. Starting with the moment you go from making love to making a baby,† we're going to explain how you can influence your child's development through this field—perhaps the most important developed in the last decade. Many of us believe that the genetics of our children are predetermined the moment that the sperm radar locks on its desired egg. But the truth is that research from various sources is suggesting that during pregnancy, you may actually be able to turn your future baby's genes

---

★ That book is two shelves over.

† In this day and age, of course, traditional intercourse isn't the only way to make a baby.

on and off. Epigenetics is not just how the musical notes of our genes are played but also how loud the volume is turned up. Since the acoustics in the womb and the real world might be different, we want these as aligned as possible. And that's where all the magic takes place, no matter where you are in pregnancy or in parenthood. You have the ability to control genes anytime.

You're also going to learn quite a bit about the key player that mediates between you and your baby, transmitting all the signals that create those epigenetic changes. That player, which gets about as much attention as a dollar bill on a blackjack table, is the placenta. This beautifully functioning organ is the place where mom and child interact, where nutrients are exchanged, and where growth and development patterns are determined.

After explaining the workings of the placenta, we'll focus more closely on nutrition (both yours and baby's), explaining how too much, too little, or the wrong nutrients all play roles in the health of both you and your child. Here you'll discover why the thought of food makes you green on some days, while other days you long for an artichoke-heart milk shake. We'll also talk about such things as fetal brain development, how to manage (and prevent) postpartum depression, and important pregnancy-related medical conditions like gestational diabetes.

In the second half of the book, we'll help you manage the wide range of side effects you may be feeling—everything from heartburn and insomnia to medical complications like preeclampsia. Finally, we're going to present a bunch of great features you can use, including:

Broadway to Birth: Our cool, interactive board game will take you through the amazing adventure that is labor and delivery to help you understand which elements you can control and which elements you need to leave to the pros (whom we'll help you choose, based on your own labor and delivery goals).

A Top Eight List of Postpartum Issues: And after you deliver your baby, you'll appreciate our chapter on everything you need to know to take care of yourself and your newborn in the first month of life. This is where the second adventure begins.

The Ultimate Pregnancy Flight Plan: Step by step, we provide the instructional dials, controls, and levers that will allow you to pilot your way to a safe landing. After all, you're carrying a very precious passenger. This plan is the shorthand version of all the best tips and strategies we give throughout the book.

YOU Tools: At the end of the book, we will give you specific advice about exercise, diet, vitamins, and the like that should serve as an action plan not only for pregnant women, but really for all potentially fertile women (that's because 50 percent of pregnancies are unplanned, and the actions you can take for your baby can start at least three months before sperm and egg mate). We also provide guidance on everything from choosing a doctor or midwife to preparing your home for a baby to recipes your partner can make for you during your pregnancy.

Yeah, Baby!

Before you get to most of the features at the end of the book, we think it's helpful to really understand the way the pregnant body works—and remember, it's your whole body that's pregnant, not just your belly. Woven throughout the book, you'll see several major themes that reflect our overall view of pregnancy:

- Your body is an amazingly resilient and adaptive piece of biological machinery. The size of your belly and the stretching of your skin aren't the only changes that occur during pregnancy: Your insides are metamorphosing too. Your heart beats faster to make sure nutrients are pumped to the fetus. Your hormone levels fluctuate to prepare your uterus for growth. Your musculo-skeletal system relaxes, giving you more flexible joints and more curvature in the back to prepare for carrying and delivering a baby. All these transformations mean that you may experience some unpleasant side effects (like constipation, for example). What's interesting is that there's an adaptive value to many of the symptoms of pregnancy, so that the nausea, breathlessness, and aching back you might feel, evolutionarily speaking, serve some value in protecting the growth of your child.

- The goal of pregnancy isn't just to deliver a healthy baby but to lay the foundation for lifelong good health for your child—not to mention that of his children and grandchildren. That's the amazing thing about epigenetics. Once you see some of the long-term effects you can have on the health of your child while you're pregnant, you'll realize that it's important to start this process with the end goal in mind. We like to call it reverse engineering.

One of the ways that you can increase your chances for a successful pregnancy is to learn as much as you can about what's happening, so you won't be anxious. Simply educating yourself about what's going on in your body is one of the smartest things you can do, because it allows you to roll with the punches rather than get KO'd by every little symptom or complication. In fact, staying calm during pregnancy has repeatedly been shown to have a positive influence on your child's health.

So we want you to take the pressure off of yourself and not to try to do it alone. The key is to have some support, regardless of whether you're married (about 40 percent of children are born out of wedlock), in a relationship, or flying solo. Your mother, sisters, friends, or even the internet buddies you meet on pregnancy websites can all become part of your support system. One of the features that has always distinguished human beings is that pregnant women have relied on other women in their communities to support them. Today, social support has been linked to improved fetal growth. (Those cavewomen knew what was good for them.)

In a way, managing your pregnancy really comes down to one overarching goal: managing stress. We're not just talking about stress management in the traditional bubble-bath kind of way, but in the big-picture kind of way. How does your body cope with the stress of housing and growing what's essentially a biological hitchhiker? How does your baby adapt to potentially stressful situations that he'll face in utero? ("Jalapeño attack, nine o'clock!") How do you calm your mind in the face of the normal and natural anxieties that often arise during these nine months? How do you tell your mother-in-law that, no offense, but you prefer not to name your child Horatio Horace Humphrey?★

That's exactly why we developed the ultimate pregnancy quality-of-life and stress quizzes. You can take them now (in this book or online at www.realage.com), as well as at various points throughout the next nine months, to see how you're coping with all of the outside influences on your pregnancy.

Although neither of us has actually experienced pregnancy (obviously), between the two of us, we've fathered six children, and if you include our entire authorship team (half of whom are women, including an ob/gyn), we've had fifteen kids and delivered or participated in the delivery of more than eight thousand little tykes. So we have a pretty good idea of what it feels like to walk in your soon-to-be-too-tight shoes.

If you're pregnant right now, we want to offer both congratulations and thanks. Thank you for letting us join you on this journey, and thank you for having the curiosity and passion for learning about what's going on under the surface, under the skin, under the elastic-waistband pants you'll soon be needing. As we step out into our exploration of this miraculous mambo, we would be impolite if we didn't ask one final question: Would you like to dance?

★ Apologies to anyone named Horatio Horace Humphrey.

Pregnancy YOU-Q:
Your Quality of Life Quiz

When somebody puts the words *pregnancy* and *test* in the same sentence, you expect to read about a little stick that gives you a yes or no, pregnant or not. We're betting this pregnancy test is like none you've ever taken. For one thing, it isn't going to give you an A or an F, a pass or a fail. This test is about something bigger: about understanding yourself and all the experiences that make up pregnancy. Some are exciting, some are stressful, and some may even be a bit painful.

This test is designed to help you get a sense of how you're experiencing your pregnancy: how you feel about yourself, your journey, and the promise of parenthood. We will give you an overall score at the end of the test that will serve as a beacon to help you navigate that journey and guide your ship to calmer waters.

Take the test as often as you like, especially as your grow and learn about yourself during these nine months. Your score may change along the way—and that's because you will too.

YOUR Quality of Life: Sex

Answer each of the following questions on a scale of 1 to 5, 5 being this is Very True of Me:

		Not at All True of Me 1	2	3	4	Very True of Me 5
1	I am not that interested in sex with my partner.					
2	I worry that my partner will lose interest in me sexually because I am pregnant.					

Now check the box that best describes your feelings about this statement:

	Much More Than 1	Somewhat More Than 2	About the Same As 3	Somewhat Less Than 4	Much Less Than 5
3 My interest in sex is _____ it was before I got pregnant.					

Sex Score

For this test, add up your scores for each question.

This score should range between 3 and 15.

Interpreting Your Score

Your interest in sex will change somewhat during the course of pregnancy. In the first trimester, you're likely to feel generally ill, not sexy. The middle trimester is the one in which most women report feeling best, so your interest in sex may go up again. By the third trimester, changes in your body and worries about hurting the baby may decrease your interest in sex again.

Keeping that in mind, if your score is:

3 to 6: Your interest in sex may actually have gone up since you got pregnant. Hooray for hormones! Remember that your body is going to change a lot over the course of pregnancy, and your interest in sex may vary during that time.

7 to 11: Your interest in sex is about what it was before you got pregnant. All of those changes in your body haven't dampened your sexuality. Enjoy.

12 to 15: You're showing less interest in sex than you may be used to. Don't be too hard on yourself. Your body is going through a lot of changes. If you are feeling a much lower interest in sex even during the second trimester, you might want to check out our strategies for adding sensuality into your life, starting on page 172.

YOUR Quality of Life: Cognitive

Answer each of the following questions on a scale of 1 to 5, 5 being this is Very True of Me:

	Not at All True of Me 1	2	3	4	Very True of Me 5
1 I have a lot of difficulty making decisions.					
2 I have difficulty remembering things, even for a short period of time.					
3 I have difficulty concentrating for more than a few minutes at a time.					

Cognitive Score

For this test, add up all of your scores.

This score should range between 3 and 15.

Interpreting Your Score

There seems to be little that is helpful about difficulties making decisions, remembering, and concentrating, particularly for women who are trying to maintain a high level of job performance during pregnancy. As frustrating as these experiences may be, think of them as evidence of the transformative power of pregnancy. Plus, they may be good for a few laughs when it's all over.

If your score is:

3 to 6 : Congratulations. Even though you're pregnant, you're sharp as a cat's claw. Somehow, being pregnant has given you laser focus.

7 to 11: Chances are, you're having a few lapses in thinking. You may feel more indecisive than you did before you got pregnant, and you may have more trouble remembering things than usual. That's quite normal during pregnancy, though it can be annoying.

12 to 15: You seem to be having a lot of trouble thinking since you got pregnant. Some moderate thinking problems are quite common in pregnancy. If you feel that you have slipped quite a bit, then you need to review aspects of your lifestyle. Are you eating properly? Are you getting enough sleep? If you have other kids already, are you getting some help taking care of them?

YOUR Quality of Life: Craving and Appetite

Answer each of the following questions on a scale of 1 to 5, 5 being this is Very True of Me:

	Not at All True of Me 1	2	3	4	Very True of Me 5
1 I find that I can eat only foods that I used to eat before I was pregnant, and no new foods.					
2 I find that there are times when I am highly interested in a particular food.					
3 I feel like I am eating less than I did before I was pregnant.					
4 I am eating mostly foods that are not nutritious.					
5 I am experiencing a lot of nausea now that I am pregnant.					

Craving and Appetite Score

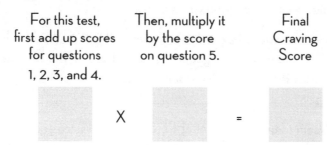

For this test, first add up scores for questions 1, 2, 3, and 4.

Then, multiply it by the score on question 5.

Final Craving Score

X   =

This score should range between 4 and 100.

Interpreting Your Score

During pregnancy, it's crucial that you get good nutrition. Your body is working overtime to keep up your energy and to help you build the brain and body of your developing baby. Pregnancy is not necessarily a time to be adventurous about food. Indeed, in evolutionary terms, there is probably good reason to eat only the foods that you've eaten successfully in the past. Morning sickness actually evolved as a protective adaptation. Early in pregnancy, your body is protecting your baby from anything that might be harmful to it. Still, even if you are experiencing a lot of nausea, you need to do your best to feed your baby and to take your prenatal vitamins.

If your score is:

4 to 30: You are probably eating fairly well. Do keep track of how much you're eating and focus on foods that will give you energy and also help your developing baby. If you do experience some nausea, remember that it is quite normal. See our plan in chapter 3 to help you figure out your diet and do your best to provide your baby with the building blocks for a healthy brain and body. And don't forget your vitamins.

31 to 50: Nausea is affecting your eating. You may not be making the best choices about your food, so it's important to listen to your body. At the same time, there may be simple changes you can make to your diet that will make you feel a bit better and will give your baby the nutrients needed for development. See chapter 3 to help you plan your diet. And don't forget your vitamins.

51 to 70: You're experiencing moderate nausea, which is affecting the way you eat. In addition, you may be having some cravings. It might be time to make a few midcourse corrections and to work on your diet to give your baby the nutrients needed for healthy brain and body development. Chapter 3 will give you some great suggestions to get started. And don't forget your vitamins.

71 to 100: Nausea is having a huge effect on what you eat. Pregnancy can be hard on your body and on your frame of mind. It's hard to think happy thoughts with your head in the toilet bowl. If you're in your first trimester, remember that that's when the nausea is usually worst. If you can get through it, you can face anything. You'll need to make the best choices you can about foods. See chapter 3 to help plan your diet. And don't forget your vitamins.

YOUR Quality of Life: Body Image

Answer the following questions about your feelings in the *last four weeks* (using the scale indicated)

	Never 1	Rarely 2	Some-times 3	Often 4	Very Often 5	Always 6
1 Are you so worried about your body shape that you feel you ought to be on a diet?						
2 Has being with women who are not pregnant made you feel self-conscious about your shape?						
3 Has eating even a small amount of food made you feel fat?						
4 Has thinking about your shape interfered with your ability to concentrate?						
5 Has being naked (such as when taking a bath) made you feel fat?						

		Never	Rarely	Some-times	Often	Very Often	Always
		1	2	3	4	5	6
6	Have you felt ashamed of your body?						
7	Have you been particularly conscious about your shape when in the company of other people?						
8	Has worry about your shape made you feel you ought to exercise?						

Body Image Score

For this test, add up all of your scores.

You should have a number between 8 and 48.

Interpreting Your Score

8 to 16: You don't seem to be at all worried about your body. In many ways, that is good. Make sure, though, that you are still keeping in shape. Eat balanced meals and nutritious foods. Exercise is good for you and for your baby. See page 310 for our exercise plan.

17 to 32: You have a small amount of concern about your body image, but it is not excessive. Pregnancy is a time of changes in your body. At the same time, you do need to make sure to take care of your body. A healthy body is good for you and your baby, and it will make it easier for you to have a body you like after you give birth. Make sure that you eat balanced meals and nutritious foods. Remember that exercise is good for you and for your baby.

33 to 48: You have quite a bit of concern about your body. It's really crucial that you exercise during pregnancy and that you eat balanced, nutritious meals. You are eating for you and for your baby. It is possible that you have gained too much weight and that your doctor may recommend ways to help solve any problems that have come up. However, it is also possible that your weight gain is quite normal. (See page 68 for guidelines for gaining weight.)

YOUR Quality of Life: Overall Score

To get a sense of how you're doing overall right now, we're going to create a total score for Quality of Life. Enter the scores from the four tests that make up the Quality of Life survey in the boxes as shown below.

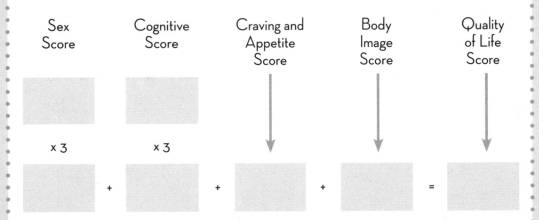

This score ranges between 30 and 238.

On many tests, you aim to get the highest score possible. This test is a little different. When your Quality of Life score is low (close to 30), your life is in balance.

Trying to maintain your quality-of-life balance during pregnancy is a bit like trying to walk on a four-inch-wide gymnastics balance beam with your pregnant body. It's not as easy as it looks, and it doesn't look easy. It is also possible you have not gained enough weight and are overly concerned about your own shape without attending to what your baby may need. If that describes you, see your OB as soon as possible, and perhaps a nutritionist, to make sure you are not underfeeding the baby unintentionally.

So most people are probably not perfectly in balance. Remember that for every gymnast who nails a perfect routine on the balance beam at the Olympics, there are hundreds who slip a little or even fall flat. The trick is just to keep getting up there and trying to balance again.

Interpreting Your Overall Score

30 to 70: Congratulations! You have achieved some real balance in your pregnant life. There's still a lot ahead of you, but you're quite centered so far.

71 to 150: Like most pregnant women, there are days when you have it together and days when things seem beyond your grasp. Keep on reading. We have a lot of tips to help keep you centered.

151 to 238: Between your nausea, your inability to think straight, and your negative feelings about your body, you're probably looking at pregnancy as more like a never-ending traffic jam than an Olympic gymnastics event. All the same, you're in the middle of one of life's peak experiences. We have a lot of tips here to make your worst days more bearable. Hang in there, and read on.

Part 1

YOU-ology

How Two Became YOU

1

Nice Genes

A New Twist on Genetics Teaches Us
How a Baby Really Develops

*B*ack in tenth-grade biology class, you were probably taught—as were we—that the unique combination of genes you received from your mom and dad (your genotype) was responsible for everything that followed: the color of your eyes, the size of your feet, your love of lasagna, your hatred for all eight-legged and no-legged creatures. To a certain extent, that's true, but over the past few years, studies have suggested that classical genetics may be only part of the picture. It's not just your genes that determine who you are, but which of those genes are turned on, or expressed, and to what degree they are expressed—a cutting-edge field called epigenetics. While you can't control which genes you pass on to your child, you do have some influence over which genes are expressed, affecting what features are seen in your baby (his phenotype). In this chapter, after giving you a brief refresher on the basic biology of what happens after your life-changing evening of romantic rasslin', we're going to introduce you to a new subject: YOU-ology—how what you eat, breathe, and even feel can affect the long-term health of your child.

Two to One: The Biology of Conception

We trust that you know the ins and outs of the process that involves his part A and her part B, so we'll skip what happens deep under the satin sheets and focus on the miracle deep below the flesh and deep inside the body—that is, how the egg and sperm come together.★

The Eggs

On the female side of the conception equation lie her eggs, which are fully formed and stowed away in her ovaries from before birth. Each mature egg contains one copy of each gene in the human genome—half the amount necessary for life. The maximum number of eggs that a woman will ever have is the number she has when she is a twenty-week-old fetus. She'll have about 7 million of them then, 600,000 when she's born, and about 400,000 at puberty. Once a woman hits puberty and menstruation begins, her ovaries release one of those eggs every twenty-eight or so days. During each cycle, even though multiple eggs start to develop, hormonal signals ensure that only a single egg will be released and the other eggs will regress.

> **Factoid:** Though it happens rarely, women who lose their corpus luteum (through a ruptured cyst, for example) might need a progesterone supplement during the first trimester to help maintain the uterine lining until a placenta forms. Other candidates for progesterone supplementation include women who have a history of miscarriages, perimenopausal women, and those having in vitro fertilizations.

(It's not wise evolutionarily to blow them all at once, so the body gives females an approximately thirty-year window in which to conceive.) Hormones also work to mature that ready-to-drop egg and to pop a hole in its sac. That hole works as an escape hatch, so the egg can slip out of the ovary and travel down the Fallopian tube,

★ Please cue "Let's Get It On" by Marvin Gaye.

where it may be fertilized by sperm.* Tissue left behind in the ovary after the egg is released, called the corpus luteum, will produce hormones essential to successful pregnancy if the egg is fertilized.

The Sperm

On the other side of the equation, of course, we have those little swimming sperm. As with a woman's eggs, each sperm contains a single copy of each gene in the human genome. Unlike women, men don't have a preset number of their reproductive players. In fact, a man produces more sperm in each ejaculation than the total number of eggs that a woman is endowed with for life. (Evolutionarily, a man can continue reproducing for the majority of his adult life, maximizing the chance of passing on his genes. A woman's reproductive life is limited to the younger years of her life because of the physical strain of pregnancy, childbirth, breast-feeding, and child rearing.)

A man's sperm, which is carried in semen that's made by glands such as the prostate, is stored in a duct called the vas deferens. When a man ejaculates, the sperm-carrying semen fires out through the urethra in a seek-and-conquer mission. It may seem that all these millions of sperm are racing one another to the finish. But just like a Tour de France cycling team, the sperm have different roles. Some are deemed the leaders of the pack, trying to be the first to cross the line. Others are designed to assist, specifically by blocking other men's sperm from making it to the finish line. Competitive little game going on in there, eh? The goal of pregnancy, of course, is for a sperm to find an egg during a precise window of opportunity and fertilize it.

* Interestingly, too little of these hormones may lead to infertility or miscarriage, while an abundance may lead to twins and other multiple sets. More on this in "Fertility Issues" on page 380.

Print Shop

The word *imprinting* may sound like something you've heard on *CSI*, but it's actually a form of epigenetics. Even though two copies of a given gene are inherited, one from mom and one from dad, in certain circumstances, one is permanently turned off. The nonexpressed copy is said to be imprinted. As of now, we know of at least eighty genes that are imprinted by epigenetic markers, causing them to be active or inactive in the offspring based on parent of origin. In general, expressed genes that are inherited from the mother conserve maternal resources and limit fetal growth, while expressed genes inherited from the father promote fetal growth, even if it means hurting the mother.

Problems can occur when genes that are supposed to be imprinted, or turned off, are not, or when the wrong parent's gene is imprinted. The gene for the chemical messenger called insulinlike growth factor 2 (IGF2) is normally turned on from the father and off from the mother. If the mother's copy is not turned off, the child can develop Wilms' tumor, a cancer of the kidney. Loss of imprinting of the mother's IGF2 gene later in life can contribute to age-related cancers, including cancers of the prostate and colon.

The Union

The purpose of an orgasm isn't solely to make you feel good or provide gossip fodder for the neighbors. The biological purpose is to better the odds that this union between sperm and egg takes place.

On the woman's side, the mucous membranes that line the vaginal walls release fluids during intercourse so that the penis can slide with just the right amount of friction. As intensity and sensations build, the woman's brain tells the vagina and nearby muscles to contract. That contraction brings the penis in deeper. Why does that matter? It increases the chance of his sperm getting closer to the target. During an orgasm, the cervix, located at the top of the vagina, dips down like an anteater and sucks semen up into the cervix (the cervix is a passageway connecting the top of the vagina and bottom of the uterus). The sperm is trapped in the cervical mucus

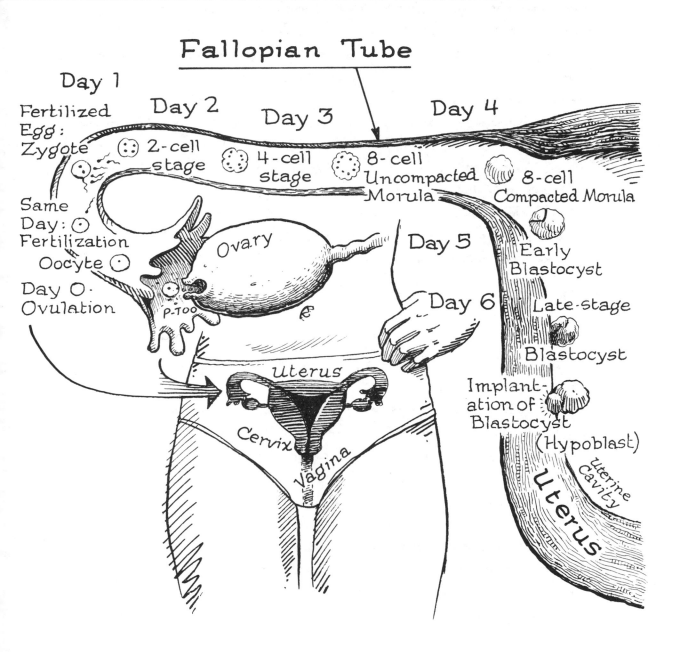

What's Age Got to Do With It?

We all know plenty of people who have made the classic clock-ticking jokes about aging women who want kids. But what does that really mean? Before ovulation, eggs have two copies of each of the twenty-three chromosomes. They're lined up waiting for the signal to divide for mom's entire life. Unfortunately, the little spindles that pull chromosomes apart don't work as well when they've been waiting for four decades. Instead of a clean break, two copies may be pulled to one side and none to the other. That's what leads to an increased risk of chromosomal abnormalities such as Down syndrome and an increase in miscarriages in older moms.

Now, that doesn't let pop totally off the hook. Older men's (as in over 35) sperm have been linked to an increase in birth defects and autism, as well as an increased difficulty conceiving. New evidence even suggests that children born to older dads score lower on various brain tests through the age of seven.

While older parents may be better equipped to handle some aspects of pregnancy and child rearing (like some of the stresses and emotional wear and tear), and may be better able to support their children financially, there are some physiological trade-offs that you'll want to consider if you are making a decision about when to have children.

until the release of the egg, and a signal then lets the sperm start the competitive swim up into the uterus.

While it's by no means necessary to have an orgasm to get pregnant, women who orgasm between one minute before and forty-five minutes after their partner's ejaculation have a higher tendency to retain sperm than those who don't have an orgasm. On the man's side, orgasm is required, because during orgasm fireworks in the brain cause involuntary contractions in lots of muscles in his body. Those contractions help him penetrate deeper and squeeze the prostate to eject sperm deep into the vagina.

Now, the actual fertilization process happens this way: After the egg drops from the ovary, it travels through the Fallopian tube, where there's about a twenty-four-hour window when it can be fertilized. Since sperm live for up to a week in the cervix (they die after a few minutes of hitting the air), it's not necessary for two people to have sex precisely when ovulation occurs, as many assume. In fact, conception is more likely to happen if sex occurs a couple days before the egg is released from the ovary. (See "Fertility Issues" on page 380 for more about getting the timing right.)

If all goes according to plan, the sperm meets the egg in the Fallopian tube, and the two half genomes unite to form a complete set of genes containing all the DNA necessary to make a new human being. The fertilized egg says thank you very much and moves along to the uterus. There it will attach to the uterine lining and begin the amazing process of becoming a baby.

YOU-ology: A New Approach to Genes

One of the most miraculous processes in nature, aside from the formation of such things as the Grand Canyon and the hammerhead shark, has to be how we grow from a single fertilized egg cell to the trillions of cells that make up a new person.

Human cells have twenty-three pairs of chromosomes, structures that hold our DNA. The DNA acts as a complete set of instructions that tells our bodies how to develop. Individual genes are short sequences of these instructions that regulate each of our traits. (See figure 1.2.) As you might imagine, given the fact that virtually every person in this world looks different from every other, the nearly infinite possible combinations of maternal and paternal DNA are what give us our individuality. When maternal brown eyes and maternal red hair get paired with paternal blue eyes and paternal blond hair, there are four possible combinations for offspring, right? Brown eyes–blond hair, brown eyes–red hair, blue eyes–blond hair, blue eyes–red hair. Extrapolate that scenario out to twenty-three chromosomes, and the possible combinations become mind-boggling, unless scientific notation is your thing: 2^{23}, or about 8.3 million, combinations—meaning that there's about a 1 in 8 million chance that the same mother and the same father would have two kids with the exact same coding (excluding identical twins). (See figure 1.3.)

But that's only part of the story. Consider identical twins. They get dealt exactly the same DNA, but they may develop different traits down the line: One may have allergies and the other may not, one may develop a particular disease and the other

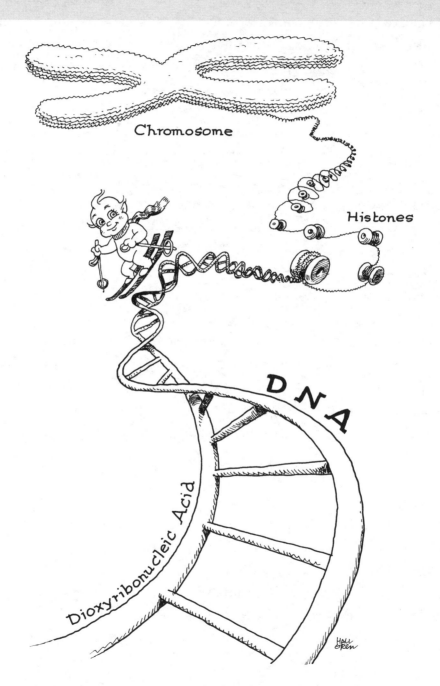

may not, one may be able to play the piano without ever learning how to read music, while the other can't carry a tune with a dump truck. What accounts for these differences? Something in their environment—potentially as early as in utero—affected the expression of their genes differently. That something is called epigenetics.

Here's how it works:

Each cell in the human body contains about 2 meters of DNA that's packed into a tiny nucleus that's only about 5 micrometers in diameter. That's the rough equivalent of stuffing two thousand *miles* of sewing thread into a space the size of a tennis ball. As with thread, DNA is wound around spools of proteins called histones. Not all of your DNA gets expressed, or used to create proteins, in every cell; in fact, most of the spools of DNA in each cell are stored away, some never to be seen or heard of again.

A good way to visualize the process: Let's say that you and your partner each comes to your relationship with a set of favorite family recipes. You may contribute a blue-ribbon chili recipe, and your significant other may bring a killer lemon meringue pie to the table. But it's not just two recipes, it's hundreds, maybe thousands. (The human genome has some twenty to thirty thousand genes, after all.) Some on index cards, some in books, some on torn-up shreds of cocktail napkins. So what do you do with all these cranberry mold recipes? Stuff each and every one of them in the kitchen drawer. Now it's hard to sift through them, you don't have access to many of them, and you really can't find what you want. Unless . . . (you knew there was an "unless" coming) you get them organized, say, by sticking hot pink Post-it notes on the recipes you really want to access quickly. You tag your favorite recipes, so you can quickly search, find, and *put them into action*.

That's the way epigenetics works.

Genes are like recipes—they're instructions to build something. Both mom and dad contribute a copy of their entire recipe book to their offspring, but for many genes, only one copy of each recipe will be used by the baby. Mom and dad have the same recipes (one for eye color, one for hair color, one for toenail growth rate, and so on), except they may have slightly different *versions* of those recipes (they're called alleles). For example, eye genes are either brown or blue or green. For such genes,

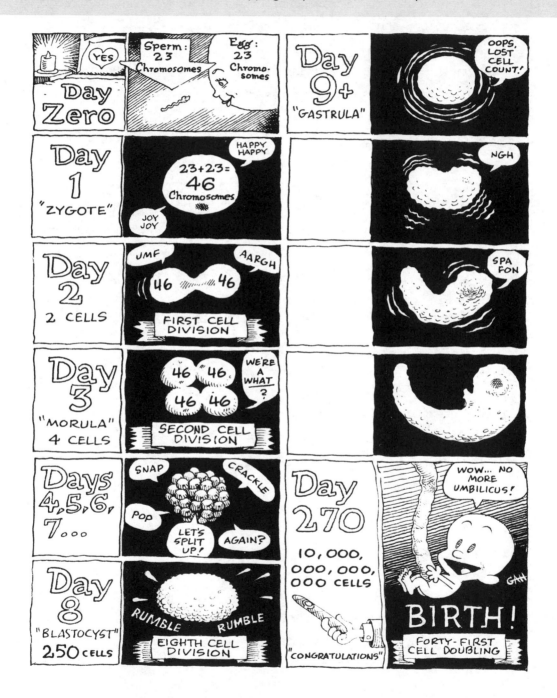

you express only the gene from your mom or dad—that is, only one copy is active, but not both. In some cases, neither copy will need to be expressed: Eye color matters only to eye cells; a liver cell doesn't need either mom's or dad's eye color gene to be cranking away.

So how does a cell turn off the 24,999 genes it doesn't need and turn on the few it does? Every cell—and there are around 200 different types in the body—needs to know which few genes are relevant for it, and, of those genes, whether mom's or dad's is going to be expressed. As with the kitchen drawer full of recipes, the genes alone are useless unless there's a way to find what you need when you need it.

There is. Your body puts biological Post-it notes called epigenetic tags on certain genes to determine which genetic recipes get used. This tagging happens through a couple of chemical processes (such as methylation and acetylation), but guess what? Actions you take during your pregnancy can influence these processes and determine where the Post-it notes go and which genes will be expressed, ultimately affecting the health of your child. (See figure 1.4.)

When DNA gets tagged, it changes from being tightly wound around those histone proteins to being loosely wound, making the genes accessible and able to be expressed. At any given time, only 4 percent of your genes are in this accessible state, while the rest can't be actively used in the body. By determining which genes are turned off and which are turned on, epigenetics is what makes you unique.

Here's a point that will help you put epigenetics in perspective: We share 99.8 percent of the same DNA as a monkey, and any two babies share 99.9 percent of the same DNA. Heck, we even have 50 percent of the same DNA as a banana.★ So genes alone cannot explain the diversity in the way we look, act, behave, and develop. How those genes are expressed plays a huge role in how vastly different we are from monkeys and how explicitly and subtly different we are from one another.

★ True statement, not a joke.

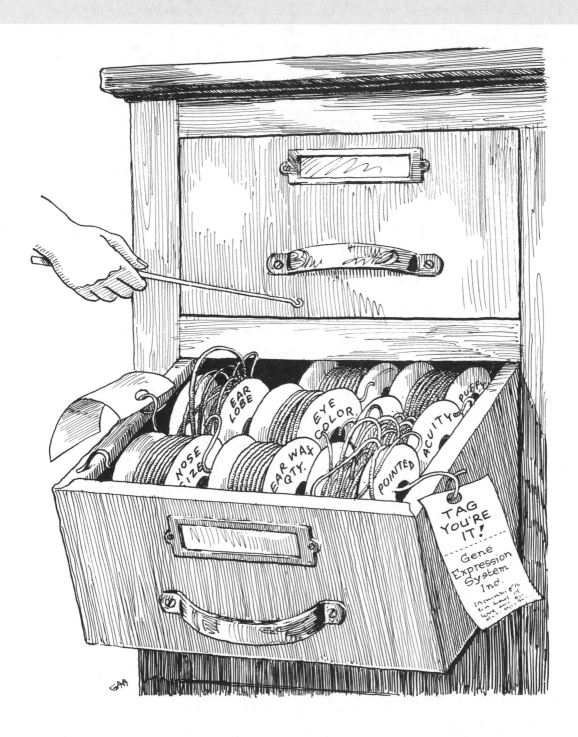

Figure 1.4 **The DNA Drawer** The way genes are expressed is a little like pulling recipes out of a drawer. They may be there, but it can take some work to find them.

Epigenetics in Action: What It Means to You

By about this time, we suspect that you're asking yourself where you can buy yourself some epigenetic Post-it notes, because they sure as heck aren't in aisle twenty-three of Walmart. The way epigenetics works during pregnancy is that stressors in the mother's environment cause changes in the gene expression patterns of the fetus. Translation: The chemicals your baby is exposed to in utero via the foods you eat and the cigarettes you don't inhale serve as biological light switches in your baby's development. On, off, on, off—you decide how your child's genes are expressed, even as early as conception. You don't have total control, though. We still don't know how you can change your baby's eye color or how old he'll be when his hair starts receding. But we do know how to influence some really important factors like your child's weight and intelligence.

So there's an important reason why we're able to turn certain genes on and off. Our bodies have to adapt to a changing environment; that's how a species survives, after all. But our ability to adapt would be much too slow if we had to wait generations for our genes to change through random mutation (the classical theory of evolution). Our bodies need some other kind of mechanism to allow us to adapt. Epigenetics gives our bodies the ability to influence which genes will be turned on—or as the scientists (and now you) say, expressed—or off, or partially on, depending on our immediate environment. Even more amazing is the fact that epigenetic changes don't occur just when a baby is developing in the womb—they can also occur throughout life and can be passed down from generation to generation.

One of the best examples of epigenetics is called fetal programming. This refers not to teaching your child to use the remote control before birth, but rather to changes in gene expression that affect the growth and functioning of the placenta, the amazing organ that filters nutrients, oxygen, and waste between mother and baby (more on the placenta in chapter 2). If a mother's genes for placental growth are turned off and the father's genes are expressed, a thicker, richer placenta develops and channels more nutrients to the fetus. This puts more strain on the mother, because it both deprives her of nutrition she needs to remain healthy and causes her to carry a larger baby, which is associated with a host of risks. (See chapter 4.) If, instead, the mother's genes are expressed, a smaller placenta develops and fewer nutrients get to the baby. In this case, the mother is protecting her interests—if this baby doesn't make it, she can always try again.

Fetal programming also occurs when a baby is malnourished in utero—either because mom doesn't eat properly during her pregnancy or because environmental toxins compromise the placenta's ability to deliver adequate nutrition (more on this in the next chapter). In either case, you get the same result: a smaller baby. You may be asking, "So what if my baby is a couple of pounds smaller than average at birth? So what?" Here's what:

Factoid: All of the epigenetic changes that you can make during the development of your fetus don't just change the way your child's genes are expressed. These changes can also be passed down from generation to generation—meaning that the small changes you make today can affect generations long after you've been said good-bye to—so your responsibility for creating a healthy environment for your offspring is even bigger than you may have thought.

In utero, if you feed your baby fewer nutrients, you're programming your child to expect an environment of deprivation ex utero. So genes that cause the fetus to be very thrifty, metabolically speaking, are turned on. Once the baby is born and the external environment is not one of deprivation, that child will conserve more of the food it gets and become fatter, exhibiting what's known as a thrifty phenotype (we refer to this in chapter 2). More fat storage equals an increased likelihood of becoming overweight and developing heart disease, type 2 diabetes, stroke, cancer, and osteoporosis as an adult. It's similar to the reason why starvation diets don't work: When your body thinks it's faced with famine, it goes into fat-storage mode and your metabolism slows. Poor fetal nutrition may also permanently change the structure and development of vital organs such as the brain. In some cases, these epigenetic changes can even be passed on to future generations as well.

We do want to make one thing clear: If this is not your first pregnancy, don't beat

Figure 1.5 **Time for Change** Through processes called methylation and acetylation, you can alter the way genes are expressed, as well as determine which genes are expressed. In other words, you can take certain actions that will influence whether some genes come to the forefront and whether others get locked away forever.

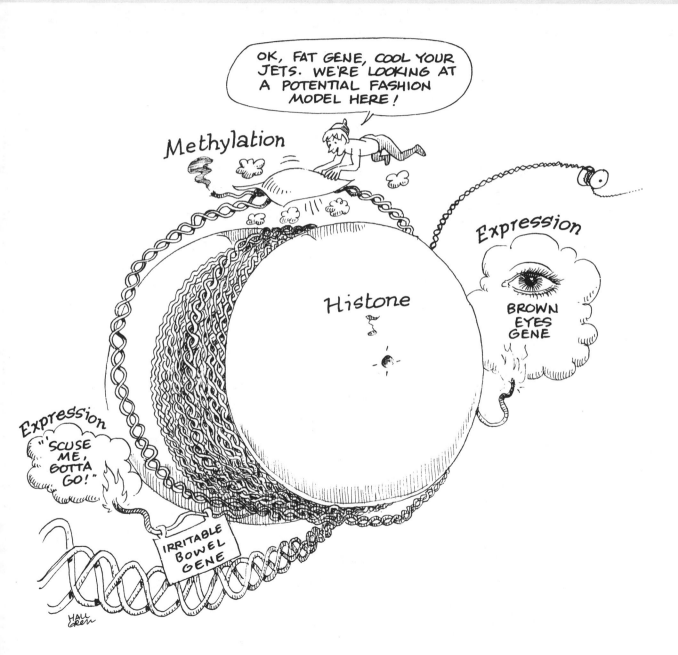

yourself up that you didn't know much about epigenetics the last time around. None of us did, either. While epigenetics plays a role in what happens before birth, as we mentioned earlier, you can actually regulate gene activity after birth—for this child, for previous children, even for yourself. Also, if you fear you've already done something damaging to this baby, rest assured that human beings are a resilient lot; otherwise we'd have died out millennia ago. Let's face it: Since 50 percent of pregnancies are unplanned, plenty of women inadvertently expose their babies to toxins like alcohol and tobacco. The key is to stop and make a YOU-turn,* reversing damaging behavior as soon as possible. Even the damage caused by smoking can be offset if you quit in the early part of your pregnancy.

Another way to think about how epigenetics works is to think about how music is created. Consider your DNA to be the musical composition that will determine the individuality of your child; after all, there are zillions of way to put musical notes together. But the catch is that there are many different ways to interpret any given song. The way Johnny Cash sang a song would be different from the way a rocker would today and is way different from how a philharmonic orchestra would perform it.† Same song, different interpretations, and different results.

You and your partner each has your own set of DNA, and through your recent rendition of a boogie-woogie-woogie, you made your own biological song in the form of a baby. That genetic coding is indeed fixed, but you still have the ability to interpret the song and change the way your offspring's genes are expressed. That, dear friends, should be music to your ears.

---

* A YOU-Turn, as we introduced in *YOU: On a Diet,* refers to the fact that it's not too late to make changes. The key is to identify when you've gone down the wrong road and get back on the right course as soon as you can.
† Not that one would.

YOU TIPS

The reason epigenetics is so important isn't because someday you'll be able to tag your baby's genes for blond hair, a composer's brain, or the ability to hurl a 98 mph fastball. It's because epigenetics teaches us this: The environment that you provide for your offspring—through what you're eating, drinking, smoking, or stressing about—is what your child will program herself to expect of the world she's entering. Based on what you're doing right now, she's forecasting her future environment. And if the programming for gene expression doesn't match that environment, problems can occur. So your challenge—dare we say your responsibility—is to provide little Dolly with a healthy environment now so that her "internal programming mechanism" predicts and can respond to a healthy environment later. Many of the tips we outline throughout the book are based on this fundamental idea, but here we'll discuss some of the major things you can do right away to positively influence the way your baby's genes are expressed.

Add Folate. Your baby needs the nutrient folate because it has a direct effect on DNA. Folate is an essential ingredient of one of the building blocks of DNA, thiamine. Without folate, your body may substitute a less effective backup building block called uracil, which can cause birth defects, primarily spina bifida. Also, a lack of folate has been shown to increase childhood cancer rates by more than 60 percent. A startling statistic, for sure, but one that reinforces the notion we just talked about: in utero nutrients influence out-of-utero health. If you're even thinking about getting pregnant, you need to supplement with 400 micrograms of folic acid (the synthetic form of folate) every day.

Detox. As we'll discuss in chapter 2, your placenta acts as a filter that allows nutrients to pass from mother to child. It's a nice system, except for the fact that it lets toxins through, too. Of course, the last thing you want is to provide your bubby an in-womb environment that resembles a landfill. We urge you to get rid of the most harmful toxins in your life as soon as you decide to get pregnant or once you find out you are. Some major toxins are:

- Tobacco (see below).
- Methylates. Found in hot dogs and lunch meats, they unwind DNA that's not supposed to be unwound.
- Alcohol.
- Marijuana.
- Phthalates. These chemicals, found in plastics and cosmetics, mimic estrogens and have been linked to feminized fish; they increase when you microwave foods in plastic.
- Aerosolized products such as turpentine, toluene, and paint thinner. Let your partner paint the baby's room. And aggressively air it out before you and the baby come near it—breast milk can carry such stuff too.
- Radon. This radioactive element comes from the ground and gets trapped in modern houses. It needs to be ventilated away if found.
- Fluorotelomers. These are found in paints and coatings and in stain repellents applied to materials such as carpets, paper, packaging, and textiles.
- Bisphenol-A. Found in hard plastic bottles; none is commonly obtained when you drink water from undamaged plastic bottles.
- Other bad hydrocarbons, such as those found in unmarinated grilled meats.
- Mercury, lead, and other heavy metals. Stay away from coal-fired power plants.

Also, if your occupation exposes you to chemicals, find out what chemicals are involved and seek advice as to their fetal safety.

Put Out the Fire. You knew you were going to get the talk at some point, so now's as good a time as any. Please don't sentence your child to nine months inside a smoky bar. Tobacco turns on genes that are later linked to the growth of cancers, as well as inflammation in arteries, which in turn leads to heart attacks, strokes, wrinkles, and impotence. Most important for you, smoking also limits blood flow to the uterus by causing inflammation in the uterine arteries, thus making it harder for beneficial nutrients to travel from mom to child. If you're currently a smoker, please see www.realage.com for our Breathe-Free, addiction-busting program.

Know the Limit. In doctors' offices, message boards, and nail salons everywhere, debates rage about the role of alcohol in pregnancy. Surely we all know that excessive alcohol during pregnancy is the biological equivalent of a lightning storm, tornado, and tidal wave all wrapped up into one. But still, many ask: Is one drink okay? While moderate alcohol has many health benefits, we don't recommend any alcohol during pregnancy. Alcohol is a toxin to developing brain cells even at minor levels, so don't take any chances. Further, a little alcohol changes brain functioning, predisposing your baby to alcohol problems later in life, as well as decreasing her brain development. A big reason to avoid it: If something does go wrong, you don't want to be guilt ridden thinking that you didn't do everything you could have to ensure the health of your child.

Squash the Radiation. To protect your baby from the toxic effects of radiation, you should avoid X-rays and other forms of radiation during pregnancy. Radiation alters the DNA of cells as they replicate, which is why it is used in cancer therapy (cancers reproduce faster than regular cells). Fetal cells reproduce the fastest and are the most susceptible to injury, which may lead to miscarriage or birth defects, or predispose your child to cancer later in life. Avoiding radiation may also mean that you should consider your flying habits. Flying for thirty hours exposes you to the same dose of radiation as one chest X-ray. Does that mean that you're automatically harming your child if you whisk off to the Caymans when you're four months pregnant? No. But if you're being diligent about taking all precautions, it's worth thinking about whether each trip you are planning can wait.

See the Dentist. You're more likely to be thinking about your appointments with your ob/gyn or midwife than you are about those with your dentist. But you should get your teeth cared for and cavities filled, ideally, six months before you become pregnant. While you are pregnant, maintain your schedule of regular checkups for dental health. However, try to wait to get any new cavities filled until after your baby is born, unless the procedure is absolutely necessary. (To be extra cautious, you can avoid breast-feeding for two weeks after dental work.) Traditional fillings contain mercury, which releases mercury vapor that you absorb, and even the composite ones have been associated with releasing phthalates (see page 38) when they harden. Even though no conclusive studies link fillings to fetal health abnormalities, one can surmise that these chemicals may be harmful to a developing fetus.

Figure 1.6 **Miracle Grow** Amazing milestones happen at every step along the way as a fetus develops. Heartbeats, taste buds, fingernails, the sense of touch—when you consider everything that develops in utero, you really can appreciate that is a womb with a view.

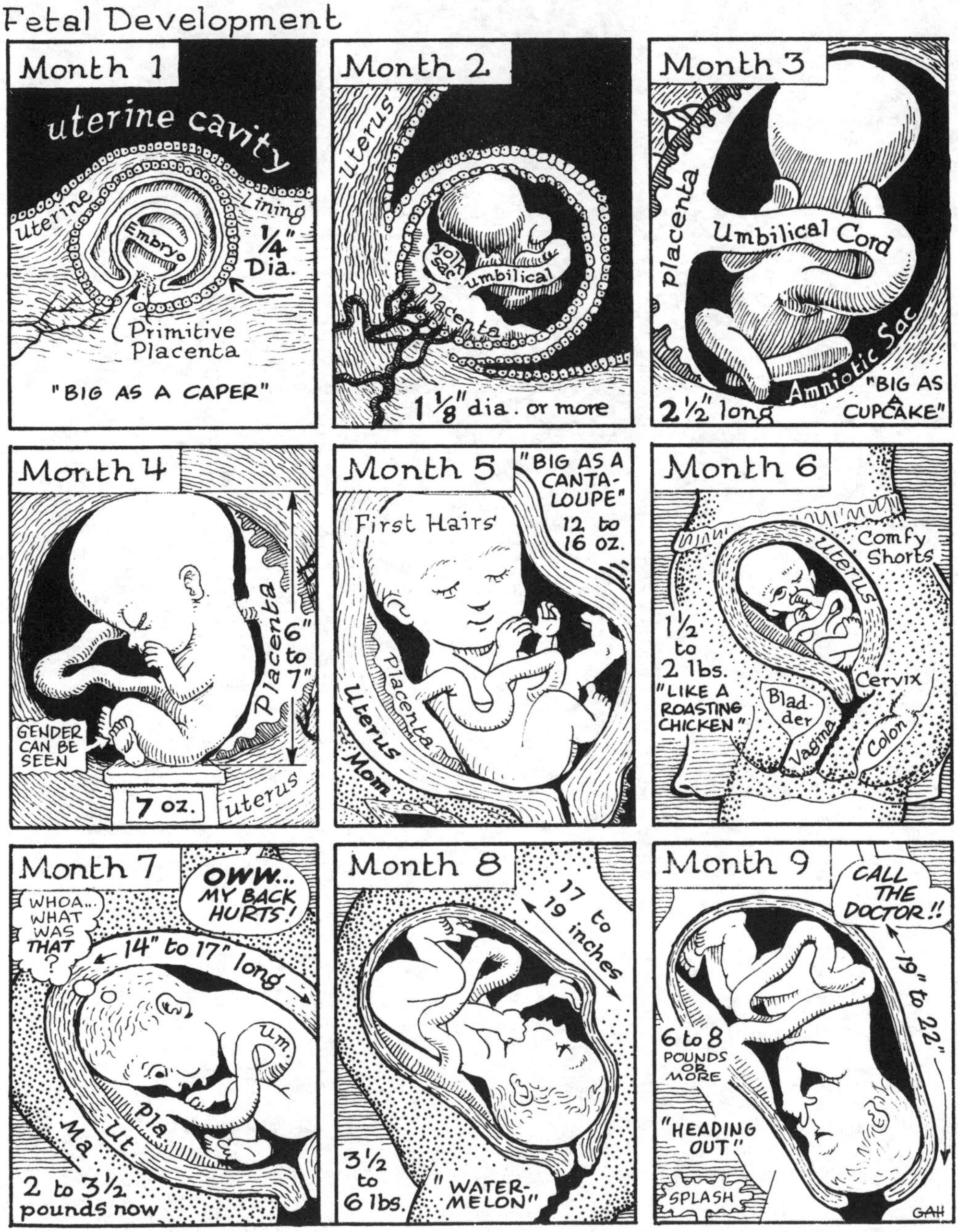

The Time of Your (in Utero) Life

Mark the milestones in your baby's development. All ages are based on clinical age; that's two weeks from the first day of your last period.

6 WEEKS

Heart is formed, circulation is established. A big part of the lungs is formed, as well as the fingers, toes, and parts of the face, like the lips.

7 WEEKS

Fetus can produce urine. Bubbles in the eye area collapse into cuplike structures.

9 WEEKS

Immune system starts to develop, with the formation of B cells, a type of white blood cell that assists in fighting infection. Nostrils are formed. Baby is the size and shape of a kidney bean.

10 WEEKS

Eyes move to the front of the face, and the eyelids form and fuse shut (they separate late in the second trimester). Fetus begins to squint, open its mouth, and make small movements with its fingers and toes.

11 WEEKS

The chin, eyelids, and arms can all sense touch.

12 WEEKS

Taste buds develop and mature. Easy on the anchovies, mom.

14 WEEKS

Immune system ramps up, with the formation of T cells. Lots of gut chemicals can be detected, including bilirubin from the liver and insulin from the pancreas. Baby starts to develop skin, hair, and nails. Swallowing begins. The entire surface of the body can sense touch. Fetus size: about that of an orange.

16 Weeks
External genitalia spotted. The 100 million neurons that form in the primary visual cortex develop between now and twenty-eight weeks. Respiration develops. Size: about that of a grapefruit.

20 Weeks
Ears stick out of the head. Downy hair covers the body. Size: 300 grams, or the weight of two iPods.

25 Weeks
Fetus can respond to sounds. Be careful what you say.

26 Weeks
Ability to suck. Ability to hear sounds. Eyebrows and eyelashes detectable. Size: 630 grams (the weight of about three oranges). Almost half of babies that reach this age will survive if delivered.

29 Weeks
Lungs with fluid in them begin to expand and compress, simulating breathing movement.

30 Weeks
Eyes can sense light, and the ability to smell begins. Fetus can suck and swallow, to help develop the gastrointestinal (GI) system. Plus, it can also hic-hic-hiccup and even breathe, which is really helpful if it is born this early, since 90 percent will survive. Size: 1,100 grams, or the weight of one pineapple.

34 Weeks
Skin is red and crinkled. Fat starts to be deposited to round out fetus. Reflexes like blinking and grasping are set, and the fetus is actually settling into noticeable sleep patterns. Size: 1,800 grams, or the size of the average Chihuahua.

36 WEEKS

If it hasn't already, baby begins the descent into the pelvis to prepare for delivery. Fingernails reach the end of the fingertips.

37 WEEKS

Lungs are considered mature, and baby is not considered premature if delivered. This is considered full-term.

38 WEEKS

With formation of more fat, body becomes more rotund, less wrinkly. Size: 2,500 grams, or the weight of a lightweight laptop computer.

40 WEEKS

Normal gestation period ends. All systems go.

2

Feeding Time

The Delicate Role of the Placenta
in the Development of Your Child

Some miracles come in the form of avoiding a natural disaster, and some come in the form of making a championship-winning shot. But we believe that one of the most miraculous processes in the human body (and there are many) is how a mother's body interacts with a baby's during pregnancy. That miracle centers around an organ that may elicit gasps of *eeeeew* from the weak-stomached men in your life: the placenta.

This amazing, essential, and delicate system of tissues plays a huge role in influencing the health of your child. How? The placenta delivers nutrients and oxygen to the growing fetus, removes carbon dioxide and other waste, and provides the fetus with its early immunities. As the physical interface between the fetus and the mother, the placenta is where you are most literally bonded to your baby.

The flip side of that beautiful bond is that everything you do—the vapors you inhale, the toxins you expose yourself to, the cucumber-and-cookie sandwich you crave—can be passed on to your child through that miraculous organ.

The placenta, as you'll learn in this chapter, has one big job: to preserve and protect the fetus. Typically, it does a darn good job, especially when facing challenges shared by our pregnant Paleolithic ancestors, such as infections and natural toxins.

But the reality is that it's not always equipped to handle all of the things that we're seeing in today's diets and environment. In this chapter, we'll explain why and how you can take an active role in protecting your baby, starting right about now.

The Point of the Placenta: Formation and Function

Unless you're starring in *Alien*, the general rule about organ development is that all of your organs are formed in utero, and that's the set you live with. There aren't too many instances of new organs or organlike substances appearing on a whim (unless you count fat, tumors, and the regenerative liver). But there is one big exception: the placenta. As we explain below, you can think of it as a kind of an organ transplant from your fetus to you that forms naturally inside you.★

Here's how the magic works. After conception, the fertilized egg (now called the blastocyst) meanders to the end of your Fallopian tube and enters your uterus, searching for the uterine wall. As we stated in the previous chapter, this trip is the most dangerous trip any human being ever takes, because if the blastocyst does not implant successfully within seven days of conception, the uterine lining will be shed, and you'll never even know you were pregnant. If it does, the placenta will begin to form at the point of attachment. Generally, the placenta starts to develop about a week after conception. If you take a look at figure 2.1, you'll see that the blastocyst is made up of two layers: an inner cell mass and an outer layer. The inner cell mass is what becomes the embryo; the outer layer is what forms the fetal side of the placenta.

When the blastocyst implants in the uterine wall, the cells from that outer layer begin to form what are called chorionic villi. These villi, which look like coral reefs, carry blood vessels that go from the placenta into the spongy uterine wall, and it's through the walls of those blood vessels that nutrients and waste are exchanged.

★ The placenta is named after the Greek word *plakos,* which means "flat cake," because of its appearance.

Figure 2.1 **Natural Resource** Shortly after conception, the cells of the blastocyst need to find a way to absorb mom's nutrients. So the outer layer of cells forms part of the placenta, while the inner layer forms the foundation of the fetus itself.

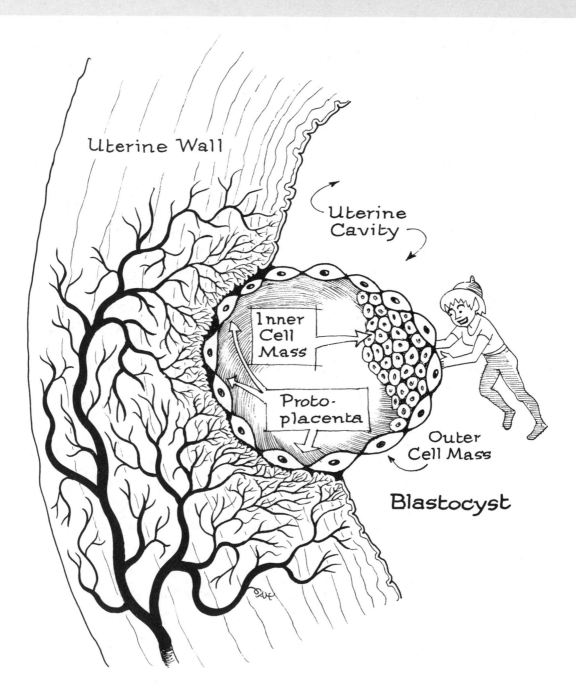

Uterine Wall

Uterine Cavity

Inner Cell Mass

Proto-placenta

Outer Cell Mass

Blastocyst

A pool of maternal blood, called a blood lake, surrounds the villi. Your blood pressure forces blood through this lake and around the villi so they can absorb and pass needed nutrients and antibodies for immunity to your baby, and transfer the baby's waste products to your circulatory system for disposal. During this process, there is no direct blood-to-blood contact between mother and child. About the same time that the placenta is forming, your hormones stimulate the inside layer of your uterus—already rich with blood vessels—to grow those vessels larger to facilitate the exchange.

Once the placenta is fully formed and attached to the uterine wall (about the end of the first trimester), you can see a distinct difference between the maternal territory and the fetal territory. The maternal side is red and bumpy, from the shape of the villi poking through, while the fetal side is like a skating rink: smooth and slick, with the umbilical cord projecting from the surface.

Factoid: The fetus needs to have oxygen continually. Its placenta supplies enough for one to two minutes, so a fetus can essentially hold its breath for that long. When a woman is in labor and having contractions, the amount of blood in the placenta lake decreases. As contractions get longer, the baby's heart rate decelerates, providing a way to gauge fetal oxygen levels during delivery.

Factoid: Despite the small size of the placenta, the surface area of the villi is remarkably large. With about 700,000 villi, the surface area available for exchange is approximately the size of a one-bedroom house.

But to think that the placenta is a one-trick pregnancy pony would be a mistake. Besides filtering and exchanging nutrients and gases, it has other duties, including making and secreting many hormones. Some of these include:

Estrogen: In pregnancy, estrogen stimulates the growth of the uterus and improves blood flow between the uterus and placenta. It also preps the breasts for milk production by enlarging a woman's milk ducts. Estrogen secretion peaks right before birth.

The Truth About Miscarriages

There are typically four broad categories of reasons why women miscarry: One, the fetus has some kind of developmental defect or genetic abnormality that is incompatible with survival. Two, the woman has some kind of medical issue that diminishes the ability of the placenta to get nutrients to the baby; for instance, conditions like the immune disease lupus and connective tissue disorders tend to destroy the placenta. Three, the woman has a hormonal imbalance that prevents the corpus luteum from successfully supporting the fetus during the first trimester. And four, the maternal immune system can overreact and reject the fetus.

One miscarriage isn't usually enough to concern docs about your future ability to carry babies. But after three miscarriages, docs will perform a full medical workup to try to get a sense of what might be causing your body to reject the fetus. They're typically on the lookout for such things as chromosomal abnormalities, diabetes, autoimmune disorders, thyroid issues, and hypertension. Infections acquired during pregnancy can also cause a bit of a resource tug-of-war in the womb, as your body tries to both fight the infection and protect the fetus.

Any loss is difficult and emotional, but we also don't believe that miscarriage means you have to panic about your possibilities of motherhood. About 20 percent of known pregnancies end in miscarriage, and it's likely that half of all fertilized eggs have chromosomal abnormalities and are flushed out before you even know you've conceived—underscoring what a truly delicate process pregnancy is.

Since many women begin to bond with their babies the moment they miss a period or find out they are pregnant, the loss of a little one, no matter in what trimester of pregnancy, can lead to feelings of sorrow, guilt, anger, and even fear that they may never be able to have a baby again. Just as we work through the stages of grief with any other loss in our lives, it's especially important to go through the grieving process to help with healing after a miscarriage. It helps many folks to seek professional help; all delivery units have resources to help you both move on and honor the memory of your little one.

Progesterone: This hormone helps maintain the inner layer of the uterus to provide support for the developing embryo. It also serves the very important role of quieting the uterine muscle, so the blastocyst can have a safe landing while implanting.

Human Placental Lactogen: Besides helping with milk preparation, this hormone also increases a mom's metabolism during pregnancy (she needs more energy caring for another human, after all), which we'll discuss in detail in chapter 4.

> **Factoid:** A substance called corin is produced in the uterus during pregnancy to help keep blood pressure low (at least in animal uteri and postulated in humans). When you don't produce it, you can develop high blood pressure and protein in your urine, both signs of preeclampsia. You need both calcium and vitamin D to activate the gene that produces corin. See page 81 for recommended amounts.

Human Chorionic Gonadotropin: This hormone stimulates the corpus luteum (the part of the follicle left behind in the ovary) to produce estrogen and progesterone in the first ten weeks after conception, until the placental cells can do so by themselves. For this reason, it is also the hormone we check in your urine or blood to determine whether you're pregnant. Levels of hCG, which have been associated with morning sickness (more on that in the next chapter), typically peak toward the end of the first trimester, then decline and level off for the rest of the pregnancy.

A Perfect Placenta: The Big Usual Picture

Very soon, you're going to be making some important decisions about what and how to feed your newborn. Mashed yams or soupy peas? Cheerios or cut-up fries? Natural or artificial nipple? While those are certainly big decisions, we think you're making a mistake if you fast-forward all of your concerns about nutrition to the moment when Homer Jr. is searching for his first sip from breast or bottle.

In fact, the time you need to start thinking about feeding your baby is the moment you know you're pregnant (even beforehand, actually), because when you're pregnant, that's exactly what you *are* doing: feeding your baby through your placenta.

The placenta, with one smooth surface and one that looks a lot like a plate of congealed spaghetti, is responsible for the exchange of all nutrients and waste products between the mother and fetus. (See figure 2.2.) It basically functions like this: Mom's blood flows into the blood lake on her side of the placenta, which bathes the chorionic villi that are threaded through with fetal blood vessels. Small molecules and nutrients (oxygen, glucose, vitamins, fatty acids, calcium, some antibodies, and so on) flow from mom to baby, and waste products (carbon dioxide, urine, and metabolic wastes) flow from baby to mom.★

Weighing in at about one and a quarter pounds when fully grown, the placenta works like a two-way filter. (See figure 2.2.) Stuff goes through it from one side to the other and vice versa. But here's the thing: The placenta is no Brita. It doesn't necessarily screen out the bad and only let the good pass through. The placenta lets *everything* through below a certain size and blocks insulin, heparin, and other large molecules that would otherwise cause immune rejection or other problems.† That means any toxins that make the size cut can get passed to the fetus, whether it's gunk from cigarettes, saturated and trans fats, alcohol, or other nasty substances.

One of the reasons we care so much about a mother's health during pregnancy is that it will influence the way the placenta functions by determining the amount of surface area of the placenta available for the efficient exchange of nutrients. For example, smoking or having uncontrolled hypertension or diabetes can cause your placenta to calcify, thus limiting the area available for the proper exchange between mother and fetus. As you can guess, that limits the amount of nutrients that the fetus can receive and can lead to issues that have a major influence on your baby's health both inside the womb and down the road.

Of course, it should go without saying that placental formation doesn't always go as smoothly as we all hope. That's because of the delicate conditions it takes for

★ After all, ain't enough room for a restroom down there.
† Some bigger substances, like immunoglobulins, can pass through by folding themselves into smaller shapes.

Figure 2.2 **Feeding Time** The miraculous placenta serves a number of functions—most important, as the bridge between baby and mom. Filtering nutrients (as well as oxygen and toxins), the placenta passes along everything that mom ingests or inhales. The placenta also serves an immunity role, helping to pass along mom's immune cells' immunity before the fetus can develop such immunity on his own.

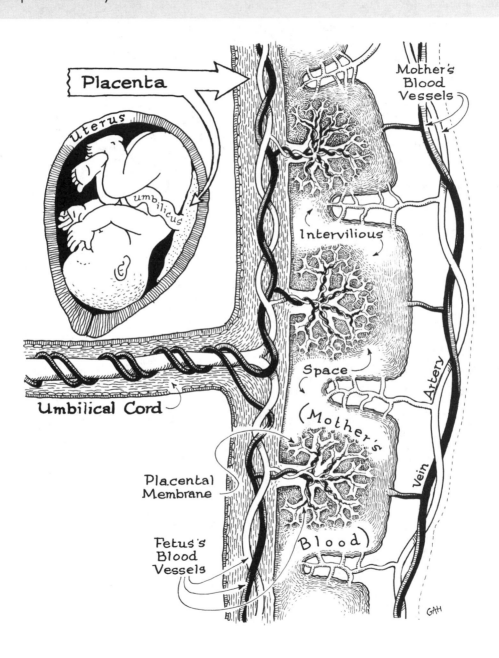

the placenta to develop and the dangerous journey that the blastocyst makes to the uterine wall. Placental issues that can threaten mom's health and lead to an increased risk of prematurity include:

Placenta Previa: This happens when the placenta attaches itself to the lower part of the uterus and covers the opening to the cervix. While it often moves up and away from the cervix as the uterus grows larger during pregnancy, it can cause heavy bleeding at the end of the pregnancy if it doesn't (in which case, you might need a cesarean section). If you have placenta previa, your prescription will include no sex and no exercise. However, if it's diagnosed early in the second trimester, there's a good chance the issue will resolve itself.

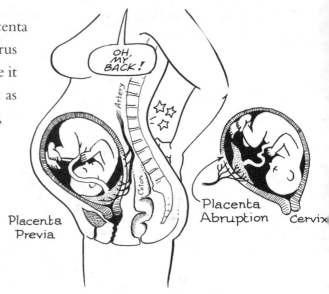

Placental Abruption: This happens when some of the placenta separates from the uterine wall, which increases the risk of cutting off oxygen from the baby. Bed rest can help if the separation is small, but if it's a major separation, the doc will determine if the child's lungs are mature enough to handle delivery. Some conditions can predispose a woman to abruption; your provider will discuss these with you if you're at risk. These include but are not limited to blunt trauma, uncontrolled high blood pressure, cocaine use, and smoking.

Immunity Granted: Mom's First Gift

The human body is designed to retaliate against invading foreign matter. That rebellion can come in the form of fever, vomit, diarrhea, and the like, as your body finds ways to expel bacteria, a virus, or a spoiled scallop. Yet in pregnancy, the mother's

The Rh Factor

Positives and negatives aren't just important for jump-starting a car battery; they're also important for determining whether a baby has blood compatibility with mom. This comes in the form of something called the Rh factor—a chemical tag that differentiates blood types. You're classified as Rh-positive if you have the factor on red blood cells and negative if you don't. The tricky part happens if mom is negative and dad is positive: If the child gets dad's type (which is likely, as Rh-positive is a genetically dominant trait), and Rh-positive cells leak into mom's bloodstream as the placenta breaks down during delivery, then her body responds by producing antibodies that fight the positive antigens. Because there is no blood-to-blood contact during pregnancy, Rh disease is rare in a first pregnancy. But once mom's antibodies have been activated, they will freely cross the placenta into the fetus's bloodstream during subsequent pregnancies and tag the baby's red blood cells for destruction, causing anemia or other serious conditions.

This situation can be prevented by giving an Rh-negative mother a prophylactic injection of an Rh immunoglobulin called RhoGam, which prevents the antibodies from forming, either midway during her first pregnancy or within seventy-two hours after delivery if it is known that the father is Rh-positive. In situations where the father's blood type is unknown, it's best for an Rh-negative woman to get the injection anyway to decrease the risk of this problem occurring. In circumstances where the mother suffers a miscarriage or has an ectopic pregnancy, it's common practice to give her the injection within seventy-two hours if she is Rh-negative, to avert the chances of her forming antibodies due to lack of information about the father's blood type in an emergency situation. Rh tests are given during prenatal visits to help ID potential problems.

body shifts from rebel mode* to ally mode, as it nurtures, feeds, and makes peace with what it *should* perceive as a foreign invader: the fetus.

Remember that 50 percent of the fetus's genes are from the father and theoret-

---

* Morning sickness may seem like a form of rebellion, but it's really more of an ally, as we'll explain in a few pages.

The Down Low on CVS

No, it's not an exposé on the drugstore chain; we're talking about the diagnostic test called chorionic villus sampling (CVS). Here's how it works: Because the placenta is made up of cells that derive from the same fertilized egg as the fetus, it's an ideal resource for DNA that can reveal any genetic abnormalities in your developing baby (or for a paternity test). Chorionic villus sampling, performed between the tenth and twelfth weeks of pregnancy, entails removing a tiny sample of cells from the placenta. The specimen is then cultured in a laboratory, and the DNA is examined for genetic content.

Because CVS is an invasive test and carries a very small (less than 1 percent) chance of miscarriage, it's generally performed when there's an indication of risk: if you've had a prior pregnancy that involved a genetic problem, if there's a history of genetic disease in either your family or the baby's father's, if you had an abnormal first-trimester screen or nuchal translucency test (see page 303), or if you will be thirty-five or older (although some do not follow the age indication) at the time of delivery and therefore at higher risk of having a baby with Down syndrome. While CVS can detect up to two hundred different genetic defects with 98 percent to 99 percent accuracy (including Tay-Sachs disease, cystic fibrosis, and hemophilia), it cannot detect neural tube defects such as spina bifida (more on page 112), which can be picked up by amniocentesis. The advantage of CVS over amniocentesis is that you can have the test done much earlier, as amnio is usually performed between sixteen and twenty weeks.

To prepare for your CVS, drink heavily beforehand (water, please), because you'll need a full bladder. Your doctor will first perform an ultrasound to assess the baby's position and the orientation of your uterus to determine whether she'll do the CVS vaginally, threading a catheter through your cervix, or abdominally, via needle biopsy. In either case, you might experience slight cramping during and after the procedure, as well as light spotting if you had it done vaginally. You should plan to have someone drive you home and you'll need to take it easy for the rest of the day. By the following day, you should feel fine; if you experience increased bleeding, vaginal discharge, or fever, call your doctor immediately. Some docs will have you come in a few days after the procedure for a follow-up ultrasound just to make sure everything is okay. Results will be ready in one to two weeks.

Take a Look

In the pecking order of things you want to look at in the delivery room, your placenta may rank pretty close to the bottom of the list. But that doesn't mean your doc or midwife should feel the same way. While you're gazing at your little darlin', your provider should be inspecting your cute, adorable, squishy organ. Why? A one-minute examination of the placenta provides info that may be important to the care of both mother and infant. The doctor will assess the size, shape, and consistency of the placenta, as well as the umbilical cord. She'll also make sure it's complete and has no missing parts, for leaving some of the tissue in the body can cause hemorrhages up to two weeks later. The delivered placenta can also give clues to future problems, and if something looks abnormal, tests can help determine the best course of treatment or monitoring in future pregnancies. A thin cord can indicate a stressed environment in utero, which may help you make different lifestyle decisions during your next pregnancy. And a placenta that has calcification may indicate a decreased delivery of nutrients and that mom may have a condition that has compromised her arterial health, such as unrecognized changes in blood pressure.

ically can carry information that could sabotage the relationship between mother and child. But the mother's immune system overlooks this fact and seeks to protect the child anyway. In a way, you can consider pregnancy an immunosuppressed state; the volume of mom's immune system is turned down as it deals with this foreign, yet welcome, invader. As we mentioned, the most dangerous time for the newly created creature is prior to implantation in the uterine wall. If mom's immune system is not suppressed when the fertilized egg tries to land, it's bye-bye, blastocyst. So exactly one day before implantation—six days after conception—the blastocyst produces a special enzyme that suppresses mom's killer T cells, preventing her from having an immune reaction to the baby-to-be's cells. Once the placenta is formed after implantation, it helps maintain the truce between these two potential adversaries.

A baby's immune system isn't fully developed before birth, so it needs a hand from mom, who passes her own immune-system warriors, called antibodies, through the

Immunity Granted

As we get older, we tend to think of lymph nodes only when they get sore or swollen, but they actually play an important role in fetal immunity. After T cells mature in the thymus, they engage the enemy on the biological battleground: the five hundred to six hundred peripheral lymph nodes distributed throughout the body. Once T cells have recognized the enemy, they head into the spleen, where B cells are made. The thymus doesn't change its responsiveness after birth, but the lymph nodes and spleen change big-time. In the fetus, about a quarter of the T cells in the lymph nodes and spleen are regulatory, meaning that their job is to prevent a child's immune system from overresponding.

Why would this happen? Immune cells from the mother that slip through the placenta into the child's body will be sequestered in the lymph nodes. After all, that's where infections collect as you grow up and overcome, for example, a sore throat and get large, tender lymph nodes in the local neck area. By not overresponding to the mother's immune cells, the fetus develops tolerance. In other words, the mother's immune cells are instructing the fetal cells to tolerate their presence. This parental guidance might not work in teenagers but works like a charm in the womb. These insights are helping scientists figure out how to perform safer transplantations so that patients do not reject the donated organs.

placenta. This is called passive immunity because the fetus doesn't make antibodies itself but accepts the mother's. Interestingly, it even turns out that some cells from mom slip through the placenta to teach the baby's cells how to tolerate foreign antigens—diplomatic cells, if you will.

This transmission of antibodies serves two roles: protecting the fetus and signaling to the mother that this foreign tissue has cleared inspection and can be safely allowed to park its behind in her uterus for the greater part of the next year. Now, a fetus's immune system doesn't start developing on its own until nine weeks and isn't up and running until week fourteen. The reason for that delay is to help the fetus to tolerate mom—after all, the fetus is 50 percent dad. If its immunity was fully developed from the get-go, there'd be the chance that the fetus might identify mom as different and reject its host.

The fetus's first line of self-defense is a primitive form of immunity called toll-like receptors (TLRs). They work a bit like an alarm system, recognizing cells as evil or friendly and then alerting other immune cells (namely, T cells and B cells, also known as T lymphocytes and B lymphocytes) to do the dirty work. By the end of the first trimester, B lymphocytes are produced in the fetal liver, while T lymphocytes develop in the thymus—a gland in the chest that is large in babies but small in adults.* By this time, the fetus is much better able to withstand sophisticated invaders and potential threats than it was when just the TLRs were in place. Along with the timing of the fetus's major organ development, the fact that the fetal immune system isn't fully functional until the second trimester is why you have to be especially careful about exposure to toxins and infectious agents during your first trimester.

T cells work by looking for bad guys in the body and creating memories of any potential invaders they encounter, such as bacteria, viruses, or parasites. It's a biological Most Wanted List of sorts. The T cells act as the captains and generals of the fetal immune-system army, deciding how many immune cells will respond to potential threats and ensuring that the body doesn't over- or underrespond. B cells serve as the privates, waiting for a signal to tell them whether the invader is a good guy or a bad guy. Once they know it's a bad guy, they start making antibodies and blasting away.

Recent research shows that the fetus's cells and the mother's immune system join forces to fight infections and other common enemies. When the fetus's cells call for help, the mother's system responds to the TLR alarm and sends reinforcements throughout pregnancy.†

So, in many ways, the placenta is the unsung hero of pregnancy, dutifully providing your baby with nutrients and immunity. That's not to say it couldn't benefit from a bit of attention. If you do right by your placenta, it'll do right by your child—with potentially lifelong effects.

---

* This gland shrinks dramatically with age; in fact extracts of thymus are injected by suspect antiaging docs, supposedly to bring vitality to aging clients.

† TLRs are the oldest immune system and the dominant system in ancient species, like the shark.

Drat, Cat

Of course, your partner is already doing everything he can to help you during your pregnancy (including making you scrambled egg tacos at four in the morning). Add this one to the list. If you have a cat, put your partner in charge of taking out the kitty litter. The litter of some cats includes a parasite that can lead to toxoplasmosis, a condition that can restrict the growth of the fetus. Your cat is the primary host of the toxo parasite and can shed egg cysts in its feces that survive for a long time. But don't worry: It's still okay to pet Mr. Moo-Moo. Just be sure to wash your hands very well in running water after doing so. The parasite can also infect raw food (via a fly that flits from the litter box to your hamburger meat). So wash and cook your food to a temperature of 145 degrees for beef, lamb, steak, and veal roasts; 160 degrees for pork, ground meat, and wild game; and 180 degrees for whole poultry. And clean all surfaces that have touched raw meat.

Toxoplasmosis causes flulike symptoms, with muscle aches, brain fog, and swollen glands. Toxo is a threat to your baby only if you're infected for the first time during pregnancy. (You may have immunity to it if you've already been exposed.) Your provider can perform a simple blood test to check whether or not you have antibodies. If not, try to avoid exposure to litter while pregnant. If you don't have an alternative to changing the litter while pregnant, either wear gloves or wash your hands thoroughly afterward. Toxoplasmosis egg cysts can survive for up to a year in soil, so wear gloves when gardening as well.

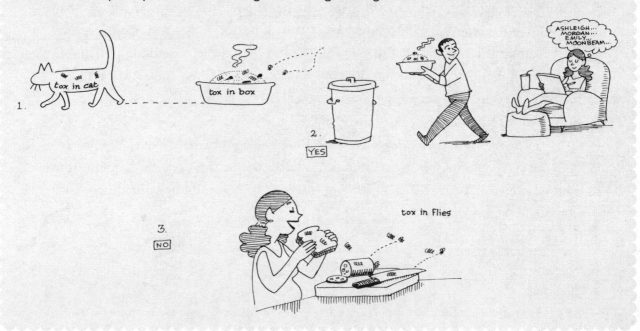

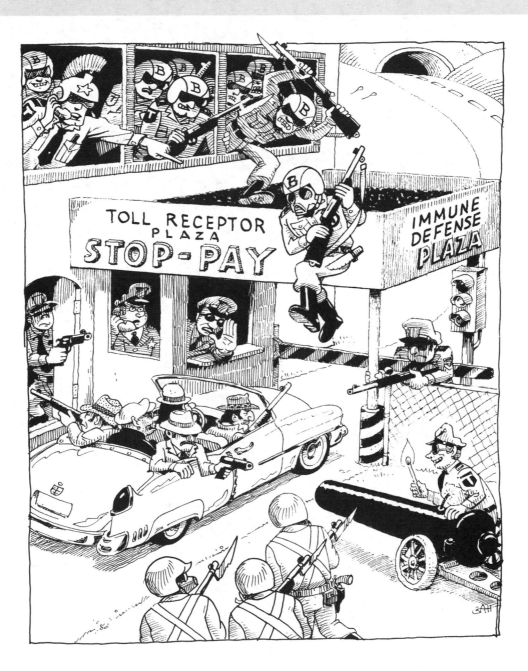

YOU TIPS

There aren't a whole lot of products out there that really tout their placental benefits. It's not like yogurt containers, cereal boxes, or jugs of OJ contain such marketing gems as "100% Placentally Fortified!" or "Boost Your Blastocyst!" So you may be unaware that there are indeed things that you can do to improve placental function. Above all, you want to maintain good arterial health yourself—namely, by doing many of the things we list below. And by avoiding exposing yourself to toxic substances, you won't risk transmitting them through the placenta to your baby.

Follow the Basics. Several things have been shown to contribute to optimal placental function. Not surprisingly, they're also good for a healthy pregnancy in many other ways. They are:

- Don't diet during pregnancy.
- Get your extra calories with extra protein.
- Exercise wisely.
- Don't smoke.
- Avoid exposure to high altitudes.
- Avoid exposure to potentially toxic chemicals such as pesticides.

Follow These Med Rules. On page 342, you'll see our guidelines for specific medications that have been deemed safe or unsafe to take during pregnancy (most are generally okay). While we recommend using that list as a guide, we also believe that you should follow these basic principles:

- Don't self-prescribe meds. Any pill you want to pop, run it by your obstetrician or midwife first.

- Don't stop any medications you're currently taking. The issue of medicine is often a risk-versus-benefit decision. If you're at high risk of developing a complication by not taking your medication, you may very well be putting your baby in harm's way by stopping.
- Don't rely on the average internet site. It's easy to get caught up in message boards and the thousands of health sites out there. When it comes to medical info, you need to make sure the source is reliable and respectable. Three sites we recommend for cutting-edge updates: www.motherisk.org, www.realage.com, and www.drugsafetysite.org.
- While your doc will advise you on medication doses, you should know that you may need a higher dose as your pregnancy progresses, because the rate that your body breaks down drugs while pregnant differs from the nonpregnant state.

Note: If you're interested in complementary medicine, choose a provider who shares your perspective on herbs and other natural remedies; you'll find our recommendations for herbal remedies that seem to work for some pregnancy-related conditions throughout the book.

Get BP Under Control. If you have high blood pressure and take medication for it, be sure to continue doing so. Why? As you just learned, a mother's blood pressure greatly influences how blood, nutrients, oxygen, and immune cells reach the fetus and also can affect the surface area available for efficient exchanges to occur. Any excessive fluctuations, both high and low, can negatively influence that process and even contribute to conditions that your child will have as an adult (remember the thrifty phenotype in chapter 1). Follow our general prescription principles from above, but always play close attention to what your ob/gyn or midwife tells you about your BP (for reasons we'll also cover in chapter 9). Your optimal numbers are lower than 115/75 mm Hg (millimeters of mercury), but BP varies greatly during pregnancy, which is why you'll want to work closely with your provider to establish ideal ranges for you.

Chill. You hear it all the time: Stress is detrimental to health, regardless of gender. One reason why it's a problem in pregnancy is that anxiety depletes the immune system. And in a situation that's already fragile because of the immune changes your body's going through, the added stress of, well, *stress* compromises your immunity even further. Moreover, stress puts you at risk of preeclampsia (high blood pressure during pregnancy) and increases your risk of going into pre-term labor. Some recommendations:

- It's a perfect time to try meditation and deep breathing. For detailed instructions, see www.realage.com.
- Find a surrogate worrier, someone who can sweat the small stuff. This is a great task for a husband, friend, or mom who insists on helping with something.
- Find a buddy who's been through it all before. (Your fertilizing buddy doesn't count.) Her experience and assurances will help take the edge off during some of your more worrisome moments.

More stress-busting tips in chapter 6 and in our Flight Plan, p. 282.

Lie on Your Side. We know you're not going to lie on your stomach as your belly grows and you enter the second trimester, but we do want you to avoid lying flat on your back. That's because when you do so, the weight of your uterus compresses the blood vessels that are feeding the placenta, creating a drought in that blood lake we talked about. Lying on your left side is better than lying on your right side because it allows more blood to flow to the uterus. Either is better than lying on your back, because when you do, you also compress a large vein called the vena cava. The pressure from that compression reduces the flow of blood back to your heart as if you were bending a water hose, and that decreases the blood flow to your uterus and to your baby.

Decide on Vaccines. When you're in an immunosuppressed state such as pregnancy, vaccinations may compromise your immune system further. The best course of action is to get updated on your immunizations three or more months before you get pregnant. We recommend that you avoid all vaccines during pregnancy, if you can. The one exception is the flu vaccine, which current data suggest has no adverse effect. The flu is more serious in pregnant women than in nonpregnant women and is the leading cause of hospitalization during pregnancy. Plus, serious flu symptoms can compromise the amount of oxygen mom and her baby are getting. Ask for the vaccine that does not use thimerosal (mercury) as a preservative. It's slightly more expensive (between $4 and $8 more) but worth the price.

Part 2

YOU

Changing the Baby

3

Eating for Who?

Manage the Moments When You Feel Like Feeding on Everything—or Nothing at All

Having a baby brings out the math whiz in all of us. There's a fair share of multiplication (8 diapers a day times 2.5 years equals about 7,000 changes per kid). There's also plenty of division (you bathe her tonight, I'll do it tomorrow). And unfortunately, we all do way too much subtraction (7 hours to sleep minus 3 feedings a night equals at least 1 whupped parent). But when it comes to the mother of all math equations, a lot of us get it all wrong.

See, when you become pregnant and think about your eating habits, the instinct—or at least the rationalization for many—is to follow this formula: My nutritional needs plus the baby's nutritional needs equals "I'll have a mashed potato sandwich with cheese, and make it a double."

Right here, right now, let's make a deal to take the "eating for two" mantra and pack it into our conversational Diaper Genie, never to see it, speak it, smell it, or think it ever again. The truth is that when you follow the science and look at adequate calorie consumption for growing a healthy baby, the more accurate principle that pregnant women should follow is "eating for 1.1." (Has a nice ring to it, don't ya think?)

Essentially, that means when you're pregnant, you need to eat only 10 percent more than the number of calories you ordinarily eat to maintain your weight. We'll explain how that formula works in more detail shortly. Then we're going to discuss how you can cope with two eating extremes: those times when you crave the contents of the entire fridge and those times when you're so sick that food is the very last thing you want to think about. The issue really becomes one of balance. You need to make sure that you get enough calories to feed your baby with the proper nutrients, but you also need to make sure you don't overwhelm her with a fat-flooded placental buffet that will negatively influence her future health. What complicates the matter is that how you feel may not be in sync with what your body needs at any given time. When you're sick and don't feel like eating, you may very well need to. And when you're famished and craving Ding Dong pizzas, it's probably time to pull the reins and slow down.

As you know from our discussion about the placenta, virtually everything you do as a mother trickles down to your baby. And from our brief intro to epigenetics, you know that your actions influence not only his childhood health but also his health as an adult. More and more evidence suggests that adult diseases and conditions such as high blood pressure, obesity, and diabetes (and even his love of salami) are linked to mom's early nutritional influence on the fetus. We also believe that it's not a coincidence that we're seeing more cesarean sections, more delivery complications, and more birth defects at the same time that we're seeing our country's nutritional habits score about a negative 37 on a scale of 1 to 10. That's why we place so much emphasis, in this chapter and throughout the book, on the fuel you use to get yourself through your day—and get your baby through to the outside.

Food for Thought:
Weight Control and Cravings

Right about now, you're likely asking yourself how in the world we came up with 1.1—and furthermore, how in the world you're supposed to keep track of that 0.1 throughout the day. Luckily, it's all pretty simple. Research shows that the ideal caloric intake for pregnancy breaks down like this: Overall, aim to increase your consumption by about 10 percent. During the first trimester, you want to shoot for an increase of about 100 calories per day more than a typically healthy intake of calories, or the equivalent of an extra glass of skim milk. During the second trimester, you'll want to increase to an extra 250 calories per day, or the equivalent of a healthy midafternoon snack of ten walnuts plus an apple. During the third trimester, you'll want to increase to an extra 300 calories per day, or the equivalent of three pieces of fruit.

As we consider those increases, though, we have to be clear about a few things. Those caloric amounts are guidelines that you'll want to hit, understanding that daily amounts may vary a bit and that there are many times when, because of nausea or exhaustion, you won't even get close to them. As long as you're in the ballpark most of the time, that's fine. Why? Because our end goal here is to make sure you maintain a healthy weight throughout your pregnancy for your own well-being and to provide the best environment for your child.

Of course, end goals do vary a bit, based on your prepregnancy size. While we're not huge proponents of the scale in most circumstances,* it is smart to use one during pregnancy to help track how you're doing from week to week. Rather than count calorie for calorie, use your weight fluctuations (up or down) to help drive your decisions about how you eat. See the next page for what you should shoot for (only a third of women manage to stay within these guidelines, so it's important to track your progress).

In most cases, the extra weight gain will occur primarily in the second and third

The Skinny on Losing Baby Fat

While some women blessed with good genes are able to fit into their prepregnancy clothes within just a few weeks, most women take longer to lose all of their pregnancy weight. Basically, it took nine months to put it on, and you should give yourself nine months to take it off. Bear in mind that if you plan to breast-feed, it is a great way to lose some of your additional fat stores, although you should also not diet while breast-feeding (more on this in chapter 10).

---

* Waist size is typically a better predictor of health risks than actual pound-for-pound weight, but as you might imagine, it's not quite so reliable once you start needing to buy maternity pants.

Your Body	Trimester Gains (in Pounds)	Total Gain (in Pounds)
Underweight before pregnancy (body mass index, or BMI,* of less than 18.5 kg/m²)	First: 4–6 Second: 14–20 Third: 10–14	28–40
Normal weight before pregnancy (BMI of 18.5 to 24.9 kg/m²)	First: 4–6 Second: 10–14 Third: 10–15	24–35
Overweight before pregnancy (BMI of 25 to 29.9 kg/m²)	First: 2–4 Second: 8–13 Third: 5–8	15–25
Obese before pregnancy (BMI of 30 kg/m² or above)	First: 2–4 Second: 4–8 Third: 5–8	11–20
Carrying twins	First: 5–7 Second: 18–22 Third: 12–15	35–44

* To calculate your BMI, see www.realage.com. Or take your weight in pounds and multiply it by 703. Then divide that number by your height in inches squared. Or use the chart on the facing page to characterize your body.

trimesters and the least in the first trimester. During the early part of pregnancy, most of the weight is in you, not the baby. For example, your body makes more blood so as to supply your baby with nutrients; the increase, about four to five pounds' worth, is complete by early in the second trimester. By contrast, toward the end of pregnancy, it's your baby who will be putting on the pounds, at a rate of about a half pound per week. Your weight will fluctuate, so you may not have the same weight gain from week to week; the important thing is to check yourself once or twice a week. Your weight gain should be steady; any huge increases or decreases may be a sign that something atypical is going on.

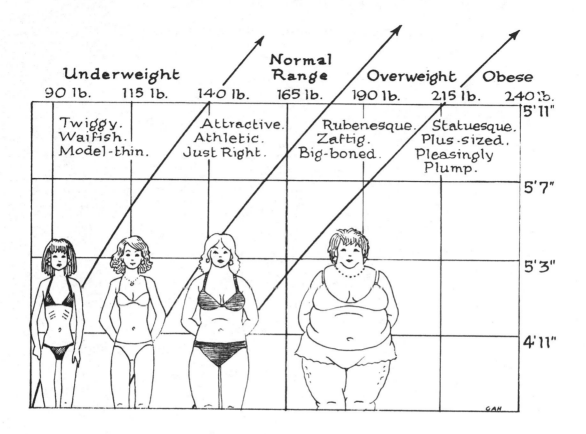

It should go without saying that now is not the time to start thinking about a weight-loss program, though it is worth mentioning that *where* you deposit excess fat is still important. It's much better to be able to store fat on your thighs; that's because fat on the thighs is much richer in omega-3 fatty acids (which the baby needs), and fat on your belly can cause a state of insulin resistance. Your baby needs you to be the opposite (that's called insulin sensitive), so that it can get as much energy from you as it can. While you can't make a formal request to the genetic gods to ask where you'd like your fat to hang out, you can use this information to adjust your behaviors a bit. If, before pregnancy, you were apple shaped (with more of your excess weight in your waist than your thighs), try to counter the effects of this omental, or waist, fat. Since waist fat causes insulin resistance, we'd recommend that during pregnancy you aim to gain in the lower end of the range for your BMI to decrease your risk of further insulin resistance or its overt manifestation, gestational diabetes (more on page

94). In addition, gaining a higher proportion of the total weight early in pregnancy throws off the metabolic environment of your baby. It makes the fetus think that you are storing weight because a famine is coming and substantially increases the risk of preterm delivery.

The ultimate goal, of course, is to make sure you gain enough weight to build the infrastructure you need to support your baby (placenta, uterus, breasts, and so on), but not so much that people are asking whether you're heading to the hospital when you're only five months along. Easier said than done, you say? There's a reason for that.

While you may fight many battles during pregnancy (over such things as crib style and middle names), there's one battle in particular that has lifelong implications. It takes place deep inside your brain. In a nutshell, your body regulates the way you eat through the communication between two hunger-related hormones: leptin and ghrelin. If you've read some of our previous work on waist management, you may be familiar with them (you'll also know that we really like nuts!), but we still think it's worth a quick refresher course, so you can understand how hunger is controlled and, subsequently, learn how to manage it.

> **Factoid:** Some women develop so much excess saliva during pregnancy that they look as if they belong in a baseball dugout rather than in a delivery room. In fact, they need to spit so much that they have to carry a spit cup around with them. They're unable to swallow it because they produce so much and because it can also trigger nausea. Since these women lose so much bicarbonate in their saliva, it disrupts their acid-base balance. It seems that chewing gum, peppermint, and hard candy can help, as can a transdermal scopolamine patch.

Lovely leptin, a protein secreted by fat (yes, fat is more than a storage tissue; it is alive and secretes stuff like leptin), helps curb appetite; recent studies show that it may be a contributor to pregnancy-induced hypertension as well. Ghrelin, the gremlin of hormones, makes you want to eat by making your stomach growl for fulfillment. (See figure 3.1.) These two heavyweights are in a constant neurological battle, pushing, pulling, clawing at each other for victory. To the victor? The dominant message that your brain receives: either you're hungry and want to chow down

Figure 3.1
Fight for Food The two hormones most responsible for the battle over hunger: leptin (the superhero) and ghrelin (the evil Twinkie-loving villain). Unhealthy foods fail to calm ghrelin, putting you in a vicious cycle of hedonistic eating. If you can learn to increase leptin by eating healthy foods, you'll score a knockout victory in the battle between your tummy and your tongue.

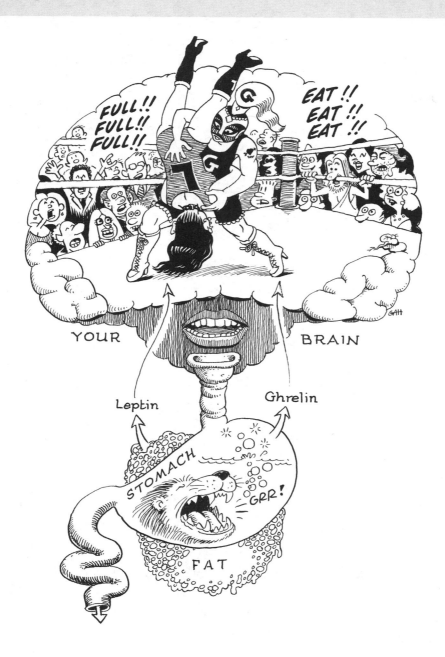

What's in Your Belly?

When you tally up pregnancy weight, you may assume that most of that weight comes from the mass of the baby or perhaps from fat accumulated during a bonbon binge. Not so. Here's how your added weight is approximately divided for a twenty-nine-pound weight gain:

Baby: 7.5 pounds

Placenta: 1.25 pounds

Uterus: 2 pounds

Amniotic fluid: 2 pounds

Breasts: 1 pound

Blood volume: 4–5 pounds

Fat: 5 pounds

Tissue fluid: 6 pounds

Total: About 29 pounds

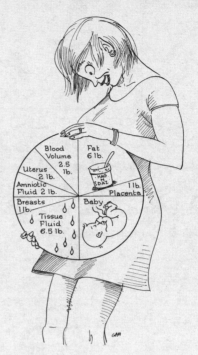

on a box of Cocoa Puffs,★ or you're perfectly satisfied and would much rather spend your time walking around the block or dreaming about what life will be like trying to get spaghetti sauce out of the carpet.

Contrary to what most people think, hunger isn't influenced by willpower as much as by the messages that these hormones send to your brain. Ghrelin works in the short term: It sends out signals twice an hour, taunting and tempting you to gravitate toward the pantry. Leptin, though, works in the long term. If you can boost

★ Preferably what's inside the box.

your leptin signals, you can ignore those ghrelin taunts—keeping your hunger (and thus your potential for dangerous pregnancy weight gain) in check.

Certainly it would be nice if we could reach our pinkie fingers into our ears, search around our gray matter, and flip some cerebral switch that would keep the leptin light on and permanently cut the power source to ghrelin. But what we do have is the ability to flip the switches (in either direction) through the foods we eat. Those foods, and the chemical reactions they cause when they enter our bloodstream, can increase or decrease the effect of leptin and ghrelin. Fructose, for example, which is found in high-fructose corn syrup and in such devilish products as soft drinks and low-fat salad dressing, can cause your sensors not to receive the leptin message. That's because many of these processed foods we're seeing today are imposters; your brain simply doesn't recognize them as real foods. The effect: As ghrelin goes up or leptin goes down, you reach for a fourth pepperoni stick. But if you eat real foods—like nuts, vegetables, whole grains, and lean animal protein—your brain gives your body a direct order: Let's close ship, sir, this one's had enough.

Under normal circumstances, you can keep these hormones in balance and your weight under control by eating minimally processed, nutritious food. But when you're pregnant, some of your hormones are in hurricane status, affecting your appetite in sometimes unpredictable ways.

Factoid: Need more evidence that junk food is just that? And addictive? Researchers found that when you feed some rats good food and some rats good food plus junk food, the rats enjoying the junk food wind up consuming 40 percent more food by weight and 56 percent more calories. Even worse: Their pups develop an affinity for junk, eat more, and gain more weight during their lifetimes than normal pups. If you want fat kids, feed yourself junk during pregnancy.

Factoid: One of the reasons you may be feeling a little hungry is because leptin, a hormone that controls hunger, is a little off during pregnancy. Receptors in the brain work to suppress chemicals that suppress your hunger—thus causing you to become more hungry—to ensure that you will eat enough to provide your baby more nutrients.

Crazy Cravings

You think that your affection for tilapia sundaes is, say, odd? That's nothing compared to the cravings that some women get. Those who suffer from a condition called pica crave nonfood items such as dirt, clay, freezer frost, paper, paint chips, chalk, sand, soap, and cigarette ashes. That doesn't mean that they're crazed; it may mean that they're suffering from an iron or zinc deficiency. (In some populations, up to 70 percent of pregnant women have pica.) While there are certainly risks associated with consuming some of these items, the biggest problem is that filling up on charcoal doesn't provide your baby with adequate nutrition. The cravings generally go away with proper iron and zinc supplementation. The other bit of good news: Though it may have an effect on how a waiter looks at you,* pica does not have an effect on baby's birth weight.

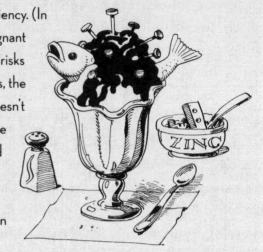

* "Yes, I'd like a salad, some soup, and a medium-rare slice of Play-Doh. Blue if you have it, but green if not."

Let's take cravings, for example, which 75 percent of pregnant women experience. Prior to pregnancy, you may have been a health food fanatic; now you find yourself craving deep-fried onion rings dipped in mayonnaise. Maybe you were a vegetarian; now you have visions of cheeseburgers dancing in your head. Hormones seem to be the most likely source of pregnancy cravings, just as they are for women's premenstrual cravings of chocolate and carbohydrates (ditto for women who take progesterone for birth control or to relieve menopausal symptoms).

Before you flip off your feminine hormones and blame them for your Almond Joy addiction, consider that a craving is really designed to help you. The scientific speculation is that women crave foods that contain the nutrients they need (like vitamin C or potassium) or simply for calories—both of which may be necessary for fetal development. Makes sense. Our bodies alert us to deficiencies so that we can better protect our offspring or take care of ourselves (so we can better protect our offspring). Consider:

- Women may get cravings for salt because sodium is needed to balance their extra fluid volume during pregnancy.
- Cravings for dry, starchy food during the first trimester may be designed to help relieve nausea.
- Similarly, many cravings may be nature's way to avert morning sickness, since women are more likely to feel nauseous on an empty stomach.

Appreciating these evolutionary advantages, however, won't do much to make you feel better if you're chin deep in a pile of potato chips. Food companies seem to try to seduce all of us to eat too much saturated fat, sugar, and salt. And sometimes we succumb. The trick is to make changes as soon as you realize you have gone off course; it's not the first cookie that destroys your plans but the ones that follow. Our tips at the end of the chapter will help you keep those cravings in check so that you can do the same with your weight.

The Sick Sense: Nausea and Nutrition

For many women, the big issue about food during pregnancy is what we just talked about: the carte blanche attitude that they're justified to eat all they want because they're carrying a baby. But just as many women (and often the very same women) want food about as much as they want a hole in the headboard. They feel sick, get sick, and are sick. And to top it off, they feel guilty about being sick because they worry that they're not siphoning up enough calories and nutrients for their babies.

The facts about morning sickness★ are this: About 80 percent of pregnancies

---

★ Morning sickness is a misnomer, because pregnancy-related nausea can, of course, happen at any time of the day.

Holy Molar

Severe nausea isn't associated with just roller coasters and frat parties. Severe nausea can also be a sign of something called a molar pregnancy. This occurs when those chorionic villi (the coral reefs from the last chapter) swell and keep functioning as if there were a fetus—even when there is no viable fetus. A molar pregnancy, which can spread beyond the uterus like a cancer and also cause heavy bleeding, can be detected by an ultrasound and treated with a small surgical procedure called a D&C (dilation and curettage) to remove the excess tissue from the uterus.

come with a side order of nausea, and 20 percent of women can't work because the nausea is so bad. Most cases resolve by fourteen weeks, and nausea usually gets better with time (and, typically, with subsequent pregnancies). Plus, it seems that there's a genetic element to it, since it tends to be passed from mother to daughter.

As is the case with most things body related, there may be a very good reason humans developed morning sickness in the first place. During a time when people ate a lot of raw food that could carry bacteria, nausea—which typically occurs in the first trimester, when the baby is most vulnerable—helped the developing fetus avoid exposure to potential toxins, since the mother would likely be able to tolerate the poisoning, while the child might not. If mom was too sick to eat or could stomach only simple, bland food, it reduced the fetus's chance of being exposed to food-borne illness. Basically, it was better for mom to be nauseous than for the pregnancy to be terminated. Even today, women who experience morning/afternoon/evening sickness are less likely to miscarry than women who do not. It's a harsh reality, but it's one of the many ways that our bodies do what we like to call biological budgeting: protecting the life of the baby at the expense of the mother's comfort.

The true biological reason why pregnant women feel and get sick isn't fully understood. It seems that something in the vomiting center of the brain (didn't know you had one, huh?) is stimulated during pregnancy to induce nausea. (See figure 3.3.) In addition, morning sickness may be linked to higher levels of estrogen and/or the high level of the hormone hCG in early pregnancy. Plus, during pregnancy, the digestive tract relaxes, which makes the muscles guarding reflux from your stomach to your esophagus less efficient, causing an increased flow of acid from your stomach into your esophagus. All those factors and the heightened sense of smell you'll

Figure 3.2 **Seeing Sickness** If you're experiencing nausea associated with pregnancy, a couple of things could be happening. The vomiting center in your brain is more sensitive and your digestive tract is more relaxed, making it more likely that foods will travel up as well as down. A number of foods can help you fight through the nausea and give your baby the needed nutrients. Tip: Try cold ones, as opposed to hot foods (hot foods heighten your sense of smell). And hang in there; it usually passes by the end of the first trimester.

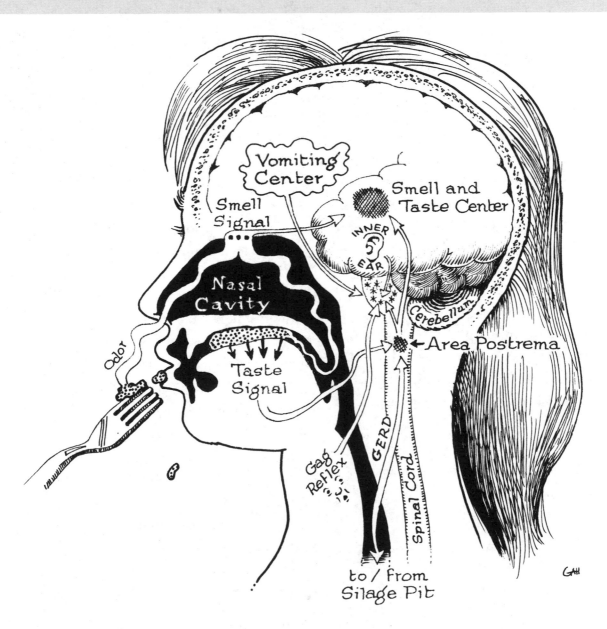

Severe Sickness

If you're unable to keep down liquids for more than twenty-four hours, it may be a sign that you suffer from a condition called hyperemesis (meaning that you vomit *a lot*). It's fairly rare (happens in about 1 percent to 3 percent of pregnancies), and some sufferers have to be admitted to the hospital to be rehydrated. Nobody knows the cause, but risk factors include multiple pregnancies, diabetes, hyperthyroidism, and a history of motion sickness. The point: Not all sickness is a "ride it out" kind of problem, and if you sense that your nausea seems unusually severe, it's worth checking out.

experience during pregnancy create a swirling GI storm that makes many expectant mothers quite literally sickened by the mere mention of food. (By the way, it used to be believed that morning sickness was psychological, which is untrue, except perhaps in a tiny, tiny, tiny percentage of women.)

Some scientists argue that morning sickness and aversions to certain foods are indeed protective. Aversions to meat or raw vegetables, for instance, can be the body's way of protecting against bacteria. Others say that there's less morning sickness in societies that don't consume meat or caffeine. Unfortunately, none of these explanations will make you feel much better as you cope with trying to feed your baby when you don't even want to feed yourself. And another big issue besides making sure that nutrients get to the baby is the risk that you'll become dehydrated; about 1 to 3 percent of pregnant women actually end up in the hospital needing intravenous fluids to correct dehydration. Fact is, you may not be able to eliminate morning sickness; your real goal should be to learn how to manage it. Even though many women have terrible memories of being nauseous during pregnancy, almost all find a way to cope.

Factoid: New research shows that maternal nutrition is important not just for the immediate health of a fetus but also for his long-term health. Just recently, in fact, prenatal nutritional deficiency was linked to developing schizophrenia in adults. It may seem like an odd association, but not when you consider how fundamental in utero nutrition is to brain development.

Your challenge is to find the subtle tricks that work for you. With that in mind, we're going to share a bunch of popular and safe tips with you at the end of this chapter.

Essential Ingredients:
The Nutrients That Both of You Need

Up until this point, we've pretty much dealt with the two extremes regarding food: getting too much and not getting enough. But the third leg of this nutritional tripod is the one that will really help you keep a balance. As you strive to eat the ideal amount of food, we also can't emphasize enough that the issue is as much about quality as quantity. If, for example, you keep a reasonable calorie count for the day, but your main caloric driver comes in the form of one triple-decker fast-food burger with a super-sized side of fries a day, you're not exactly creating the ideal nutritional environment for your child.

Instead, now is the time to really start thinking about food as medicine (if you don't already). Everything you eat will be broken down into smaller molecules that will be transported from your blood to your baby's via that blood lake and placenta interface that we outlined in chapter 2. So, we ask you, which would you rather your child's blood be made of: the vitamins, minerals, and nutrients that are the components of whole foods or the toxins, fat, and artificial junk that's masquerading as food and committing some of the worst health crimes the world's ever seen? We thought so.

The basics are pretty easy. (More details in our tips below.) For the best pregnancy outcome, follow this handy nutritional traffic signal:

> Factoid: When women are obese during their first pregnancy, then lose weight via diet or bariatric surgery before getting pregnant again, the children born before the weight loss end up being heavier than those born afterward. Why? Thank epigenetics, as the environment in a heavy mom lowers a baby's metabolism and teaches his body that it needs to store fat to survive.

Green Light	Red Light
Fruits, vegetables, low-mercury-content fish (domestic salmon and trout are the ones with the healthy fats in the USA), lean meat, poultry (nonfried), legumes, nuts, dried beans and peas, cereal grains, low-fat dairy products, soy, whole grain bread	Saturated fats (some animal fats, plus palm and coconut oil) and trans fats, simple sugars, syrups, enriched or bleached flour, anything fried, sweetened beverages, high-fructose corn syrup, fish identified by the U.S. Food and Drug Administration (FDA) as at risk for high mercury content

While we're on the subject of nutrition, it's also worth talking a bit about vitamins and minerals—specifically, the important role they play in child development:

Vitamin A: Vitamin A aids in both cell development and brain growth, but this vitamin does have a drawback. There have been links between excessive amounts of vitamin A and an increased risk of birth defects, especially neural tube defects. (Be careful of eating too many meal-replacement bars, each of which may have 100 percent of your daily value of A. Get into the habit of checking the FDA nutrition labels on everything you eat.) You should consume no more than 15,000 IU (international units of A) a day while pregnant or just before becoming pregnant, as opposed to limiting yourself to about 3,500 IU a day from supplements and packaged foods when not pregnant.

Vitamin B6: Low levels of B6 are associated with a delay in the development of the baby's nervous system. Plus, low levels are linked to problems for mom, such as morning sickness, preeclampsia, and complications during delivery.

Vitamin B9: You know it as the all-important prenatal nutrient called folate, which in adequate amounts reduces the risk of specific birth defects like spina bifida (an incomplete spinal cord). Getting the right amount during pregnancy—at least 400 micrograms (mcg) from supplements such as a prenatal folic acid vitamin pill and a total of at least 800 mcg including the amounts from food—also reduces your infant's cancer risk for the first six years of life.

Calcium: A full-term baby accumulates 30 grams of calcium in bone mass, so a mom needs to make sure to get three or four servings of calcium-rich foods every day to maintain her own bone strength and get those necessary bone builders to her baby. We recommend taking 600 milligrams (mg) of calcium citrate supplements three times a day, plus 200 mg of magnesium twice a day. (Calcium without one-third the amount of magnesium leads to constipation, so choose your combo carefully.)

Iron: Because a mom transfers about 1,000 milligrams of iron to a growing baby and increases her total number of red blood cells by 20 to 30 percent, it's important to get adequate iron during pregnancy.

DHA: The omega-3 fatty acid DHA (docosahexaenoic acid) is a major structural component of the brain at a time when a fetus's brain is doing a lot of growing. A minimum of 200 mg to 300 mg of DHA per day through fish, fortified foods, or supplements is what you should get to support a healthy pregnancy and grow a healthy baby. Recent research indicates that 600 mg to 900 mg may be even better. We recommend 600 mg.

Zinc: Low levels of zinc have been shown to be related to increased birth defects, low birth weight, miscarriage, and even behavior problems down the road.

Now, the truth is that you don't need to count every milligram of every nutrient of every food that you eat. If you take a good prenatal vitamin every day with DHA, you likely have the basics covered. But that doesn't give you a free pass to eat "whatever" for forty weeks straight. Make your best effort to eat healthfully, but accept that you're going to deviate a bit over the course of your pregnancy—nobody's perfect. In fact, slight deviations here and there are preferable to the alternative: stressing out over every single stray chocolate chip that somehow finds a home in your belly.

YOU TIPS

During these next few months, we know that you're not always going to make decisions as you normally would. That's because shifting hormone levels can steer you in directions you never thought you would go. And that's okay. While it is your job to provide a good nutritional environment for your growing baby, you don't have to feel bad if you occasionally stray from our recommendations. The important thing is to eat well most of the time. Let good decisions comfort and satisfy your body, and they'll do the same for your mind.

Shoot for Balance. We know that your eating habits can flip-flop more than an inexperienced councilman. And as we've outlined, you should expect times when you'll feel like feasting and times when you feel like fainting. That said, it's smart to be aware of what your basic nutritional goals should be (though not to feel guilty if you don't hit them every day). You should strive for:

- nine or more serving (fistfuls) of fruits and vegetables
- three or more servings of whole grain and other grain products
- three or more servings of lean protein in the form of lean meat, skinless poultry, low-mercury fish, eggs, nuts, beans, lentils, and tofu

Your overall philosophy should be this: Eat foods that look like they did when they came out of the ground. (Last we checked, potatoes don't grow with a layer of grease.) Why? Because those are the foods that the placenta recognizes as real food, and those are the foods that contribute the most to a healthy pregnancy.

Adopt the YOU-Turn Mantra. Along the dietary journey, you may make some wrong turns. Sometimes they're A-OK. We just want you to make sure you don't make a habit of it. Acknowledge that you will face obstacles, but instead of falling into the avoidant and defeatist mentality by drop-kicking healthy eating the moment you make one bad choice, act like a GPS system and tell yourself, "At the next available moment, make an authorized YOU-Turn." That is, if you have a day of indulgent, crazed eating, tell yourself that one day won't hurt you and that you need to get back on track. What kills any regimen of healthy eating—whether for 1 or for 1.1—isn't the occasional dessert or pizza binge, it's the cascade of behavior that happens after the initial indulgence.

Eat Often. "Eat often" may sound like a contradiction when we're asking you to be conscientious about any big changes in weight, but the truth is that it's smarter to eat five or six *small* meals throughout the day rather than the traditional three squares. That will help you avoid drops in blood sugar, which can cause cravings. Maintaining an even blood sugar level will also help you avoid nausea. Mainly, though, it will help you feel satisfied so that you don't have the urge to dive headfirst into a gallon of caramel-infused nougat. When you do, search for a food that will satisfy your craving without doing the damage. Some examples:

Instead of . . .	Have . . .
French fries	Roasted sweet potato (see page 362)
Ice cream	Kefir or yogurt with live culture or spore bacteria
Potato chips	Baby carrots or celery sticks
Fried foods	Grilled, baked, or roasted foods
Chocolate chip cookies	½ ounce high-quality dark chocolate
Potato chips	Air-popped popcorn
M&M's	Edamame beans
Toffee, caramel	Nuts or or cut-up fruit
Cheez Doodles	Low-fat string cheese, walnuts
Corn chips	100 percent whole grain pretzel sticks, celery sticks, or cut-up apples
Store-bought salad dressing	Extra-virgin olive oil and either vinegar or lemon juice or both

Stay Away. We know how hard it can be to stay away from foods when your brain is telling you that you have to have them. And every once in a while, it's okay to indulge a craving; the damage really happens when you keep indulging. But we do think it's important for you to familiarize yourself with a few nutritional demons* that you should avoid during pregnancy, in addition to alcohol, which we discussed in chapter 1. Be careful of these:

- **Caffeine:** Restrict soda, carbonated beverages, and all caffeine, especially during the first trimester, when miscarriage rates are highest. After that, up to 200 mg of caffeine a day (one cup of coffee or two cups of black tea) is considered okay.
- **Risky Fish:** Expert bodies such as the FDA have advised pregnant and nursing women to limit their consumption of certain types of fish due to potentially high levels of toxins such as mercury, a contaminant that when present at high levels can harm the developing nervous system of fetuses and newborns. All fish have traces of mercury, but large, bottom-dwelling, fatty fish like sharks, swordfish, king mackerel, tuna, and tilefish contain more mercury than other kinds because they eat smaller fish and live longer, thereby accumulating more of the toxin over time. And fish caught in the waters near coal-powered power plants are the worst. Pregnant women should avoid high-mercury fish and eat up to 12 ounces (two average portions) a week of a variety of fish (salmon and trout are the best commonly available for their omega-3 fat content) and occasionally shellfish that are lower in mercury. If you plan on eating fish caught in local rivers, lakes, or coastal areas, check local advisories about industrial or agricultural pollutants at the U.S. Environmental Protection Agency (EPA) website (http://epa.gov/waterscience/fish/states.htm) before eating. It's important to note that farm-raised fish can also be high in contaminants, so it's best to choose "wild" varieties when available.

Know the Sweet Truth. Many of you surely have questions about the use of artificial sweeteners; those no-calorie, pretty pink and baby blue packets sure are tempting. And the truth is that we can't say much good about artificial sugar substitutes, but we can't say much bad either. While the evidence doesn't show that they're harmful to developing fetuses, we would simply make the point that virtually everything can pass through the placenta, so why would you want to muck up your baby's blood with a bunch of chemicals?† We know you want to watch calories and avoid

---

* An oxymoron if we ever heard one.
† Aspartame hangs out in your body for thirty-six hours. Blecch.

sugar, and that's good. But now can also be a time for creativity in the kitchen. In many cases, fruit juice can be a nice substitute that helps curb your craving for sweets without pumping you full of chemicals or filling you with fat. Another good option: agave nectar, which isn't fermented; otherwise, it's called tequila. Unfermented, it has a cup of sweetness for a half teaspoon of calories (even fructose calories).

Go Organic. If there's one time in your life when you should consider splurging on the often more expensive organic food, it's now. Eating organic will help you avoid the toxins and pesticides that may be present in nonorganic foods. Even so, wash organic fruits and veggies three times in a salad spinner to remove all the natural stuff used as fertilizer. One other helpful tip we live by whether pregnant or not: Avoid waxed foods. You can tell if something is waxed by smelling the stem; if it doesn't smell like the food, then it's likely waxed. The problem with wax is that it locks in pesticides that can be found on fruits like apples, pears, and nectarines. Other big pesticide offenders include berries, potatoes, peppers, peaches, spinach, lettuce, and celery; during pregnancy, it is better to buy them organically grown. And while we're talking about the produce aisle, we recommend that you choose frozen fruits and vegetables in the winter, since the fresh kind would be coming from remote locations. Frozen produce is picked at its peak and frozen immediately, often containing far more nutrients than out-of-season fresh produce that is trucked long distances. Freezing stores nutrients better than canning: Fruits and veggies often lose as much as 20 percent of total nutrients in the canning process.

Here are the fruits and vegetables with the highest and lowest pesticide contents, if you're not going to go organic:

Highest		Lowest	
Peaches	Strawberries	Onions	Asparagus
Apples	Cherries	Avocados	Sweet peas
Bell peppers	Kale	Sweet corn	Kiwis
Celery	Lettuce	Pineapples	Cabbage
Nectarines	Imported grapes	Mangoes	Eggplants

Control Your Sickness. In life, long lists can keep you organized. In magazines, long lists might sell copies. In medicine, a long list of solutions means that there's no surefire one. Such is the case when it comes to morning sickness and nausea. A lot of things *can* help you feel better, but that doesn't mean they all will. So, unfortunately, this is one of those areas in which you may have to play mad scientist and experiment a bit to see what therapy may be best for your body. Here are some things that have been shown to relieve the misery:

- Keep 100 percent whole grain crackers by your bed and eat a few as soon as you wake, to get something in your stomach before you start moving around.
- Eat a diet high in protein and complex carbohydrates.
- Chicken broth, to help you get some calories in along with the liquid.
- Cold foods; hot foods have a stronger smell, which can trigger queasiness.
- Vitamin B6 (10 mg).
- Leafy greens, because they're rich in vitamin K, which seems to help.
- Brown rice.
- Acupuncture (forearm needles for two days).
- Acupressure wristbands to stimulate pressure points.
- Fresh gingerroot in a cup of tea (or a 300 mg capsule).
- Light exercise.
- Use a mouth rinse after vomiting (and after each meal) to keep your mouth fresh, reduce nausea, and reduce the amount of tooth decay that can occur from the interaction of stomach acid with enamel.

- Meditate to help control stress. Morning sickness is more common in women under a lot of stress.
- Homeopathic remedies are hotly debated within the medical community but are unlikely to cause harm. Nux vomica seems to help with nausea and irritability.

Consider Meds. If your morning sickness is really bad, talk to your doc about prescription medications like scopolamine (Transderm Scōp, Scopace), promethazine (Phenergan), prochlorperazine (Compazine), and trimethobenzamide (Tigan). You can also consider Diclectin, an over-the-counter (OTC) remedy available only in Canada. Each capsule contains 25 milligrams of vitamin B6 (pyridoxine), 5 milligrams of Unisom (the OTC sleeping medication that is not Benadryl), and 250 micrograms (.25 milligram) of folic acid. The manufacturer of Diclectin voluntarily withdrew the drug from the U.S. market (where it was known as Bendectin) in 1983 due to some safety concerns that were not borne out through study. As a result of all the accusations about Bendectin, it is now the best-studied agent for treating nausea, and lots of substantial research shows it may prove to be the safest antinausea agent. You should of course consult with your doc, but if you want to re-create Bendectin at home, take a combination of one 25 milligram tablet of vitamin B6 and one 5 milligram tablet of Unisom orally three or four times a day. (You're already getting 400 micrograms of folic acid from your prenatal vitamin.)

Decide if You're Nuts. Not nuts as in crazy, but nuts as in walnuts or even the legume, peanuts. There's been a lot of talk about whether eating peanuts during pregnancy contributes to childhood peanut allergies or asthma. The research suggests that avoiding peanuts doesn't seem to have an effect on nut allergies except when there's a family history of extreme cases of the allergy. Eating peanuts during pregnancy has, however, been related to an increase in asthma rates. If you want to be supercautious, you can avoid peanuts and peanut butter, but generally, it's okay to eat both during pregnancy. The more important issue is to make sure that you eat apples, fish, and omega-3 fatty acids like DHA, found in salmon and trout, fortified foods, and supplements, because they've been shown to help prevent asthma and avert allergies that can run in families. Eating them during pregnancy will help strengthen your child's delicate immune system before the environment starts taking shots at it.

4

Growing to Extremes

How to Make Sure Your Baby Isn't Too Plump or Too Puny

At this moment in your life, we can guess what curves you're likely obsessing about: your growing tummy, your fuller breasts, your figure in a maternity bathing suit. Now, though, is the time to shift gears and consider another kind of curve: the bell curve. We know, we know. Graphs and charts are about as compelling a topic as laundry detergent. But as we build on our discussion of nutrition from the last chapter, the classic bell curve helps make a vital point about how your baby's weight in the womb will influence his lifelong health.

You already know how the bell curve looks and works. (See adjacent illustration if you need a refresher.) For whatever the given criteria, you have a small number at the two extreme ends and a big number in the middle; hence the bell shape. The traditional example: A school course that fits a bell-curve model would have a few students who earned A's in a class, a few who got slapped with F's, and the vast majority residing in the B, C, D world of the majority, the norm, the average. In pregnancy, the bell curve teaches us about what's happening to your developing baby. Here's the difference between the pregnancy model and the classroom one: The extreme ends of the bell curve don't represent excellence and failure, as they do in the A and F example. Instead, your baby's optimal grade rests right in the middle of the bell curve. Why? Because, at the risk of annoying our literature-teacher readers by adding a

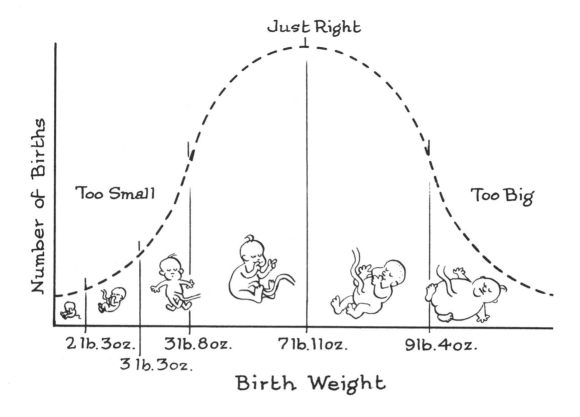

Just Right

Number of Births

Too Small

Too Big

2 lb. 3 oz.
3 lb. 3 oz.
3 lb. 8 oz.
7 lb. 11 oz.
9 lb. 4 oz.

Birth Weight

metaphor to a metaphor, Goldilocks was right about your baby's size. You don't want *too big* and you don't want *too small*. You want *just about right*.

The fact is that even if you're eating perfectly well and following all the guidelines for a safe pregnancy, something else could be causing your baby to receive the wrong amount of food—resulting in either undernutrition or overnutrition, both of which can put your baby at risk.

What's at stake? For underdeveloped babies, there's the risk that vital organs and tissues won't develop enough to fully prepare them for life on the outside. For the plumper peeps? Too much baby fat can put both you and them at greater risk for developing complications from pregnancy. Why? For one thing, big babies raise your risk of stalled labor and cesarean section. For another, remember from chapter 1 that kids learn to forecast their future environments while in your belly. Not enough nutrition means they come to expect an environment of scarcity (there's that thrifty phenotype again), thus sending the message that they should load up on Ding Dongs

Testing, Testing

It can be hard to tell from the surface whether you have gestational diabetes, so you should pay special attention if you have the risk factors or the main symptoms: increased thirst and urination, blurred vision, fatigue, and/or infections of the bladder, vagina, and skin. This issue is important: 25 percent of women with gestational diabetes will go on to develop full-blown diabetes, and the greatest risk is within the first five years after delivery, especially in overweight mothers.

Today all pregnant women are screened for diabetes, even those at low risk (under twenty-five, not obese, white, and no family history of diabetes). For a fasting blood test (no food within eight hours), blood sugar should be under 95 mg/dl.* In your doc's office, you'll also be given a test called a glucose challenge, in which you'll consume 50 grams of sugar. It's why you get that cup of orange soda, an admittedly nasty concoction called Glucola. If your blood sugar level is higher than 135 mg/dl after an hour, it's a sign that you're not clearing glucose fast enough, and you'll be given a second challenge with 100 grams of sugar.

In this case, after consuming a load of sugar (in a soda or candy bar), your blood sugar will be monitored over three hours. Your goal is to be less than 180 mg/dl in the first hour after eating, less than 165 after two hours, and less than 145 after three hours. If not, your doc will talk to you about the first line of treatment: controlling blood sugar through diet and exercise. If that doesn't work, she may consider prescribing antidiabetic drugs for you.

* Normally, it's 100, but pregnant women have lower blood sugar, so the norm is lowered to 95.

and store every excess calorie they can as fat to prepare for future famines. Too many calories condition them to expect overabundance and to indulge in a fat-filled life that comes with all of the fixings that complicate it.

Most times, kids fall in the middle of that bell curve; right in the normal range. That's why the middle of the baby-weight bell curve is bigger than a septuplets' grocery bill. But you also need to be aware of what happens when you teeter toward the extreme edges of fetal weight, because that's when your provider may need to intervene.

To examine these ends of the bell, we're going to look at how babies get their nutrition and how metabolism influences that process. Through that discussion, you'll learn about why some children grow too much, why some don't grow enough, and if that is the case for you, how you can guide your baby back to the middle.

Metabolic Magic:
How Your Nutrition Influences His

Remember from our introduction about how pregnancy is a lot like a ballroom dance, with you and your partner nudging each other in different directions? Nowhere does this dance play out more than when it comes to metabolism. As your hormones surge during pregnancy, your body changes too. It changes the way it processes energy, it changes the way you store fat, and ultimately it changes the way you deliver nutrients to your baby.

Considering the torture you've already put your body through at various times in your life,★ you're already pretty aware of how amazingly responsive human metabolic processes can be. For example, our

> Factoid: How often does your baby move? Unless you've got a counter, it's hard to keep up. At twenty weeks, the average is about 200 times a day. At thirty-two weeks, it's 575. At forty weeks, that number drops to about 300. The reason? There's less room for the tyke to move around as it grows.

bodies are able to weather all kinds of biological storms, adapting to such things as high altitudes and extreme climates. Your metabolism also makes adjustments when it sees another kind of biological storm: pregnancy.

In a nonpregnant person, metabolism typically works this way (see figure 4.1). When you eat food, your body converts it to energy in the form of the sugar called

★ All-day mountain hikes, all-night study sessions, weeklong cabbage soup diets.

Figure 4.1 **Energy Efficient** When you eat, your body takes the calories and converts them to glucose, your body's energy source. With insulin serving as glucose's carrier pigeon, that glucose is shuttled throughout the body to help all of your muscles and organs function smoothly. In pregnancy, that system often is much more resistant, as your body needs to make sure to provide the glucose to your baby.

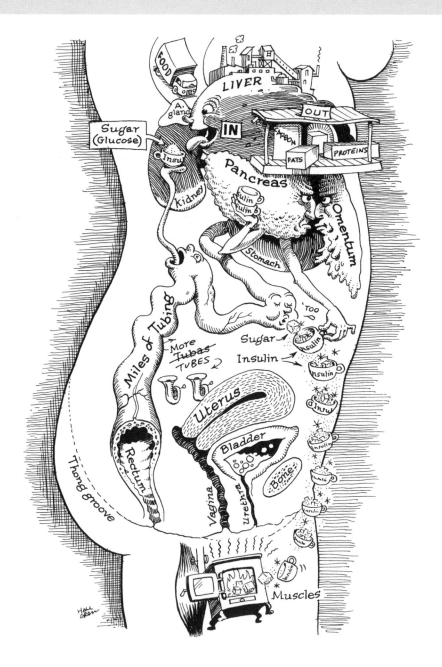

glucose. That glucose goes through the liver, where it's processed into fat, proteins, and carbohydrates, and gets shuttled around your body to help your muscles and tissues function.

Glucose, like underage airplane passengers, can't travel alone. It needs some assistance: specifically, something to help it get from the bloodstream into the cells to provide the energy you need to breathe, to make your heart beat, and even to do the missionary mambo that got you into this condition in the first place.

The pancreas provides the hormone insulin, which chaperones glucose throughout the body and facilitates its entry into the cells. It's a nice, efficient system that allows the food you eat to provide the energy that all parts of your body need to function. In a perfect world, there's the right amount of glucose, the right amount of insulin, and life is simply swell.

Now, consider what happens when the metabolic storm comes rolling in, in the form of—bada-bing—little Leonard. Lenny's not quite ready for smashed turnips when he's doing laps in amniotic fluid, so he needs some of mom's chemical nectar to keep him growing in utero. And yep, that energy-giving and baby-growing nectar comes in the form of—you got it—glucose.

Because the baby's brain depends on glucose, the placenta's mission is to make sure that the glucose cupboard is never, ever bare. In fact, if the fetus's blood sugar drops below the magic number—90 milligrams per deciliter of blood (mg/dl)—for even a few minutes, the fetus can suffer irreversible brain damage. So the placenta produces a hormone called human placental lactogen (hPL), which inhibits mom's insulin from getting glucose into her cells, thereby increasing mom's bloodstream glucose levels available to baby. Big-time. The hormone hPL is almost identical in structure to the growth hormone present in all women. But in pregnant women, it can reach a thousand times the equivalent normal concentration. And you can see why: no glucose for baby, no development; no development, no birth. Human placental lactogen acts like maternal growth hormone, helping all the mother's structures grow appropriately as well.

When hPL blocks insulin's ability to transport glucose into your cells, it allows your baby to get the glucose he needs to grow. This hormonal dance, delicate and subtle as it is, ultimately influences whether your baby will achieve a target weight during pregnancy or not. And when this dance gets a little bit out of sync—oftentimes through absolutely no fault of the mom—that's when we start to see issues that can influence both the development of your baby as he grows inside you and your baby's future health after birth.

The Plump Position: When Big Is Bad

In some circles, there seems to be a sort of badge of honor that comes with carrying and delivering a big baby. We celebrate with—and even admire—moms who can carry and deliver kids who enter this world the size of dishwashers. But there are many reasons why you don't want your baby to be too big at birth. As we said, you're programming your child to store weight later in life. Plus, you're opening yourself up to more potential complications at birth as well as the risk of future conditions such as adult-onset diabetes.

One of the reasons we see XXL babies is because of a metabolic problem in mom called gestational diabetes. Many of us assume that the only way to get diabetes is by pummeling your insides with a four-a-day cheesecake habit, but gestational diabetes works a bit differently. (See "What's Food Got to Do with It?" on page 96.)

To see exactly how it works, let's take a closer look at glucose metabolism. When hPL causes the changes that increase maternal blood glucose, this leaves more glucose circulating in mom's bloodstream, available to satisfy the glucose-greedy fetus. That's a good thing. Bubba needs glucose to grow. But it comes with a price.

To counteract those rising sugar levels as your pregnancy progresses, you secrete more insulin. So the placenta responds by pumping out even more hPL, which limits the effectiveness of that extra insulin. If your muscles and liver cannot easily use up all that sugar, you may end up with too much glucose floating around in your blood. That's called insulin resistance, and in some moms, the vicious hPL-insulin cycle escalates into full-blown gestational diabetes (a risk factor, by the way, for prenatal and postpartum depression).

One problem with gestational diabetes is that mom's excess sugar freely passes through the placenta to the fetus. In response to this excess sugar in its blood, the

The Thyroid Puzzle

Many women already know all about thyroid hormone problems; too much or too little can slow down or speed up metabolism and cause a host of symptoms that can make you feel out of sorts in an all-around kind of way. When you add pregnancy to the mix, thyroid issues can get even more complex.

Typically, a mother's level of thyroid hormone increases between 10 percent and 30 percent during pregnancy, most likely due to the increase in estrogen. Extra estrogen during pregnancy stimulates your cells to make more proteins with binding sites for thyroid hormone. To fill those binding sites, you make more thyroid hormone, but the amount free in your bloodstream, which stimulates your cells, should remain normal, as the increase in production should balance the increase in binding sites. Sometimes, however, the adjustment is imperfect, and you end up with too much (hyperthyroidism) or too little (hypothyroidism) circulating thyroid hormone, which can cause you to experience metabolic chaos. Thyroid conditions are difficult to diagnose because they share some of the same classic symptoms associated with the hormonal changes in pregnancy, such as frenetic or low energy, excess weight loss or gain, and emotional fluctuations. In addition, hyperthyroidism can occur during pregnancy because two of the hormones produced by the placenta—hCG and hPL—mimic thyroid-stimulating hormone (TSH), which does exactly what its name implies—stimulates the thyroid to produce thyroid hormone.

It'd be nice if you could just pop thyroid medication to handle these problems, but it's not so easy. Because tests used to determine levels of thyroid-stimulating hormone in your blood often cannot distinguish among TSH, hCG, and hPL, it's hard to be sure that the thyroid is causing your symptoms and, if it is, to determine the optimal dose of medication.

In pregnancy, women who start out with hypothyroidism typically need to increase their thyroid hormone dosage by 50 percent because the increased estrogen produces an increased level of a protein that binds thyroid hormone, meaning even less thyroid hormone is available for the mother.

Another interesting note: There are talks about requiring a thyroid test for pregnant moms because there seems to be a strong link between undiagnosed hypothyroidism during pregnancy and reduced IQ in their offspring.

What's Food Got to Do with It?

You probably know that diabetes is typically associated with too many calories, so you may be asking yourself how you can become diabetic in pregnancy without overeating. Good question. Normally what happens in an insulin-resistant state is that your appetite increases when glucose can't get into your cells—especially your liver cells and the satiety center of the brain. In response, you'll crave and eat simple carbs (chocalert!) to combat those cravings. However, that only increases the glucose surge and starts the whole cycle over again. In gestational diabetes, insulin resistance starts because of the surge of hPL, which increases your blood glucose levels, so it's not overeating that's to blame. However, you may still experience cravings for carbs, which exacerbates the situation and, if you're susceptible, may push you over the line to a full-blown case of gestational diabetes. That's why we say that even if poor nutrition isn't the cause per se of gestational diabetes, eating smart will certainly lower your risk of developing it. See our food recommendations throughout the book.

fetus must increase production of its own insulin. This insulin increase acts like a growth hormone. The result is that your baby gains weight too quickly and ends up on the heavy end of the bell-shaped curve.

While it may seem as it's no big deal for your baby to pack a few extra pounds at birth ("A future offensive lineman!" shouts the uncle), a chunky fetus makes more fat cells in utero. So now the husky baby is not only prone to being overweight as a child, he's also prone to storing fat as he gets older. (And a baby whose mom had gestational diabetes is also prone to delays in language development.) In addition, immediately after birth, the newborn tends to develop dangerously low blood sugar because his body has been overproducing insulin to cope with his diabetic mother's sugar, which was leaking into his body. If this occurs, baby has to be monitored closely for the first few days after birth until he can adapt to an environment outside mom's body.

There are other risks with gestational diabetes as well: Your ob/gyn may want to deliver a bit earlier than your due date if she thinks the baby is getting too big for your britches. And because lung development may not be complete if the baby is delivered early, premature delivery places him at risk for breathing problems after birth.

Gestational diabetes can also pose problems for mom. Without insulin's ability to move sugar into your cells due to the aforementioned insulin resistance, the extra sugar in your bloodstream acts like shards of glass, scraping up the walls of your arteries and potentially inflaming the blood vessels that go to the placenta. In this case, you can actually end up depriving your baby of oxygen and vital nutrients, and when diabetes predates the pregnancy, it can lead to the opposite extreme of the bell curve with a condition known as intrauterine growth restriction, which we'll talk about shortly. At the same time, a series of hormones produced by the uterus and mom's body—namely cortisol (the stress hormone), leptin (the high blood pressure hormone), and adiponectin (an inflammation-reducing hormone)—all flood mom's bloodstream and contribute to higher glucose levels floating around in a biological never-never land. And all that continues the vicious cycle of too much glucose and insulin resistance.

Considering that up to 10 percent of pregnant women get gestational diabetes, you're probably wondering who's at risk. Because of the surge of hPL, all pregnant women are put into this hypermetabolic state of insulin resistance, and most women's bodies are able to adjust and handle the storm just fine. The problem happens when women have additional risk factors, stemming from either a family history of diabetes or gaining too much weight during pregnancy. (Nearly 30 percent of women who gain forty or more pounds during pregnancy have heavy babies, compared to less than 15 percent of women who don't gain that much weight.) If you're already overweight, have had a large baby in the past, have a strong family history of diabetes, or are over twenty-five, you might be more susceptible to responding poorly to hPL and developing gestational diabetes. (See page 90 for how you're tested.) If you are diagnosed with gestational diabetes, your doc will put you on a special diet, encourage you to exercise, and teach you how to monitor your blood sugar level, which you'll have to test several times a day.

Thriving and Well: How Is He Growing?

If a glucose-rich baby is one end of the spectrum, you don't need to be a biological brainiac to guess the other end: when something either prevents nutrients from reaching the fetus or makes the fetus unable to use energy properly to grow.

There are many reasons why you need to make sure your baby is getting enough calories. Among other things, lack of growth in the womb can cause a decrease in brain development and immune deficiency, as well as short stature. If vital organs don't get the nutrients they need, they're not going to grow to and function at maximum capacity. And there's evidence to show that this can contribute to a wide range of problems when these babies become adults, including hormonal problems such as thyroid issues, metabolic problems (obesity), and even cardiovascular problems (heart disease and hypertension).

Like so many other conditions, there can be many causes of intrauterine growth restriction, which affects the smallest 5 percent of babies. IUGR is just a fancy name for saying that the baby isn't gaining enough weight. On the one hand, it can occur when there are maternal nutritional concerns. Perhaps you're not eating enough or you're suffering from so much nausea that you are losing weight and can't keep nutrients down. Another reason could be that you had babies too close together, so your body may still be recovering and repairing itself after baby number one, making fewer resources available for baby number two.

On the other hand, you may eat a perfectly balanced and nutrient-rich diet, have no nausea problems whatsoever, and still have a growth-restricted baby. In this case, something else might be causing a kink in the link between your nutrition and your baby's. Infections, exposure to toxins, and genetic conditions all increase your baby's risk of IUGR. Cigarette smoke, uncontrolled hypertension, and other serious coexisting maternal diseases, for example, cause arteries to constrict, so there's less

Factoid: It seems that social support isn't just good for you, it's also good for your baby. Research shows that moms with strong social connections, be it friends or family, have babies that are at less risk of having low birth weight.

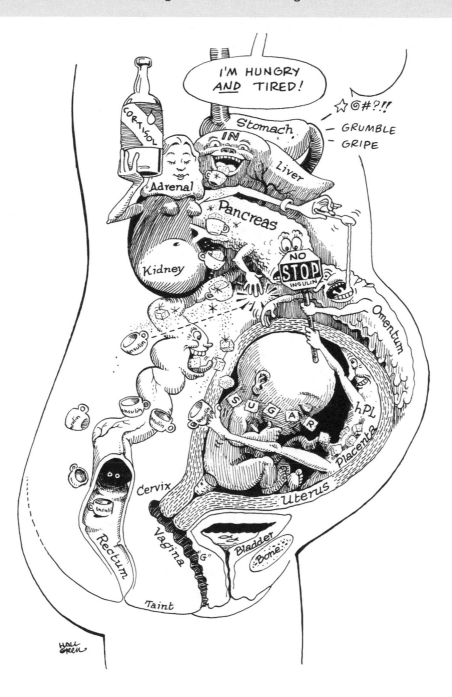

blood flowing to the uterus. Restricted blood flow may also be caused by inadequacy of a chemical called nitric oxide, which opens up the arteries.

When arteries are too constricted to deliver adequate nutrition to the fetus, they also can't deliver adequate oxygen, so many of the tests used to diagnose IUGR actually evaluate your baby's oxygen supply. Docs can get a good idea of fetal growth by looking at the size of the fetus, as well as for signs that it might not be getting enough oxygen. If your child is not growing at a proper pace, your doc will try to identify the cause. In many cases, if the problem is fixed, the baby can catch up.

As you may have guessed, it's not as if you're going to step on a scale, look at a number (which can vary pretty mightily from day to day), and let that be the sole determinant of whether your baby is growing properly or not. Typically, you and your provider will go through a multistep process to try to pinpoint growth problems (and their severity) so you can then take actions to improve the situation. To help prepare you for the prodding, poking, and testing that can go on during pregnancy, we've outlined some of the tests that will take place if your doc has a clinical suspicion that your baby is not developing at the pace he should be. While ultrasounds (in the doctor's office, not at the mall) give us a lot of data about how your baby is growing, there's no one best test to determine definitively if there is a developmental issue. That's why docs use a number of different methods to help them evaluate fetal size, growth, and well-being.

The Doc Check:
How We Determine Growth Rate

Now, the tricky part about determining fetal weight is that we can't exactly get a scale inside the womb, so we docs need to rely on a number of other methods to determine whether your baby is sliding down from the middle of the bell curve.

Midway through your pregnancy, your provider will start measuring the size of your baby. By twenty weeks, the uterus as measured from the pubic bone to the top of your belly should be about 20 centimeters in length and grow 1 centimeter every week for the next fourteen to sixteen weeks. (The 1 cm a week doesn't hold up late

The Twenty-Week Ultrasound

Of all the monumental moments in your child's life (first walk, first tooth, first date), the first ultrasound ranks right up there as one of the biggest. While it's traditionally thought of as the "find out the sex" test, that's not always the case; the little rascals often close their legs, making it difficult to tell the gender, so don't get your hopes up. Instead the twenty-week test is used to detect whether your baby is headed in the right direction. After checking the size of your belly to make sure your doc or midwife has predicted the right gestational age of the baby, the sonographer will look at things like the volume of amniotic fluid, the anatomy of the brain and heart, the face, kidneys, limbs, and bones, and the blood vessels in the umbilical cord to make sure they're all developing healthfully. He's also looking for more ambiguous things like the baby's general tone; for instance, if your baby is lying down in a froglike position, it could be an indication of Down syndrome. This ultrasound is one of the places where your provider can first start to see markers for growth retardation or a hint that further testing for chromosomal problems may be necessary. At this ultrasound, the doc will also be checking for what's called an incompetent cervix. That's a condition that typically shows up early in the second trimester in which the cervix is too weak to stay closed—thus increasing the risk of preterm labor and miscarriage.

in your third trimester.) Your doc can estimate the size of the baby by measuring from the top of the pubic bone* to the top of the uterus. You can also do this yourself; just ask your doc or midwife to help you locate the top of your uterus, so you know what to feel for.

Now, keep in mind that a full bladder and belly fat can change this measurement, so it's not perfect, but it certainly can offer a clue as to whether you're on the right track. If things aren't looking quite up to par, that's when your provider may try a few other tests to figure out what's happening on the inside.

* That's at the site of a disc of cartilage called the symphysis pubis.

The Beautiful Bodily Fluid

No matter your fluid of choice (water, tea, a venti pumpkin spice latte), it's time to appreciate another. The most important fluid that moms need to know about is the one that acts a bit like an air bag for your developing baby: amniotic fluid. A product of fetal metabolism, amniotic fluid serves several purposes: It helps exchange substances between mom and baby, it acts as a physical barrier that protects the fetus (a sort of cushioning against trauma, such as a car accident), and it also works as part of a baby's immune system, as it contains immune chemicals that fight viruses and bacteria. Another cool fact: The fluid coats both sides of the tympanic membrane in the baby's ear, which allows sound to pass through from the outer ear to the inner one.

Babies also need amniotic fluid for lung development. A newborn's lungs are like crumpled Saran Wrap. When a fetus inhales amniotic fluid, it stimulates the lung tissue's production of surfactant, which lubricates the airways and allows the lungs to mature. By the way, too much insulin in the child, as in the case of gestational diabetes, inhibits the production of surfactant; this can slow down lung development and stress a newborn child.

Amniotic fluid is a great diagnostic tool because it gives us clues as to what's happening developmentally in utero. Besides bathing in amniotic fluid, which helps the fetus train to balance himself in space, like a gymnast, the fetus is constantly swallowing and inhaling the fluid—about 340 milliliters a day, or a little less than a pint. The fetus regurgitates about half of that and pees out the rest. Amniotic fluid turns over completely every three days, as opposed to being the same old broth for the entire pregnancy.

There are several reasons for varying amounts of amniotic fluid, and docs estimate its volume to identify potential problems. For example, if we see too much fluid in an ultrasound, it could be a signal that there's a problem with fetal swallowing and digestion. Too little fluid could mean that the fetus's kidneys aren't working the way they should.

Nonstress Test

Performed in the third trimester, this test monitors the fetus's heart rate. You'll have a monitor strapped around your waist, and your doc will look for two or more accelerations of fifteen beats per minute above the normal baseline reading, each lasting

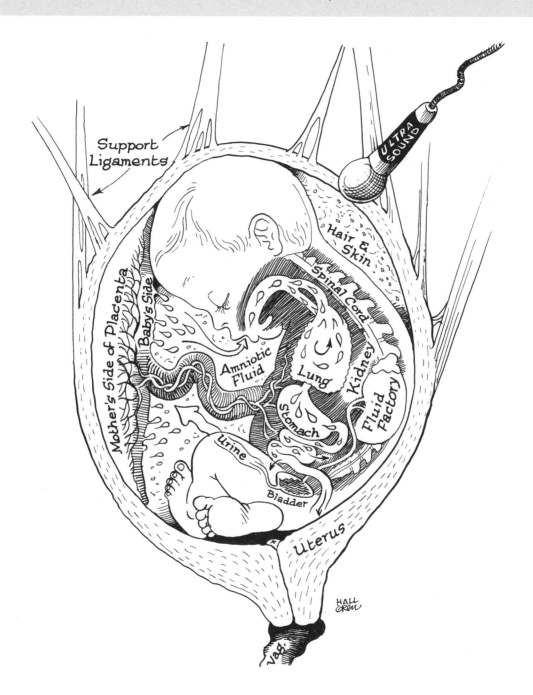

Figure 4.3 **Fluid Check** Among the many functions of amniotic fluid, two main purposes are to help develop a baby's immune system and to help mature a baby's lungs. Plus, it provides a nice cushioned environment in the womb; sort of like baby's first waterbed.

for fifteen seconds or more during a twenty- to thirty-minute period. If your baby doesn't move, he could be sleeping. To stimulate him, you will usually be given a sugary or bubbly drink, or the nurse will make a loud noise. If you pass this test, you typically don't need to move on to the next ones.

Contraction Stress Test

This test is one way to tell if your baby is experiencing a stressful environment. After contractions are induced (either through intravenous administration of the hormone oxytocin or through stimulation of the breasts), your doc will look for a decrease in fetal heart rate occurring with more than 50 percent of your contractions. During contractions, the pressure of amniotic fluid increases, and because no blood is entering the uterus, there's less blood flowing into the space between the placenta and the uterus. So the capacity to maintain oxygen levels depends on the amount of working surface area available in the placenta. If there are placental problems, you'll see the fetal heart rate slow down more than normal, as the amount of oxygen delivered becomes dangerously low for your baby's heart. This is often used if no ultrasounds are available where you are getting care.

> **Factoid:** Maybe you've seen boutique ultrasounds, offered at the mall and pitched as an opportunity to frame your baby's first pictures. Resist the temptation. Amateurs are doing them, and they often have the settings way too high—a dangerous risk for your child. The FDA has issued a warning about these, as the energy used might permanently harm the baby's hearing and may even cause burns, with subsequent permanent scarring.

Biophysical Profile

If you have an abnormal nonstress test or other high risk factors (and sometimes your doc will skip from the nonstress test to this profile), your doc will perform a biophysical profile, which measures several elements of fetal development and thus gives a more complete picture of the duress facing a fetus. Here's how it works: In each of the following categories, you get a score of 2 or 0, then the individual scores are added to determine your overall risk.

Test	Score of 2	Score of 0
Nonstress test (described above)	Two accelerations of fifteen beats per minute for fifteen seconds within twenty minutes	0 or 1 acceleration
Fetal breathing (doc will monitor your baby's chest wall movements)	One episode within thirty minutes of rhythmic breathing lasting thirty seconds	Less than thirty seconds
Fetal movement (looking for vigorous movements, but will slow down closer to term because there's less space to move around)	Three body or limb movements within thirty minutes	Less than three
Fetal tone (how the baby extends or flexes limbs)	One episode of flexing within thirty minutes	No movements or extensions/flexions
Amniotic fluid volume (measured in pockets of fluid via ultrasound) (see "The Beautiful Bodily Fluid," page 102)	Single vertical pocket of greater than 2 cm	Largest single vertical pocket, 2 cm

Your Score: If you score an 8 or above, the baby is typically in a normal state. A 6 or below indicates that he may be experiencing some stress, and you and the doc will discuss how to manage the situation.

Managing Risks

The next question, of course, is what the heck happens if your doc decides that your baby is bringing up the rear when it comes to growth. The answer really depends on how far along you are, and the decision about how to manage the situation comes down to weighing risks versus benefits. Essentially, if you're far enough along (say, thirty-eight weeks) but the baby is showing some signs of distress, your doc will probably suggest that you deliver. But if you're at a point in your pregnancy when your baby's lungs may not be fully developed (say, thirty to thirty-two weeks), your doc may want to take other precautions, such as retesting a few hours to a few days later or putting you on bed rest. While bed rest may help you catch up on Bravo channel marathons, it also helps your situation by minimizing the need for your blood to provide energy to your body—thus maximizing the blood delivery to your baby. That's the theory, at least; bed rest may have no benefit, but docs (like most humans) feel they have to do something for you, and this is a pretty benign option.

If you are identified to be at risk for IUGR, you'll likely increase your doctor visits and monitoring through the last several weeks of pregnancy, and you can even do some self-tests. For example, look for about ten fetal movements in the two hours after a meal; fewer than that, and you might want to check in with your doc. The good news is that if the problem is related to inadequate fetal nutrition, as opposed to a genetic condition or inadequate blood flow to the uterus, the prognosis is usually good. The following tips will help maximize your chances of optimum nutrient delivery throughout the pregnancy.

Factoid: During labor, the minute the placenta is expelled, all insulin resistance starts to diminish. That's why you may experience a very abrupt decrease in sugar supply, and that's why a baby may experience low blood sugar too. The sugar your baby got because you had insulin resistance and passed sugar to him goes away, but your newborn still produces a lot of insulin. So all sugar is escorted into the baby's cells, leaving the baby with a deficiency in the blood. While your baby will use some of his energy-giving brown fat to sustain himself, it's also why he needs the calories from frequent feedings early on. Brown fat is a kind of fat that's found along the upper back and spine in newborns (as well as in hibernating animals) to help them generate body heat. Most of this fat disappears as we grow up, unless we live in especially cold climates.

YOU TIPS

We've said it before, and we'll say it again: It's detrimental for moms to shoulder two tons of worry about every movement, stage, and milestone that happens in utero. You control the controllables to help the process, but you also need to allow the biological miracle to play itself out. In the "do what you can" category, here are our recommendations for increasing the chances that you'll sit in the middle—and not slide down the sides—of the all-important nutritional bell curve:

Don't Keep It Simple. In your diet, you want to avoid simple carbohydrates (for instance, white foods such as refined sugar, pasta, white rice, and white bread). These foods raise your blood sugar level, which requires your body to make more insulin. Since insulin is already pushing as hard as it can, this can contribute to the insulin resistance already caused by pregnancy and tip you over the edge into gestational diabetes. Instead stick to more complex carbs (think high-fiber foods, 100 percent whole grains, Jerusalem artichoke pasta, or brown rice). It's also smart to avoid saturated and trans fats (four-legged animal fat, palm and coconut oils, hydrogenated oils, fried and processed foods), since they cause inflammation, which can mess up the metabolic miracle of delivering the right nutrients to the fetus at the perfect moment. Your child wants nutrients rather than calories, so concentrate on eating foods that don't come with labels.

Watch Your Waist. We know it's growing *now*, but in pre- and postpregnancy, make sure that your waist measurement at your belly button is not wider than half your height. So if you are five foot four, or sixty-four inches, you should keep your waist size at or below thirty-two inches to decrease your risk of health problems. If your waist measurement is greater than half your height, you have too much belly fat. As you know, this type of fat blocks the ability of insulin to work on muscle, so sugar can't get into and be metabolized by your cells. Slimming your waist size before and after pregnancy with less food, more physical activity, and stress management is the best way to prevent and treat diabetes.

Adopt a Chia Pet. Add whole grain chia, which contains omega-3 fats as well as fiber, to your diet. Unlike flaxseeds, you don't need to grind chia seeds to absorb their precious cargo of healthy fats. And chia keeps moisture in foods, making them taste better. More important, when you eat chia seeds, they form a gelatinous substance in the stomach. This helps to inhibit the speed at which sugar is absorbed, which may benefit diabetics. Mix chia seeds into yogurt, sprinkle them on cereal in the morning, or add them to salads. Make sure not to eat the clay pot, just the chia growing through the holes—or just purchase it in its pure form.

Mention the Meds. There's no question that the best defense against gestational diabetes comes in the form of smart food choices and exercise, and nearly half of women can get gestational diabetes under control by making these behavioral changes. But if they don't seem to work, it certainly is worth talking to your doc about prescription medications that can alter your blood sugar levels. First in line is usually metformin (Glucophage), which stimulates the liver to listen more carefully to the insulin. Second in line is glyburide (Micronase, Diabeta), which increases the release of insulin from the pancreas. Insulin itself is typically given if nothing else works. (All but insulin cross the placenta.) It's also worth noting that if you're at high risk of developing gestational diabetes, you may want to consider consulting a physician who is a maternal-fetal specialist. Such a doc has more experience with the disease and can advise your primary doctor.

Get a Lift. Most pregnant women are so used to adding weight, adding inches, and adding stress that the last thing they want to do is add something else. But we have one more thing to add to the list: muscle. While now is not the ideal time to shape your body into that of a contestant on *American Gladiators,* it's generally a fine time to add a little lean muscle mass by doing some resistance exercises with light weights. (See our plan starting on page 310.) Why? Muscle speeds your metabolism, which lowers your risk of gaining extra fat and developing diabetes; muscle mass also serves as a reserve that will burn extra calories whenever you eat them. Just as important, muscle itself loves to chew up surplus blood sugar—and that will keep those particles from floating around and gunking you up.

Being less active during pregnancy can cause you to lose muscle mass, which underscores the importance of making an extra effort to maintain and add muscle during pregnancy. Another good reason to take up weight training is to prepare yourself for the physical demands that come with carrying, holding, and picking up your baby. (That's one of the reasons why we recommend asymmetrical exercises in our workout on page 310, unless perhaps you're carrying in multiples of two.) Pregnancy yoga and water aerobics are great ways to burn calories and prepare your body for delivery.

Walk and Stretch. Walking for thirty minutes every day will provide you with a base level of fitness. We also believe that you should add some flexibility training to your routine. (See our plan on page 310 to help prevent injuries when you are working out.) We should also emphasize that low-impact activities are a lot safer than you think; remember that, historically, moms had to do a heck of a lot of chores while pregnant, so your pregnant body is designed to withstand some physical stress. Also, if you were running, biking, or swimming before getting pregnant, it's generally considered safe to continue those activities once you get pregnant, just as long as you take your usual safety precautions. Pregnancy is not considered a good time to start an intense new activity or to substantially increase the intensity of one that is in progress.

Get a Family History. Since your health history is one of the major predictors of gestational diabetes, it's important that you undergo a thorough history with your doc—not just your parents' medical history but yours as well, especially when it comes to previous pregnancies. The lifetime risk that a first-degree relative (sister, brother, son, daughter) of someone with diabetes will develop diabetes is five to ten times higher than that of a person with no family history of diabetes. If you had gestational diabetes in one pregnancy, the chance of developing the problem with future children is 50 percent. If you're at high risk, your doc may decide to test you and provide treatment during your first trimester.

5

Makes a Lot of Sense

The Fascinating World of Senses Teaches Us About the Amazing Development of the Brain

Surely, not a day goes by that you don't bathe your senses in the world around you, whether you savor chocolate (dark, please), jam to Kanye, or ooh and aah over a fireworks show. Now, you may think that as your baby grows inside of you, he's living in an alternative world—floating around in a muted, dark place that's basically the wet and warm equivalent of solitary confinement. No windows, no light, no TV, no nuttin'.

While it's true that your baby doesn't have a tricked-out womb complete with surround sound, wireless internet, or an oceanfront view, don't make the mistake of thinking that his senses are lying dormant until he's born. In fact, in utero is the exact time when his senses start kicking in, not only in response to what he needs now but also to help prepare him for all the things he'll need to do once he relocates to the outside world.

Sensory development is one of the more amazing processes of pregnancy, especially because your unborn baby's senses serve as a proxy for his overall brain development. While senses manifest themselves through such things as mouths, ears, eyes, noses, and fingers, the real sensory magic happens inside the skull. So join us as we perform a verbal ultrasound and take a look at what's happening inside your baby's brain, and then explore ways you can best stimulate it during pregnancy and in the weeks and months after birth.

The Brain in Training

In the world of fetal development, the ten-fingers, ten-toes test gets all the attention,★ but we all know that this digital obsession is a mere symbol of the bigger picture: making sure that everything's humming along perfectly during the forty weeks of gestation. That's especially true when it comes to the newborn noggin.

To understand brain development, it helps to take a look at something called "critical periods." As the name implies, the learning that happens during these sensitive developmental phases has long-lasting influence on future behaviors and cannot, as of now, be reversed later in life. One good example from the animal kingdom: Baby ducks have been known to follow a scientist's yellow boots as if those boots were their mom, because that's what they were exposed to directly after birth. This learned response is called indiscriminate bonding.†

Now two examples from the people kingdom that will help you see how these critical periods work: The capacity to process a language proficiently requires early exposure to the language, and the capacity to form strong social relationships and manage stress requires early (and positive) interactions with a primary nurturer. Of

> Factoid: Want to see the interaction between the senses of smell and taste, and the fetal environment? Unwashed newborns are more successful at bringing their hands to their mouths in the first hour after birth and initiating self-calming behavior than newborns that are washed.

★ Mike's wife, who is a developmental pediatrician, even assigned Mike the counting task when their kids came out. Mike used his own two hands to count to ten.

† Perhaps one explanation for why we sometimes date the wrong person.

Why Folic Acid?

If you're pregnant or thinking about getting pregnant, you probably have heard the instructions: Get folic acid. That's because folate is essential for fetal development. Specifically, it helps prevent spina bifida, which happens when the neural tube—a structure that encases the spinal cord—doesn't fully close. That incomplete closure can happen near the neck or the buttocks and lead to walking problems. Because the spinal cord fuses so early on, you need that folic acid in the first six weeks of development—a time when many women might not even know they're pregnant. Ideally, you should take folic acid supplements or make sure you're getting enough folate from food if there's even a chance that you could become pregnant or be pregnant already. That's why we like you to start taking a prenatal vitamin with DHA at least three months prior to becoming pregnant—or, to be safe, during all years when you might become pregnant. (When Canada added folate to flour and bread to increase its intake among women who might not know they're pregnant, the country saw birth defect rates drop over 65 percent.) You should get 800 micrograms (400 micrograms from your prenatal vitamin) of folic acid a day; some women need extra supplementation because their bodies aren't able to convert it to the form that's needed for DNA production, and docs may prescribe up to 4 milligrams.

course, babies may have genetic predispositions to certain talents, traits, and emotions, but early exposure—or lack thereof—to various stimuli can influence whether that predisposition is accentuated or diminished.

You're probably asking when the critical periods for sensory development happen. Well, it's not like a department store sale with set hours (get your cello-playing neurons from nine o'clock to ten o'clock Thursday only!), and nobody's quite sure how long these critical periods last. But they most likely start in utero and continue through the first few months after birth. Our point isn't that you should replace your baby's rattle with a violin bow or brainwash your son into becoming a Yankees fan by piping play-by-play into his room. Rather, it's that even though it may appear that your newborn does nothing more than sleep, blink, and do a mighty fine job of transporting milk to diaper, there's a heck of a lot more going on. So go ahead and

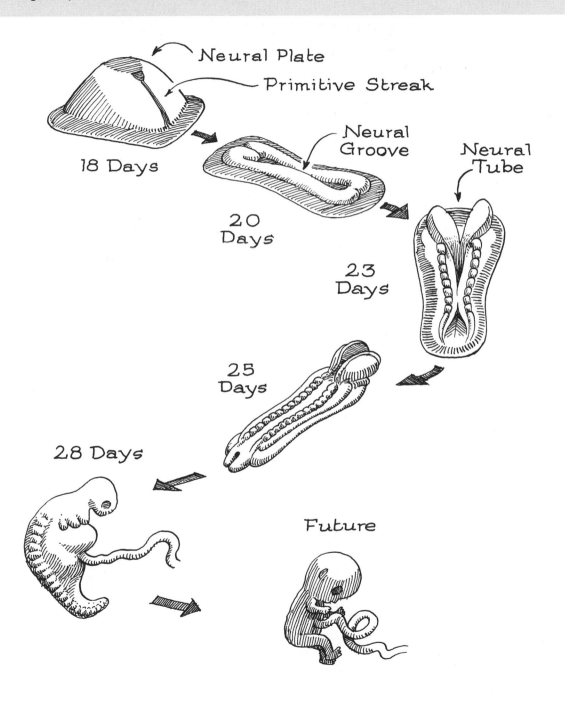

Figure 5.1 **Back Brace** One of the first parts of the fetus to develop is the neural plate, which forms the structure of the spinal cord as well as the brain. It's not long before the reptilian image morphs into a human one.

Neural Plate

Primitive Streak

18 Days

Neural Groove

20 Days

Neural Tube

23 Days

25 Days

28 Days

Future

talk to yourself (positively, even loudly if you want) when you're pregnant to establish that voice bond early on and expose your infant to all kinds of stimuli (visual and auditory) in utero and after birth. Your kids may not remember those experiences consciously, but their neural circuitry will.

Now let's see how some of that circuitry is formed by looking at brain development in three distinct areas.

The Basic Structure

During the first thirty days of pregnancy, the neural plate—a flat structure that will become the central nervous system—forms a groove and rolls up into a tube that runs the length of the entire embryo. One end starts to swell; this is where the brain will form. The rest of the tube becomes the spinal cord. By eight weeks, as the spinal-cord part of the tube is fused together, we can already see three distinct parts of the brain: the forebrain, midbrain, and hindbrain. All of this swelling has started to form the basis of some of the neurological structures that you may have already heard of—things like the medulla, the basal ganglia, the thalamus, and the cerebral cortex.

> **Factoid:** Avoid raising your core temperature above 39 degrees Celsius (102.2 degrees Fahrenheit) in the first month of pregnancy. The increased temp has been linked to neural tube defects. Steer clear of saunas, hot tubs, and long, hot baths, and make sure that you are well hydrated before and during exercise. Treat high fevers with acetaminophen (Tylenol).

Interestingly, since the spinal cord is further advanced in development than the brain, for most of your pregnancy it's what's responsible for the fetal movements and reflexes that you feel as kicks. In the last few months, the hemispheres of the brain grow and thicken and start taking more control over the rest of the baby's body.

Figure 5.2 **Connect the Spots** The way we all learn is to develop connections from one set of neurons to another. These neural structures are shaped like a tree and root system. A baby's brain (both in and out of utero) is extremely plastic, meaning that it can constantly adapt and make new connections between trees. And if that's not a good enough reason to start reading *Hop on Pop* well before birth, we don't know what is.

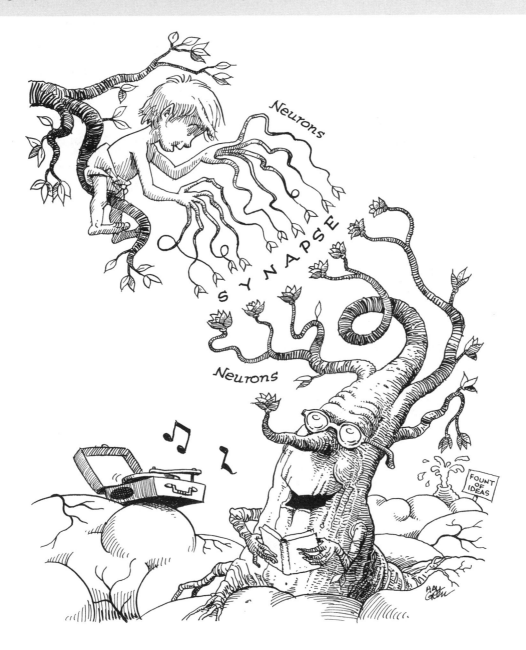

The Neurons

The brain structure without neurons is like a soup bowl without soup. Neurons, the nerve cells of the brain, carry information that allows us to act, think, learn, and feel. Think of a neuron as a tree with a strong root structure as well as branches. The roots (or dendrites) receive information from other neurons and send that information through the trunk of the cell and out to the branches. Those branches pass the message to the roots of another neuron, like a game of telephone. Between the branches of one neuron and the roots of the next lies a space called a synapse.

Factoid: The preference for sucking a particular thumb in utero correlates with right- or left-handedness, and this preference is visible as early as fourteen weeks.

When information is passed from one neuron to the next, a chemical messenger called a neurotransmitter crosses that space. Establishing and reinforcing connections between neurons is the key to learning and brain development.

Neurons, which rely on other support cells called glial cells to be built, are created at a pace that's hard for even the finest of minds to comprehend: 500,000 per *minute* to reach the end result of about 100 billion neurons per baby. (The entire planet has only 6 billion people.) Wow, wow, and double wow.

The importance, though, isn't in the sheer number of neurons, it's in their function. The brain is an amazingly plastic (meaning changeable) organ:* It can adapt, it can change, and it can learn. For example, in babies born blind, the brain recruits neurons from the underutilized visual part of the brain to help bolster hearing. While neurons are formed after birth only rarely, the dendrites continue thickening after birth into a dense forest of connections, in response to whatever stimuli a baby is exposed to.

So what's really happening inside a baby's brain? Early experiences—being exposed to both English and Russian as an infant or constantly interacting with a

---

* It's also very greedy. Though the brain takes up only 2 percent of our body mass, it uses up 25 percent of our body's energy.

caregiver—lay down neural circuits that are actually customized for every individual. So while a newborn baby might have the neurological capacity for learning violin, being a history whiz, or even developing nurturing relationships, the neurological circuitry is not yet hooked up. The neurons are waiting for the signals that will enable particular information to be processed in the brain. The more frequently the experience is repeated, the stronger these circuits grow. The less common the experience, the weaker they become, until they are eventually pruned away. The reason the "old dog new tricks" mantra is largely true is because children's brains are more plastic than those of adults. Neural pathways are like freeways through the middle of cities: Once they're established, it's much more difficult to change their direction or increase their lanes (except in China, where it's done regularly).

At first, brain development in a fetus is concentrated on making neurons without much networking going on. After birth, though, the rate of neuron creation slows down, while the rate of connections skyrockets. It's normal for each neuron to have one thousand connections. Over time, neuron formation stops altogether, then actually goes into reverse as nerve cells gradually die. The brain can still be fine-tuning its internal network well into our twilight years. On average, only 10 percent of the messages to a neuron come from the rest of the body or from lower parts of the brain's hierarchy of operations (the "unconscious" part of our brain, which controls things like breathing and heartbeat). The rest is taken up by an enormous network of relationships with fellow neurons in the "conscious" part of our brain, all constantly providing feedback to one another—the brain's almost round-the-clock conversation with itself.

Factoid: You probably know this from the fact that you can ID another woman's perfume from three blocks away, while a dump truck could park in your living room and your husband wouldn't have a clue. From birth onward, women are more sensitive to odors than men. That's because testosterone decreases olfactory sensitivity, while estrogen increases it. Although women sense smell more during ovulation and pregnancy (because of the increase in estrogen), the sense of smell at birth is higher than at any other age and declines after age eight. Why? Upper respiratory infections and pollution damage the structures that enable us to smell.

It's important to expose your baby to many different stimuli (music, language, pictures of horses, your favorite college fight song) early on, while his neural pathways are still forming. Neural connections that help children develop happen when there's a need for them. The reverse is also true: If the brain has no reason to make connections for, say, Chinese language, it won't make them and eventually will prune away those branches.* Because kids have more neurons actively creating new connections than adults, they can do things like learn to play tennis or memorize the multiplication tables or learn to play video games or fix a computer much more easily than adults can. So it's much better for you to expose your kids to lots of different things—ideally repeatedly—to allow those connections to be formed, rather than trying to catch up later.

Myelination

If you go back to our image of the tree, information travels along the trunk (or axon) in order to hook up with another neuron and pass along the message. Info travels the length of the axon via an electrical impulse, and it is important that the

---

*Yes, you can learn Chinese or piano when you're older, but it's much more difficult for this reason.

Figure 5.3 **Brain Booster** To send and receive messages fast, neural connections need to be protected by a myelin sheath—it helps those messages move fast and keeps the neural structures from getting tangled. What keeps the myelin sheath healthy? DHA. We recommend that you get 600 milligrams a day.

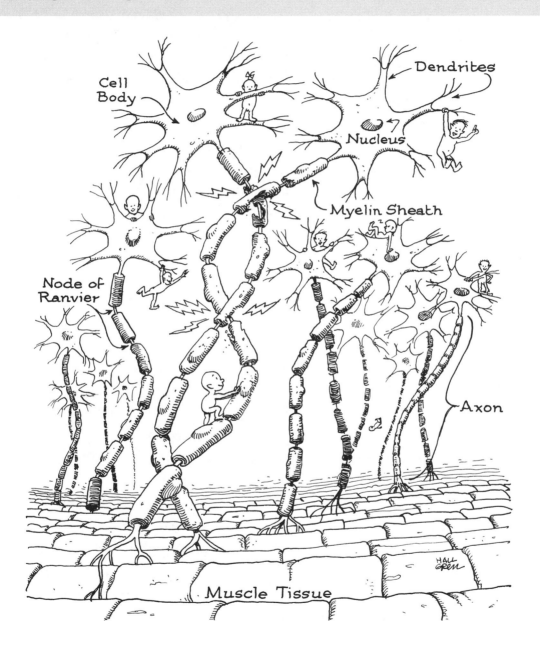

The Male and Female Brains

Because the male fetus has more testosterone than the female fetus, the male fetus typically lags three weeks behind the female fetus neurologically at birth. (This early testosterone poisoning does come in handy later because it helps some coordination neurons develop better, thus making males better at catching moving objects such as animal prey and baseballs.) So when babies are premature, females are usually much better off neurologically and survive more commonly. The evolutionary reason for this? Females are much more precious to a society because of their childbearing potential, but men are expendable, since one man can impregnate multiple women.* Because of this, brain development is built more to spec and much more precisely in females, meaning that there's less variation in how girls' brains develop. On the other hand, nature doesn't have to be so meticulous when making the male brain, so there's a wider variety of ups and downs during boys' brain creation—a variability that manifests in more autism and a broader intellectual curve. Nature, in effect, can roll the dice more during male brain development; sometimes the results are better, and sometimes they're worse.

* Though they do need to rise to the occasion when they're mature and fight off enemies.

trunk not get mixed up or tangled with any other axons. To move the message faster and avoid wrong connections, the axon has to be protected by a myelin sheath—think of it like the bark of a tree or the coating of an electrical wire; it protects the fragile stuff inside.

Myelination, the formation of this protective coating, starts at about five months of gestation in nerves extending to our organs and extremities from the spinal cord, but much later in the brain. Because myelin is made up of about 80 percent fats and 20 percent proteins, healthy fats (such as DHA, which makes up over 97 percent of omega-3 fat in brains) are essential to aiding the myelination process. That importance continues from before birth until eight years of age, with DHA helping to increase brain function and IQ. This is why all infant formula made in the United States includes DHA. It's not a law, but the research is so abundantly clear.

Common Senses: The Inside Story

These days, we tend to associate our senses with pure pleasure: the taste of our favorite food, the smell of our favorite flower, the touch of our favorite lover. All great, no doubt. But when you think about senses and how they develop in utero, it's time to go back to basics. As you know, our babes aren't using their senses to enjoy sunsets, sonatas, and sangria. They're developing them to better prepare themselves to survive in and to adapt to their new world. Let's take a look at how these sensational senses develop.

Touch

The first sense to emerge, touch happens as early as seven and a half weeks, when your baby can first sense touch on the lips and nose, and quickly extends to the rest of his body, as he goes from touching his lips or nose to touching the uterine wall, his face, and the rest of his body. Touch is a critical survival sense, as it not only enables a baby to suck, swallow, and cough at birth, but also to take in amniotic fluid while in the womb.

Now, it's worth noting here that the fetal response to touch takes place in the spinal cord and brain stem, which are the lowest and most primitive, or reptilian, levels of the central nervous system. So? Well, that means that fetuses don't process touch—and by extension, feel pain—in the intellectual part of the brain known as the cerebral cortex, so they don't experience pain the same way that we do. That fact

Factoid: Innumerable environmental factors influence the formation of fingerprints, including the exact position of the fetus in the womb at a particular moment and the exact composition and density of the amniotic fluid that's swirling around the fingers as they touch surrounding structures. And that's what decides how every individual ridge will form. The entire development process is so chaotic that, in the entire course of human history, there is virtually no chance of the same exact pattern forming twice.

may comfort you if your baby goes through a stressful delivery, for instance.[*] In other words, the peripheral nerves that scout out sensations throughout their bodies are sending messages that pain might be occurring, but the fetal brain cannot understand them or put them into perspective. Fetuses may experience nonspecific stress, however. Neurons sense painful stimuli and communicate with the spinal cord. While this doesn't register in the brain as pain per se, it may bother them.

Smell

Scientists used to believe that fetuses had about as much of a sense of smell as they had a sense of fashion; that's because smelling typically depends on such basics as air and breathing. Now, though, it's believed that amniotic fluid jets through the nasal and oral cavities to help a fetus smell, beginning at about 30 weeks; until then, tissues plug up the nasal cavities.

How does this sense of smell develop? Olfactory epithelial cells[†] form at nine weeks along with nostrils. These connect to molecules that bind with the olfactory nerve, which leads to the brain. After your baby develops a sense of smell, he can actually smell everything that you eat or inhale. Most important, because a mother's

---

[*] In fact, electroencephalograms (EEGs) at birth show minimal activity, indicating that there's not likely to be much suffering on the baby's end during delivery.
[†] Olfactory epithelial cells are the only neurons known to be continually generated throughout life; they're replaced about once every sixty days.

milk, sweat, and saliva contain some of the same odors as her amniotic fluid, your baby will recognize your smell after birth, which makes breast-feeding easier. The lesson: Mom should eat what she wants her baby to like to smell.

Sight

Most of us assume that the womb is like grandma's off-limits closet: dark and mysterious. But the truth is that there might be just enough light coming through to give the fetus some visual stimulation. It typically happens when mom herself is in any kind of bright light.

By seven weeks, the baby has developed cup-shaped structures to hold specific parts of the eye: the retina and the lens, which are attached to the brain. And by the fourth month, synapses start forming in the part of the brain where vision is perceived (called the visual cortex, oddly enough). This continues for a year at the rate of ten billion new synapses a day. The simple act of seeing demands half the neurons of the brain.

Hearing

Though we're sure you wouldn't want your babe to hear everything that you do (hide the Chris Rock DVD!), the truth is that the fetus can hear. The predominant sounds include the churning, whirring, and whooshing of things like blood running through your blood vessels and the movements of your stomach and intestines. That sound actually reaches the level of about 90 decibels—about the level of background

> **Factoid:** Bottle-fed babies do not recognize their own mom's underarm odor after two weeks of age. If you do not breast-feed, it may be better to bottle-feed while holding a baby bare chested or under your shirt. And if you do breast-feed, consider this: Babies prefer to nurse on a mother's unwashed breast, so don't use soap on your nipples, just water.

> **Factoid:** Until ten weeks, every brain is female. Then, in boys, a huge surge of testosterone hits the brain, killing cells in the communication center and growing them in the sex and aggression center.

noise in an apartment next to an elevated train.★ The way that babies' hearing works (and ours too) is that sound waves stimulate little hairs attached to nerve cells in the cochlea, a tiny shell-shaped structure in the inner part of the ear, which send impulses to the brain. Any damage to those hairs—from loud noises, for example—can affect the functioning of the inner ear. That's why you should protect yourself and your baby, especially if you work in a factory, on the subway, or on the tarmac. That also means you should choose recorded drum solos over live ones.

While fetuses hear much the way that we hear a next-door stereo (lots of bass, not a lot of high frequencies), they are able to hear voices filtered through tissues, bones, and fluid. And by week twenty-four, they recognize—and are calmed by—their mothers' voices. Of course, they can't distinguish words from one another; rather, the rhythm and melody of voices they hear serve as their foundation for language.

Balance

The ability to balance doesn't come in handy just for gymnasts and tightrope walkers; it's essential for babies too. Most of our vestibular system (which is responsible for giving us our sense of balance) comes from the structures of the inner ear—called such because it is right next to the cochlea—specifically, semicircular canals and otolith organs, which are lined with tiny hairs called cilia that transmit electrical impulses to the brain. You may think that babies don't need to have balance at all, since they're not exactly standing or walking in the womb, but the vestibular system allows them to somersault into a head-down position right before birth.†

Now, the really interesting thing about balance is its connection to other issues. There are some data to suggest a link between balance problems, as measured by dysfunction of the vestibular system, and children with emotional problems, attention deficits, learning disabilities, and language disorders. (There is no data on autism yet.) One possible cause of balance problems: antibiotics such as streptomycin and

---

★ This was measured by researchers who inserted a hydrophone into the uterus.
† Those babies with vestibular problems are more likely to be born breech, in the head-up position.

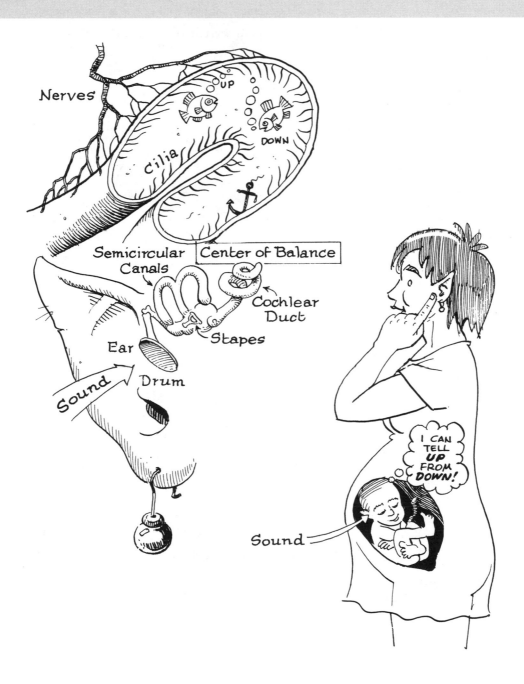

Doing the Flip

There are lots of explanations for why your baby might be in breech position (head up) before delivery, including structural limitations in your uterus and carrying multiples (so there is no room to flip). Another reason: Slower development of the inner ear or inadequate blood supply to the brain can hinder balance. There are exercises you can do at home to encourage flipping, like these:

- **Pelvic rocking:** Get on your hands and knees, arch your back, and tilt your pelvis gently. Return to a flat position. Do thirty repetitions several times a day.

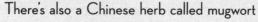

- **Knee to chest:** Kneel on a steady chair (or on the floor) and place your elbows on the floor. Your partner can help you get into position and steady you. This shift in gravity may help float your child out of breech position.

There's also a Chinese herb called mugwort that has been reported to help change the position of a baby. We still need formal trials to gauge its effectiveness, but it's worth a try if your doc agrees. Docs may also try to flip the baby externally by massaging the mother's abdomen with baby oil. An ultrasound will be used to help monitor the position and the baby's heart rate during the movement.

gentamycin, which in utero (and even out) can damage hair cells in the inner ear and cause both balance and hearing problems.

Taste

Though it will be a few years before your baby starts ordering shrimp cocktails, we actually start seeing taste buds in utero by week eight, and they actually start communicating to the brain about five weeks later. Located primarily around the perimeter of the tongue, each of the fetus's 4,500 taste buds★ has about forty receptor cells, which bind with food and send information to the brain. And that's what activates reflexes for feeding, salivating, and swallowing.

The fetus can taste some flavors by two months, and by fifteen to seventeen weeks, the amniotic fluid can reek of curry, cumin, garlic, onion, or other strong tastes from a mom's diet. The taste of that fluid changes all the time, depending on what you're eating, and that may strongly influence what your child prefers to eat after birth. More important, though, is that the sense of taste develops so early for a very big reason: Taste helps a baby recognize his mom after birth, since many of the same flavors in her amniotic fluid turn up in her sweat and breast milk.

Other Reflexes

You already know what reflexes are: involuntary movements (think blinking or taking your hand away from a hot stove). A fetus develops plenty of reflexes, and all of them depend on the central nervous system. These are the main ones:

Movement: Fetuses develop the ability to flex and extend their limbs and suck their thumbs in utero, but these reflexes usually disappear by eight months after birth, when gross motor skills start to take over. At this point, movements such as thumb sucking become more voluntary than reflexive. By the way, even moderate alcohol

---

★ Fetuses have more taste buds than infants or adults.

use during pregnancy seems to impair a child's sucking reflex at birth, a potential feeding problem.

Walking: Before babies learn to crawl, they pretend to walk (you've surely seen that infant kick-kick-kicking motion). They practice that movement (more kick-kick-kicking) in utero and continue it for the first three months. (The reflex has to be lost before they gain the ability to walk consciously.) It's also called the stepping reflex; you see it in action when you hold a baby upright by her waist and watch her flail her legs as if she's trying to walk.

Factoid: If you are using formula in addition to or instead of breast-feeding, make sure to get the kind with the most DHA. Most major brands have 32 milligrams per bottle, but check the label to be certain.

Moro reflex: You know the sensation where you feel as if you're falling even though you're lying securely in bed. Babies feel this in utero when a mom's sudden movement causes them to fling out their arms and legs reflexively. This startle reflex starts in the third trimester and continues after birth (see our tips for a swaddling technique that will help ease that flailing feeling), and some parents may confuse the reflex with seizures because it's often accompanied by trembling.

We know that you spend a lot of time dealing with side effects of pregnancy and the daily struggles that can make life tough, but we hope that this discussion of a baby's developing senses gives you something to really hold on to and think about, knowing that a song here or a conversation there can be the little touches that make the experience for all three of you (mom, dad, and baby) that much more special.

YOU TIPS

It may seem that sensory development is simply a standard feature of pregnancy: If your child develops normally, she's surely going to grow the eyes, ears, nose, mouth, and fingers that will give her access to enjoying everything the senses have to offer. While that's essentially true, that doesn't mean that there aren't things that you can do to help along the process—not merely so she can appreciate the sweet taste of fruit or enjoy the compositions of Mr. Ludwig van B. Improving your child's sensory development means you'll be improving her brain development as well.

Pop It. The greatest thing you can do for your child's brain isn't reading physics textbooks to her while she's in utero, though there's nothing wrong with doing that. One of the keys to strong brain development is taking a supplement of DHA, which helps create the myelin sheath that speeds up connections between neurons. We recommend that you get 600 milligrams a day; supplements derived from fish oil are generally purified, but if you're worried about methylmercury contamination, vegetarian sources are also available.

Stimulate, Stimulate, Stimulate. It's already well established that the womb isn't some noise-free vacuum. That's why so many moms read aloud to their child even before that first night in the crib. We strongly endorse that practice too—not just for brain development but also to allow your baby to hear your voice and establish an auditory bond at an early age. We also encourage you to listen to all kinds of music, not because we think Petey boy needs something to pass the time but because music will help stimulate his senses and improve his brain development. During and after pregnancy, you want to expose your child to as much pleasant stimulation as you can (as long as he's not sleeping) in all kinds of settings. Exposure to different sounds and scenes is essentially what helps establish those neural connections.

Take Your Time. Because stimulation is so important for brain development (and obviously for bonding), we recommend that you try to spend as much time with your newborn as possible in the weeks immediately after birth. We know that financial and family situations don't always allow that, but if you can take six weeks—the average paid maternity leave allowed by law—and another two weeks through vacation, sick days, or personal time, your child will benefit greatly from that motherly stimulation. The typical working woman in America takes ten weeks, so try to shoot for at least eight weeks as a fair and reasonable goal. One of the great challenges if you do go back to work is to try to avoid playing catch-up with housework and bills when you're at home. Dedicate after-work time to bonding with your baby, and come up with a plan to divide the household responsibilities or handle them when he's dreaming away.

Take a Buffet Approach. Hold on just a second: We don't mean the buffet approach in terms of pumping your gullet with dozens of different foods at one time. But we do think it's important to eat diversely (as diversely as you can depending on your nausea levels, with healthy food choices, of course). Doing so will help stimulate your child's taste buds. The long-term effect: a more adventurous eater who might actually utter the words "Please pass the broccoli" in a couple of years.

Swaddle. You've likely heard all about swaddling, that seemingly mathematical formula for wrapping a blanket around a baby. Some people think that swaddling is done for warmth, and some think it's for comfort. (Still others think that the full-body swaddle seems more like a straitjacket than anything else.) But the major reason swaddling is so important is that it helps limit the startle reflex, so babies don't wake themselves up. You can swaddle your child for much of the day when he's sleeping or resting and loosen the reins as he stays awake longer and seems curious about moving around, starting at about three months. In cultures where women swaddle their babies for more than a year (Eskimos and Andes Indians), there's a slowing of motor development by up to a month, but kids are extremely adaptive and catch up developmentally. Swaddling is very effective for cranky babies, since the reason they're fussy is often that they actually want to sleep but can't calm themselves down. Follow these step-by-step illustrations for creating a secure swaddle:

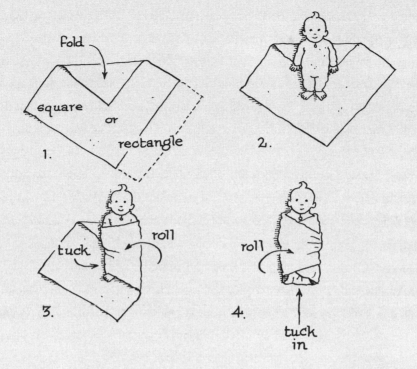

- Fold down the top corner of a blanket and place baby in the middle, with her feet pointing down toward the middle of the triangle.
- Pick up a side corner and wrap it over baby's opposite shoulder and tuck it under her back.
- Fold the bottom corner of the blanket up to baby's stomach or chest.
- Fold the last remaining corner over baby's other shoulder and tuck it under her back.
- Instant cocoon!

Watch Who's Watching. If you're opting for child care after your baby is born, we know you're probably feeling a lot of stress about the decision. Now's the time to start nailing down who's going to play this essential role. While there are many factors to consider, one of the things that you want to screen for is how much stimulation your caregiver will give your child. If she's on her cell phone (the caregiver, not the infant), or watching TV, or otherwise distracted, she's not a good match. So check references, and don't be afraid to check up on her. (Web cameras aren't cheating.) You should expect a caregiver not only to feed and change your baby and handle emergencies, but also to help with his neurological development. A side note: You also want to pay some attention to language and accents. While there's nothing wrong with hiring a foreign-speaking caregiver to help your child learn a second language (after all, it's easier to learn languages earlier in life because your brain is more plastic), you should also consider that in some cases, the first language might not develop as perfectly and quickly as possible.

Shop for Toys. Get a few that are black and white. A newborn's vision is worse than a bad referee's. While they can't see color (babies, and maybe referees too), they can see contrast because the cells in the retina that perceive details and colors (the cones) are kind of stubby for a while. Now, don't run out and redecorate your entire house with noncolor items. By ten weeks, babies start to see big objects and bright colors (red, oranges, and greens, especially), but in the first few weeks, it wouldn't hurt to outfit your crib with a few pandas or zebras. Babies' attention to contrast is one of the reasons why your areolas get larger and darker during pregnancy. (See page 177.)

Be a Massage Therapist. Okay, we know that you don't have the flexibility to perform in utero massage, nor should you, but once your baby is born, we recommend that you regularly engage in infant massage. We're not talking the deep-tissue variety. Instead you're going to apply firm pressure and use long, rhythmic strokes. (See the You Tool on the next page for details.) Skin-to-skin contact is an ideal way to bond—it's especially nice for dads who feel out of the loop with breast-feeding moms—and it's also been shown to have innumerable other benefits, such as teaching babies to deal with stress, calming colicky babies, stimulating nerves in the brain that facilitate food absorption, improving immune function, and helping babies fall asleep more easily.* Some research shows that touch is crucial to neurological development, so you should make this ritual part of your everyday baby care routine.

* Woo-hoo!

YOU TOOL

INFANT MASSAGE

In a few years, you'll bond with your baby on car rides, shopping trips, and Sunday morning snuggles. Once the baby is born, one of the best ways to bond is a daily massage routine that will help relax her (and you). Do it when she's quiet, yet not ready to fall asleep. And pick the same, soft music each time; she will connect the sound of the music with the relaxation of the massage. Sit on the floor with your feet together and knees apart (diamond shaped), so you can lay her on a blanket between your legs. If that isn't comfortable, place her on your lap. Be sure she's warm, and use a pure, light oil to increase the glide of your strokes. Some tips for getting started from the American Massage Therapy Association (please note that the adverbs *slowly* and *gently but firmly* should precede every verb):

Legs: Hold her foot with one hand and pat the length of her leg with the other. Stroke up and down from her toes to her hips and back. Then massage the sole of her foot and pull each toe. Use your thumbs to stroke the bottom of her foot from heel to toe and massage around her ankle using small circles.

Belly: Use your fingertips, massaging in small circles.

Stretch: While she's on her back, hold her feet and knees together and stretch her knees up to her belly. (Fair warning: This move might help her expel gas.) Also, hold her legs together with her knees bent and rotate them in a circular motion, both to the left and the right, to loosen her hips. This also helps ease a tummy ache.

Arms: Hold her wrist with one hand and pat the length of her arm with the other. Stroke up and down from the bottom of the arm to the top, and then massage her palm and squeeze and pull each finger. Repeat with the other arm.

Back: Lay her facedown on the floor or across your legs and move your hands back and forth from the top of her back to her buttocks. Massage in small circles up and down her spine. Hold your fingers like a rake and stroke down her back.

Head and Face: Hold the back of her head in your hands and stroke her scalp with your fingertips. Then rub her earlobes and stroke her eyebrows, her closed eyelids, and from the bridge of her nose across her cheeks. Massage her jaw in small circles.

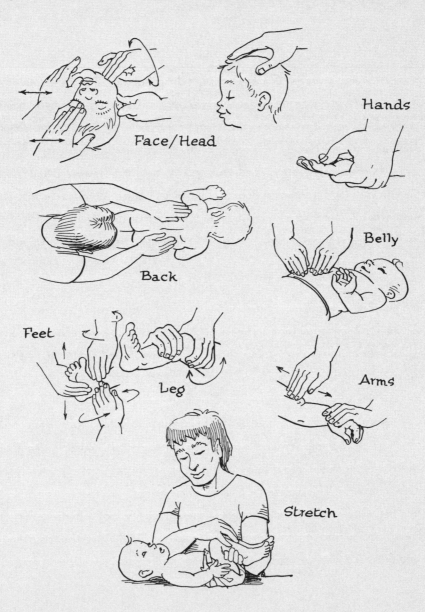

Part 3

The Baby Changing

YOU

6

The Mind of Mom

Manage Your Stress, Sleep Better, and Find the "Om" in Mom

*N*ow that we've discussed the developmental issues associated with your child's brain, we're going to dive into yours by explaining the way your pregnancy-changed brain affects you (as well as your child) when it comes to such matters as stress, anxiety, sleep, and depression. The reason we've grouped all of these issues together is because, like dominos, a vicious cycle, or a chain-reaction fender bender, they're all interconnected in a cause-and-effect kind of way. If you don't get enough sleep, you get stressed. If you're stressed, you don't get enough sleep. Now throw depression into the mix: You don't sleep because you're depressed, or you're depressed because you don't get enough sleep and are stressed. Or better still, you're stressed, can't sleep, feel depressed, and are infinitely PO'd because your husband snores his butt off for eight and half hours a night while you ricochet like a highly caffeinated pinball.

Even though we all know that they're big issues for most pregnant women, there's still a stroller-sized stigma attached to mental health problems. As a consequence, moms-to-be tend to internalize all worries, mood changes, and emotional challenges with an "I should suck it up" attitude. Our job: to burst that blasphemous bubble, encourage you to acknowledge these feelings, and teach you how to manage your stresses—even to embrace them. Our mantra here is "Just say know." The more you know, the more you'll feel at ease. And the more you can create almost autopilot behaviors that allow you to handle day-to-day stresses automatically, the better off you'll be. By taking our Worry and Anxiety Quiz on page 163, you can get a realistic look at where you fall on the anxiety scale and discover what you may need to adjust to get your stress level into a healthy range.

It's easy to dismiss mental issues as being "all in my mind," but what occurs between your ears powerfully influences what's going on in your belly and in your baby after he is born. How so? Quickly, here's some of the research: A mom's anxiety and depression during pregnancy are associated with preterm delivery, lower birth weight, and admission of her baby to a special care nursery. And babies exposed to a mom's anxiety and depression after birth score lower on developmental scales, have more sleeping and feeding problems, and have less interaction with mom. So to be clear, your anxiety may affect your child in ways that *should* make you anxious. We can't always predict the individual risk; some babies are very resilient and won't be affected much by stress. But until we can, it's best to assume that your stress could negatively affect your baby.

On the positive side, human beings are remarkably adaptable, so putting a baby into a healthy, low-stress, nondepressed family postpartum can reverse some of the problems that might have resulted from a stressful pregnancy. So if you are anxious or depressed during pregnancy and get treated, you can reverse any damage that might have been done. We say that not to scare you or blame you but to help you realize that anxiety and depression are real health issues—as real as gestational diabetes or preeclampsia. The key to handling stress successfully is to distinguish between normal, healthy stress and overwhelming, negative stress—and to seek treatment for the latter.

Negative stress leads to tension, anxiety, depression, and all of their associated health risks. But healthy stress is a normal psychological state that can lead to positive growth and change. In our day-to-day lives, we may associate stresses with tension, with headaches, with deadlines, and with the overwhelming sense of being bowled over by a neurological dump truck. The typical response: We want to burn our to-do lists, rub our temples, retreat under a goose down comforter, and dream of the Caribbean life.

But in many cases, stress gets a bad rap, we tell you. It's not that we don't appreciate stress, tension, and anxiety as real health risks, as we'll explore in this chapter, but before we do, we have to take a step back and think about what stress does to our lives on a deeper level.

The very best experiences in our lives—the peak experiences, as we call them—are typically motivated by positive stressors, which we strive to overcome. In fact, we seek out challenges, excitement, and pressures because they give our life meaning, even though they come with a side order of stress. The bigger the challenge, the greater the opportunity for growth (and pleasure). And isn't that really what pregnancy is? It's one of the top ten stressors in life, but it's considered to be a top rewarding experience—a peak time, no doubt.

It may help to think of pregnancy and stress as a hot-air balloon ride. The balloon fills up with air, which stresses the balloon as it stretches, just like the pressures of life. But the air is also what helps you get off the ground to see the world in ways you've never seen it before—to elevate you to a higher level of experience and appreciation. Now, the challenge is to make sure that you have the right amount of air. Too much air (too much stress), and you lose sight and can't see through the clouds; too little air, and you never get off the ground to experience the beauty of your journey. As much as we claim we want to ease stress in our lives, we also don't want the opposite: to stay anchored to the ground and never see the world or enjoy the opportunities around us.

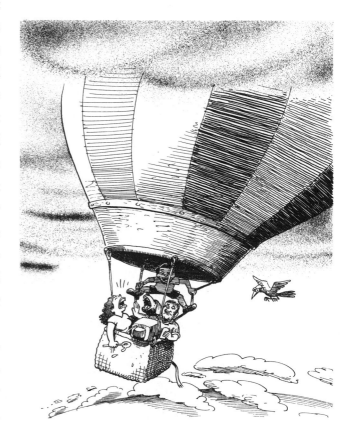

But stress and depression during pregnancy can interfere with your ability to bond with your baby. If untreated, anxiety and depression develop a life of their own and linger postpartum, making it even harder to cope with your newborn. There's no "toughing it out" until the end, knowing that the reward will be worth the misery. The misery will just go on.

The best way to deal with the stresses of pregnancy is to learn techniques to ease as much as possible whatever causes you discomfort or frustration, and to know when you need to ask for help. The trick is not necessarily to eliminate them but to find the sweet spot that allows you to manage stress, rather than the other way around.

All Brains: The Biology of the Mommy Mind

In most cases, people are pretty good at prioritizing stress. We all know the difference between big stresses (mounting debt) and small stresses (mustard stains). And even though small stresses can seem big at the time, we know deep down that at no time and in no world do condiments ever trump credit scores.

Factoid: The fetus sleeps almost all day—95 percent of the time for first thirty-two weeks and about 85 percent of the time just before delivery.

That all changes in pregnancy. Every stress feels like a big one, as your brain swirls and twirls and somersaults with more questions than a prosecuting attorney. We imagine that this sampling sounds a bit familiar to that voice in your head: Is my baby healthy? How hard is labor going to be? Can I afford child care? Will my mate look elsewhere now that I've lost my figure and I'm not as interested in sex? Does he really want to name the child after his favorite football player? Why are my parents hounding me to be in the delivery room? How are the siblings going to handle another child? Will I be like—*gasp!*—my mother?

These questions are meant to reinforce the fact that we know you have a lot of important issues on your mind, and it's no wonder that you're feeling such a psychological burden. These are tough questions, but one thing there's no question about:

Everyone has anxiety during pregnancy, especially during her first one. Of course, that's because there's a fear of the unknown the first time around (but also because there's less time to be worried when you have other tykes to chase after). Moms explode with tension when presented with so many questions—and so many possible answers.

While you may already know what's happening emotionally because your feelings and questions are as tangible as the slats on a crib, have you ever thought about what may be going on physically? Specifically, what happens deep inside your brain when you get pregnant? Lots of things, actually.

For one thing, your brain actually shrinks during pregnancy. That's not surprising for those of you who've experienced mommy brain: You dump chili powder on ice-cream sundaes or make some other kind of mental mistake; it's a kind of subtle forgetfulness. Your brain doesn't lose cells per se, but as your metabolism changes, your brain restructures the connections between cells and changes in preparation for motherhood. Typically limited to the third trimester, this might actually have evolved as a way of preparing you to focus on your baby and block out lots of other worrisome thoughts, but it can be discomfiting just the same. In the final one to two weeks before birth, your brain will begin to increase in size again and build new maternal neural circuits, eventually becoming stronger than it was before and helping you to better understand and cope with your newborn.

For another, your brain requires additional fuel during pregnancy. The major chemical player here comes in the form of DHA, the critical omega-3 fatty acid in both your child's brain, as mentioned in the last chapter, and your own. Fetuses are pretty assertive when it comes to taking those omega-3 fatty acids. Because the brain is 60 percent fat,★ you'll be depleted of those important neuron-protecting fatty acids unless you make a point of getting them through diet or supplements. DHA seems to help repair your brain cells or connections damaged by stress: Studies of stressed-out cab drivers show that they coped better when they took extra omega-3 fatty acids. We recommend that you take DHA supplements to help replenish your supply. DHA will help you prevent or cope with stress and manage depression as well.

★ Proving once and for all that we're all fatheads.

Throughout pregnancy, a woman's brain marinates in neurohormones manufactured all over her body, including her placenta, and those hormones wreak havoc on a mom's senses and emotions. In the first few months of pregnancy, these chemical messages cause a woman's sense of smell to change, making her sensitive to anything that might hurt the baby. This is one of the reasons why pregnant women get nauseated so easily. The brain gets used to those hormones, typically after the first few months, helping her want to eat again.

Two hormones in particular—progesterone and estrogen—go into overdrive during pregnancy. Progesterone provides a tranquilizing effect to protect against stress, one of the reasons why women can handle so much heavy thinking and anxiety during pregnancy.

Increased estrogen, which you may associate with more sexy topics (we'll cover them in the next chapter), also plays a role in brain function. How? First, estrogen seems to protect neurons, preventing them from being damaged by outside influences (oxidative stress, for instance). Second, estrogen increases the effect of nitric oxide, a gas that widens blood vessels. Unlike many other organs, the brain doesn't store excess fuel to any great degree. So your brain relies primarily on blood vessels to receive the fuel it needs to function. More estrogen means better blood flow; better blood flow means there's a smaller chance that you'll try to clean the bathrooms with banana peels.

In addition, during delivery, huge bursts of oxytocin run through the brain. Oxytocin is the feel-good hormone that helps us bond with others. In the days and weeks immediately before delivery, many women experience mild euphoria and also strong nesting behavior (inexplicably washing walls, baking, and so on), and this may be linked to oxytocin as well as to other hormones and steroids. After delivery, when a woman holds her newborn, she also gets what's called "baby lust," a chemical reaction that happens when a baby's pheromones stimulate the production of additional oxytocin—thus augmenting that bonding feeling.

The effect of all the hormonal and neural changes during pregnancy is that the brain is really receiving a loud and strong message: Baby's a-comin', and you need to be prepared. One of the side effects may be a bit of mind fog, and this may lead to a bit of stress: If I can't remember where I left my shoes, how in the world am I going to care for a baby or function at my job when I go back to work? But take comfort in the fact that all of these changes not only are reversible, but are preparing you to be the best parent possible.

Under Pressure: The Science of Stress

On this roller-coaster ride of pregnancy, you can't always control the ups and downs. But as long as you pick a safe park and a good seat and get strapped in, you can take the ride, enjoy the ups and downs, and stop fretting over every loop, drop, and twist that may crop up along the way. One way to do that is to learn a little bit more about the human stress response and why a little bit of stress can do a lot of good.

Worry helps with problem solving, and the stress reaction, also known as the fight or flight response, traditionally is what helped us deal with life-threatening problems such as saber-toothed tigers. The problems with stress typically happen when we go to extremes of the anxiety scale. Here's yet another example of the bell curve–Goldilocks principle in action: Some anxiety is good because it helps keep you on your toes, but too much anxiety can be destructive, and no anxiety at all can mean that no decisions ever get made, and you end up as a saber-toothed snack.★

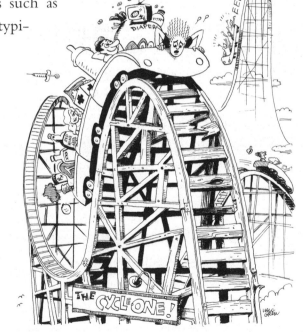

The evolutionary difference between acute stress (tiger charging) and chronic stress (famine) helps us understand how this all works, especially in relationship to pregnancy. In times of acute stress (like trying to fit thirty

★ Athletes, musicians, and other performers know this as well. A little bit of stress helps them focus and ultimately perform better, but too much can derail their efforts.

minutes of work into the twenty minutes before a deadline or running through an airport to try to make a connecting flight), your body reacts by helping you survive the situation:

- Your stress hormone cortisol goes up, which helps raise your blood glucose levels, which provides energy for all your cells and muscles to move so that you have the power and strength to deal with the situation (awfully handy in the tiger scenario).
- Your adrenaline goes up, which redistributes blood flow to your heart and brain and away from your uterus, so that you can make decisions about how to survive (imperative in the short term for both you and your baby).
- In cases of extreme and unexpected periods of acute stress, decreased uterine blood flow can cause the fetus to panic, triggering premature delivery.

Now, all of that makes sense if the stress lasts for short bursts. But if the stress switches from acute to chronic—nagging bosses, overbearing relatives, constant worry about which color to paint the room—you can probably figure out that that's not a good thing. Why? Because chronic stress diverts resources from baby to mom over the long term. And when you restrict nutrients and oxygen through either depleted glucose or diminished blood flow, organ development decreases and growth restriction develops. Our bodies have evolved to handle the onetime anxieties; it's the chronic worries that we have to worry about.

Factoid: Research shows mom's anxiety is associated with mixed-handedness in her child. So what if your kid can throw a baseball with either hand? Great for a sports future, you say. But it seems that mixed-handedness is also associated with neurodevelopmental problems such as dyslexia, autism, and attention deficit disorder.

How our bodies handle stressful situations involves a circuit of chemicals called the hypothalamic-pituitary-adrenal (HPA) axis. This axis essentially represents the relationship between your brain and your stress hormones as they interact in what we call a feedback loop. A feedback loop in your body works the same way it does in relationships: Your body's system doesn't act like a robot; it reacts, depending on what information it is receiving (hence the feedback). In the case of this axis, what happens is that stressors cause the hypothalamus (the part of your brain that's the *H*) to release certain stress hormones, which then stimulate your pituitary gland (that's the *P*, also in your skull) to release more hormones. That cascade of chemicals signals your adrenal glands (the *A*, located on top of your kidneys) to release the biggest stress hormones of all: cortisol and epinephrine (otherwise known as adrenaline). These chemicals are designed to help you: Adrenaline raises your BP and heart rate, and cortisol increases glucose, giving your muscles the energy to move more swiftly and suddenly. That's helpful when a lion is approaching, but not so much so when the reaction lasts nine months.

When you're pregnant, the feedback loop affects not just you but your child as well. How? The increased cortisol in your bloodstream challenges the integrity of the whole system, and that can lead to very subtle changes in your baby's development, including his brain. Adrenaline, on the

Factoid: There's a theory—repeat, *theory*—floating around that maternal stress is linked with sexual orientation. It goes something like this: While genes have a huge influence, there may be some evidence that stress hormones like cortisol can interfere with the production of testosterone. And in a stressed mom, those stress hormones may cross the placenta, interfere with testosterone, and nudge the male fetus's brain to develop along feminine lines.

other hand, doesn't seem to cross directly from mom to baby. But researchers believe that it may have an indirect effect: By changing a mom's vascular system (adrenaline redistributes blood flow and decreases the amount that goes to the uterus), increased adrenaline production can alter the way in which nutrients pass to the placenta.

Now that you have the biological picture, let's think about what is happening behaviorally. In a pregnant and stressed state, you may gravitate toward unhealthy ways to handle that anxiety, such as overeating, smoking, drinking, using drugs, or avoiding doctor visits. Those unhealthy choices simply increase the guilt that a depressed, stressed pregnant mom already feels. Our tips at the end of the chapter will help you manage the connection between what's going on in your mind and what's happening in your belly.

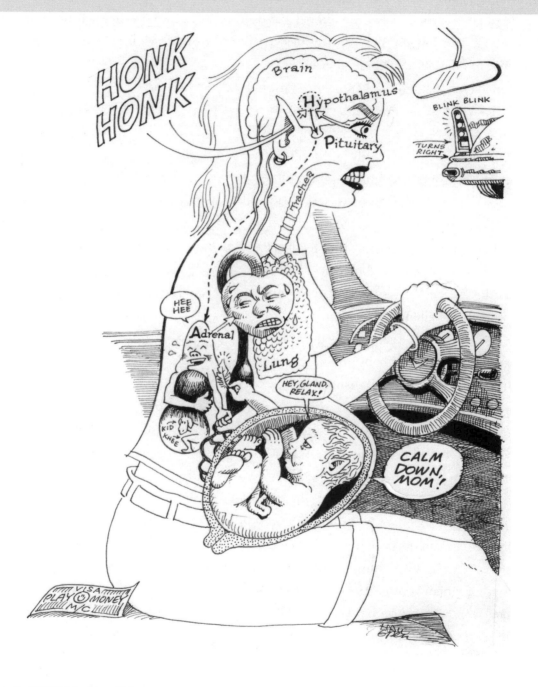

Slumber Party: Get Some Rest

While your bed may be the source of serious fun and serious bonding, it is—and will be—the source of some serious stress. Most pregnant women worry about how they're going to cope with being awakened every couple of hours every night for several months after the baby is born, and most women already develop sleep problems during pregnancy. Some experts theorize that frequent awakenings during pregnancy are your body's way of preparing itself for postpregnancy.

You certainly know that your body needs sleep, for all sorts of reasons. Sleep helps improve your immune system, your skin, and your mood, as well as your brain function. Neurons need ninety minutes of uninterrupted sleep to recover normal activity. Plus, sleep helps boost growth hormone, the ultimate rejuvenating hormone that helps you keep an ideal body weight and shape. But growth hormone isn't just important for our own bodies; we also need it for growing the placenta and uterus. In a way, growth hormone helps counteract many of the stresses of pregnancy by ensuring fetal development during tough times.

Here's how the normal sleep cycle works:

Your brain works almost like a computer. If you clean out and trash old files you don't use, your computer can work more efficiently. Sleep cleans out your neurological database, allowing you to feel rested and think more clearly. Our bodies go through several stages of sleep every night, ranging from early sleep (stages one and two) to a deeper level (the dreamy REM, or rapid eye movement, sleep). The deepest levels (stages three and four) are where most of the rejuvenation occurs. If you don't get to REM, you won't feel as rested and won't enjoy refreshed brain function.

Your body cycles through these ninety-minute cycles several times a night—unless something disrupts you, like pain, heartburn, or getting up to use the bathroom. If you're always getting awakened before that ninety minutes, you're never getting into deep sleep and never restoring your brain properly.

The problem is that the pattern of nighttime awakening can snowball: You wake up at night, so you're never fully rested. Then you're tired during the day, so you sneak in naps when you can. Still exhausted, you retreat to bed so early that before you know it, you've missed the whole season of *Dancing with the Stars.* But then you wake up before midnight because you have to pee, and on and on and on.

Up to 95 percent of women say they experience sleep changes during pregnancy. The biggest changes: a decrease in REM sleep and an increase in vivid dreams. Many pregnant women (and especially postpartum women) report that their dreams become extremely vivid—even nightmarish. This vividness may result from the extreme range of emotions that pregnant women experience, as well as from disrupted sleep patterns in pregnancy and postpartum. It's also believed that the prevalence of the hormone oxytocin may intensify dreams. So your brain and subconscious may be in overdrive when you have that very vivid dream about Aunt Fleda driving an old Chevy down to your neighbor's pond to bury machetes that were used to carve pumpkin pies for a dinner that included you, your first-grade teacher, your high school crush, and Ozzy Osbourne.* But it could also be a symptom of a mood or anxiety disorder, and you may need some interventions (perhaps even a sedative prescribed by a doctor) to help break the pattern of bizarre dreams and get your sleep back on track. Some of the other more common patterns or symptoms when it comes to sleep changes include:

First trimester: A decrease in total time and quality, and an increase in daytime sleepiness and insomnia.

Second trimester: Tends to be somewhat normal, but about one-fifth of women do experience some disturbances.

Third trimester: Women wake up up to five times a night and report taking naps for over an hour a day, plus insomnia and daytime fatigue get worse.

It should be no surprise why pregnant women wake up so frequently: As pregnancy progresses, you have to go to the bathroom more (more pressure on the blad-

---

*You've had this dream *too*?!? Thank God we're not the only ones.

der from your uterus), the baby moves more (the ultimate biological alarm clock), you have more breathing problems (the weight gain and the big thing below your diaphragm push your lungs up, causing your airways to narrow), and you have more side effects that rustle you out of slumber (backaches, heartburn, leg cramps).

We're concerned about the quantity and quality of sleep that you get, not only because of the health implications we discussed a few paragraphs ago, but also because of the bigger picture when it comes to your mind. Lack of sleep is perhaps the most important stressor for a mom—and the most easily treated.

Our mission here isn't to fight your biology but to find ways to work with it. So our goal is really to help you rest more comfortably and sleep a little better—even though you may wake up throughout the night. At the end of the chapter, we'll review some actions you can take to improve your sleep quality throughout your pregnancy and beyond.

Down, Not Out: The Bright Side of Depression

Since we've covered hot-air balloons and roller coasters, why not just make it a metaphorical trifecta and talk about the most basic of pleasure rides: the swing. Back and forth, back and forth, we fly high, we sink low—just the same way our moods do. Any woman knows that mood swings are simply a part of her normal hormonal cycle. Sometimes you feel good, and sometimes you feel like hot-waxing his forearm hair just . . . so . . . he . . . feels . . . your . . . pain.

Take those normal mood swings and multiply them by any double-digit number of your choice, and you've come upon what happens during pregnancy. Much of the time, you're going to feel happy. Other times? You could cry when you read a restaurant menu. It's normal to swing from happy to sad to mad to every emotion in between because your hormones are basically playing drum cadences throughout your system—always changing pace, always changing rhythm, always keeping you moving.

While mood swings are indeed normal, you need to recognize when normal crosses into destructive, as is the case with full-blown depression. How can you tell?

One way is if you seem to bring down the mood of others around you. That's how docs sometimes diagnose it—if they leave the room more depressed than when they came in, it's a good indicator that their patient is depressed. A depressed mom-to-be tends to feel disconnected from her baby, whereas moms usually bond with their babes. And if they're seriously depressed, they may even feel as if the baby is a stranger. Risk factors for depression during pregnancy include a personal history of depression (especially if you have been taking antidepressant medication), a family history of depression, poor social support, relationship problems, and high stress.

That bit about family history is an important point, since you're three times as likely to suffer from depression if you have a family history. If you are genetically predisposed to depression, pregnancy can trigger it, just as it may with diabetes. That's what pregnancy tends to do: cause problems that may lie beneath the surface to bubble up to the top.

You can also help diagnose whether you have a problem by doing this self-check. You likely have depression if:

- You have one or both of the following symptoms during a two-week period: (1) a sad, depressed, or irritable mood all day long on most days. (2) sharply decreased interest or pleasure in your activities on most days.
- You've drastically changed the way you viewed the world.
- You have had any thoughts of hurting yourself or your fetus (you need to seek professional help).

(See Appendix 5 for the official depression scale that medical professionals use.)

If you answered yes to any of the above questions, you should see your doc, who should conduct various tests, including a blood count and thyroid test, to diagnose possible causes and discuss possible treatments, such as "talk" therapy and/or, if needed, medications.

About 10 percent of pregnant women suffer from depression (and at least 10 percent suffer from postpartum depression; more on that later). No single factor has been determined to cause depression, making it difficult to explain what happens neurologically. However, changes in brain chemistry are thought to play a big role.

We know that in depressed people, levels of the feel-good neurotransmitters serotonin and dopamine are down, as are steroid hormones—all of which help you cope with stress.

At a time when logic would tell you that you should be depressed—you're laid up, your body's changing, you can't do many of the things that you normally do—it's actually pretty amazing that about 90 percent of women are *not* depressed. There's something overriding those messages, and we believe that something is estrogen. The hormone plays a protective role in depression by negating messages that you should be depressed, so that you can focus on the baby.

So why, despite all this extra estrogen, do some pregnant women get depressed? Well, in some women, high estrogen and progesterone levels can actually *cause* depression. Other women, despite estrogen's protective effect, may be experiencing slight (but important) alterations to what's going on along the HPA axis. In this case, just the slightest stressors or emotional changes you feel after a doctor visit or a talk with your mom or a fight with your spouse trigger chemical changes that lead to sharp mood swings. The effect: A hormonal symphony turns into a cacophony. Typically, stress induces more steroid hormones and alters the amount of circulating epinephrine (aka adrenaline) in the HPA axis that cross-talks with brain hormones. Even minor changes in the amount of neurohormones can disrupt your rhythm and send you into a psychological mess.

The downside, of course, isn't just that you're no fun to hang out with or that you want to curl up in bed all day. It's that depression has been linked to health problems. Depression can lead to loss of appetite and weight loss or self-medication through overeating, tobacco, or drugs and/or alcohol. Depressed women may also skip prenatal visits. So let's be clear: If you're depressed enough for it to affect your health, it will also affect the health of your child. The good news is that if you recognize depression early enough and get treatment, most babies show no noticeable effects.

Now, the last thing we want you to do is become depressed about being depressed. So it's a good time to consider the adaptive value of depression. Why would our bodies want us to go into a depressed state? One theory is that depression may be an evolved response to a loss of status (it used to be that our ancestors became de-

What's a Doula?

You may have heard of a birth doula before; that's a person who provides all kind of support for a mom to prepare her for childbirth. A doula gives emotional support, has lots of information about pregnancy, can be a spiritual companion, and even can be an advocate in health care situations. Many people find that having a doula gives them additional support and info they need to help make the birthing process easier. But you don't have to limit a doula's experience to just birth. Many doulas offer support both before and after birth. That's especially helpful for women who need to go on bed rest for a significant amount of time before birth; the doula takes care of tangible needs but also helps mom emotionally during this difficult time.

Now, a doula doesn't take the place of a husband or partner, so don't feel as if you're trampling on his territory if you would like to use one. It's just that women often feel that it's extremely helpful to have another woman (kind of like the village expert) who's been through similar experiences to provide additional informational and emotional support. In the context of emotional issues, having a doula may be one of the best answers there is to reducing stress, anxiety, and depression. Just be sure you find one who's compatible with your philosophies. For example, if you're planning for a natural, unmedicated delivery, you want to make sure that you don't have a drill sergeant for a doula, in case you change your mind and decide you want an epidural. Remember, it's your birth experience, not hers. Plus, it's not a bad idea to introduce your doula to your doctor before your delivery if they haven't worked together previously, to make sure they're comfortable with each other. You want them working as a team, not as rivals. Find one in your area by going to DONA International at www.dona.org.

pressed after losing the throne),★ and that forces us to make different decisions. What once worked isn't working any more, so you'd better move your butt and switch strategies. Depression actually serves as a signal: Change up or lose out.

In a way, the same can be said for pregnancy-related depression. If you're feeling

★ Not that one, but the real one.

down, certainly there are hormonal influences that are affecting your mood, but it can also serve as a cue that perhaps you need to make different decisions or change some of your life strategies; that's where talking out issues and problems with other people plays a huge role. One of the treatments for depression comes in the form of medication combined with counseling. Although antidepressants do have some risks, the dangers of depression—to you and to your unborn child—usually outweigh those risks. We'll outline our stance on antidepressant medications in our tips, but most of all, we want to make sure you realize that if you are suffering from depression, you need to discuss it with your doc and take steps for the health of your baby and your own peace of mind.

YOU TIPS

FACT: Pregnancy is remarkably safe, or else the human race wouldn't be here.

FACT: Pain management is better than ever, and deliveries are becoming much easier than they ever have been.

FACT: Most of the time, your job is to just get out of the way and let this remarkable process work naturally.

We call attention to these facts because they help reinforce our "just say know" mantra. As knowledge goes down, anxiety goes up. If you can flip those trajectories, you'll feel much better about some of the issues you may be facing.

How to do that? Well, for one, you want to try to automate your life a bit—to be prepared to handle the everyday stresses as easily you can; that way, your body and brain will be ready when bigger ones hit. After all, a lot of stress management really comes down to managing your energy levels. If you can live a balanced, healthy life, you will undoubtedly have more power and energy to cope with stressors. You can start by following some of these tips, which we have divided into three categories: stress, sleep, and depression.

STRESS

Tackle the Problems Head-on. Look, we totally understand that you feel as if you've got more things to worry about than a bankrupt CFO. Being the center of attention of all your family and friends can be a wonderful thing, but it can also be stressful, as you try to manage the questions, the issues, and the family squabbling that come as surprising side effects of pregnancy. While massages and music can certainly help reduce the load, the only way to really manage the stressors is to deal with them and move on. We certainly can't address every stress you may face over forty weeks, but here's some advice for managing a few of the biggies:

- **Stress About Baby's Health.** Knowledge is the best defense, and we hope that what you learn in this book helps ease some of your mental burden. The truth is, almost all of your vices will be forgiven—we humans are a resilient lot. So while there's no guarantee for a 100 percent perfect birth, you can take comfort in the fact that many health issues are genetically predetermined and not something for which you should accept blame. Your job is to optimize the fetal environment.

- **New-Mommy Stress.** If this is your first child, chances are that you feel a little anxious about how healthy the baby is going to turn out, although the odds are greater than 90 percent that you'll have a baby with no short-term, life-threatening birth defects. Instead of obsessing about the big picture, you can reduce some of your anxiety by dealing with lots of little pictures. Some tactics:

  - Take a class on baby basics. (See page 190 for more details.)
  - Keep regular playdates with other moms-to-be—for yourself.
  - Get the nursery ready; stock the shelves with diapers.
  - Plan for child care.
  - Cook some meals and stick them in the freezer. A well-prepared life tends to be a less stressful one. If you have a friend or coworker who's throwing you a baby shower, drop the hint that perhaps a most welcome gift would be for your colleagues to make dinners for you and your family after the child is born.

- **Long-Term Work Stress:** If you're worried about how to deal with your job, it's best to have the talk with your boss sooner rather than later. When you're ready, tell your employer about your prenatal visits; many women tell only one friend until after the first trimester is completed. Also ask how you can help manage the burden that will come when you're on maternity leave. Because it won't be easy for your coworkers, who may have to cover for you while you're away, start lining up options a few months in advance. This kind of planning helps ease their worry and, in turn, makes it easier for you. And be up front: If you think you can financially handle a three-day week instead of five, just ask, ask, ask. Most bosses would rather have frank discussions in advance than have you ignore the issue and try to make up ground later. Plus, it's not a bad idea to go over family leave policies and options with the human resources department.

- **Day-to-Day Work Stress.** Besides the big picture of dealing with your job, there are also plenty of little nags that can eat at you during the day. You're worried about resting, about performing, about getting enough to eat, and about so many other issues—especially during a time when nobody may even know that you're pregnant. Some little strategies that will help you cope:

  - Spread out your lunch hour and rest breaks to create fifteen-minute relaxation periods that calm and recharge you. The amount of time is less critical than how well you spend these precious moments, so work out a soothing ritual like a shoulder rub, meditation in the sun, or a walk (exercise helps). Using this time wisely will increase your productivity and ensure that you're getting enough rest. Stash small meals and healthful snacks in your desk to keep up your energy levels.
  - Keep plenty of water on hand so your reflex response to irritation becomes sipping something that is good for you.
  - Confide in one close colleague, if possible, before you tell the whole crew. Having one person who can understand why you need to go to the bathroom so often, for instance, and who has your back can help ease the anxiety that comes from trying to hide your pregnancy from the entire office for the first few months.

- **Mother-Daughter Stress:** Maybe you're a first-time mom; maybe your mom is a first-time grandma. Just as you're longing to care for this new life, your mom or mother-in-law is also longing to help, to pass along wisdom, to share her little secrets for burping success. Intentions may be good, but those words of wisdom can be more annoying than a broken remote control—and that can cause some serious tension. Because these cracks can become caverns, you may need to think about strategies for dealing with your mother. Of course, one option is to talk about the issues. But here's another thought: Sometimes it might be okay to put some distance between you to help reduce anxiety during a naturally stressful time. At the opposite end, if you, for instance, are not close to your mother or have lost your mother, that can be a source of stress too. That's why it's important for you to find a surrogate—like a sister, aunt, or friend—who can help fill in a bit of the emptiness you may feel during this time.

Buddy Up. You may be thinking about baby playdates a few months down the road. But how about this? Schedule a mom-to-be playdate right now. Joining a support group of moms going through the same thing (along with those who may have recently gone through the same thing) is one of the best things you can do for your state of mind. In fact, studies show that handling a pregnancy with little emotional support is associated with greater emotional distress, anxiety, and depression. Those who cope with the aid of support? They tend to take better care of themselves in all aspects of their health.

Move It. If you know us, you know that we think the mind-body relationship is as close as the mom-baby relationship. What you feel in your head influences what you feel in your body and vice versa. So it should be no surprise that a physically strong body is also going to make you feel mentally strong. In fact, even moderate exercise or physical activity is associated with fewer pregnancy pains and problems—and thus serves as a huge mechanism for stress relief as well. Swimming is a great activity, especially toward the end of pregnancy, since the baby is buoyant and you can move comfortably while floating. Exercise also helps relieve depression.

Get in Touch. In the last chapter, you learned about how your soothing, gentle strokes pay huge dividends for your infant. Don't scrimp on that kind of lovin'. You too need some physical comfort. As you pass this passage to your partner (Read this, buster!), understand that massage works by stimulating feel-good endorphins and oxytocin, and decreasing blood pressure. It's also been shown to reduce stress during labor. So whether it comes from your mate or a professional, make it a habit to be on the receiving end of a rubdown.

Get Your iPod Playlist Ready. Whether you like Mozart or Metallica, music has been shown to reduce stress in pregnancy and even reduce pain during childbirth. It seems that listening to tunes for about a half hour a day substantially reduces stress and depression. The added benefit of piping it through the house: You stimulate your baby with various sounds in utero.

SLEEP

Find Comfort. Telling someone to get better sleep or more sleep is like telling someone to lift a car over her head twelve times. When it comes to sleep, you just can't impose your will on your body. Our goal here is to help you find the little things that will make you more comfortable, so that your body follows what your mind wants. Some suggestions:

- If you have difficulty breathing (from the weight gain), try multiple pillows, which will pull the baby away from your diaphragm so it can move your lungs up and down.
- Don't drink water after six in the evening to reduce the need to get up to use the bathroom. And no caffeine, either. Make sure that you do get your two quarts of fluid a day before that, especially if you're in a hot climate.
- Don't try to suffer through all the aches and pains you might be experiencing. It's better for your mind and body to quiet the pain (through Tylenol) so that you can get the restorative sleep you need, rather than grit your way through the aches just to avoid taking medicine.
- Try a small glass of warm skim milk, but not after six o'clock. The lactose in the milk is a sugar, which stimulates insulin, which helps proteins like tryptophan in the milk enter the brain—and that can help people fall asleep. If you develop lactose intolerance, which many moms do during pregnancy, try soy milk or rice milk.
- Create a dark, quiet environment in the bedroom, using the bed for sleep and sex only—and not for work or surfing the web.
- Ratchet up the air conditioner. It's easier to sleep in a cooler environment; plus, pregnant women are extra hot.

Try Sleep Meds. If you want to try the pharmaceutical route, you should talk to your doctor. Benadryl is considered safe for pregnant women to take for sleep. It's sometimes even given to newborns. You can also consider an over-the-counter medication called Unisom, which has been shown to help promote sleep during pregnancy. Just don't use it for more than a week.

Quiet the Kick. Many pregnant women suffer from leg cramps and restless leg syndrome, which occurs when your leg reflexively spasms in a kicking motion. The problem isn't that you risk bruis-

Figure 6.2 **Huff and Puff** You can make adjustments in your sleeping position to help open your diaphragm and make breathing easier. This will both help relax you and ensure that an optimal amount of oxygen is getting to the baby.

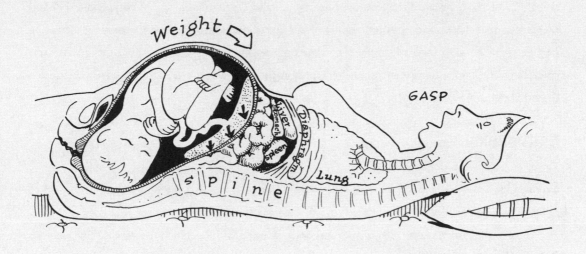

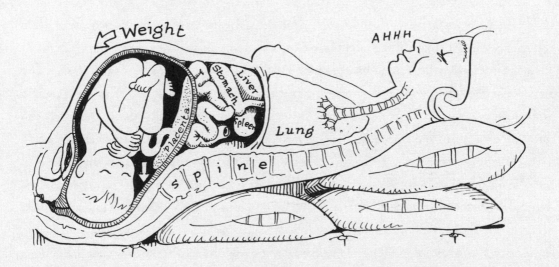

ing your bedmate; it's that the motion can wake you out of a good sleep. The syndrome is also associated with that creepy-crawly sensation; your leg feels as if it's being pinched. It seems to be caused by irregular levels of the chemical dopamine. Some treatments include making sure you get 800 micrograms of folate a day during pregnancy (400 micrograms) in a prenatal pill and 400 micrograms in food or supplements and 30 milligrams (mg) of iron. Applying a heating pad to the area also seems to quiet the disturbances. Also, magnesium (400 milligrams) and calcium (1,200 milligrams) can help leg cramps, as these minerals are naturally used by muscles to contract normally.

DEPRESSION

Speak Up. The fact is that most women suffer in silence. They assume they're just supposed to pull up their socks, move on, and be strong. And by the time they actually say that they're feeling depressed, they're really far down the road and suffering from significant distress. For reasons we mentioned earlier (about how emotional support helps people cope), it's important to talk about how you're feeling to people close to you, your doctor, or your midwife.

Add DHA. As we discussed, DHA omega-3 fats are essential for helping restore some of those fatty acids that get stolen by the fetus. Take 600 milligrams a day during pregnancy and breast-feeding because it helps a child's brain development and also may reduce mom's depression. The reason we need the DHA form of omega-3 is that it helps protect nerves. Now, some people who might be afraid to get DHA from fish (because they fear the toxicity of fish) think they can get their omega-3s from flaxseed or walnuts instead. But flaxseed contains alpha-linolenic acid (ALA), another form of omega-3. ALA converts poorly to a form called eicosapentaenoic acid (EPA), which is the predecessor in DHA, which is present in baby formula because the fat is essential for brain growth. But ALA doesn't convert perfectly to DHA, so you should get at least some DHA through fish or the vegetarian DHA source algae (which is where fish get it from anyway, so you're just skipping the middleman). By the way, the EPA thins your blood, but don't worry about taking DHA omega-3 fats right up to delivery.

You can also take 2 grams of cod liver oil—gulp!—if you prefer, although its smell often exacerbates nausea. Two grams of fish oil contain approximately 600 milligrams of DHA.

Figure 6.3 **Fat Stance** Healthy fats come in different forms and serve different functions, but they do play a crucial role in a baby's brain development—and help to stave off a mother-to-be's depression. The most important is DHA, which makes up 60 percent of our brains.

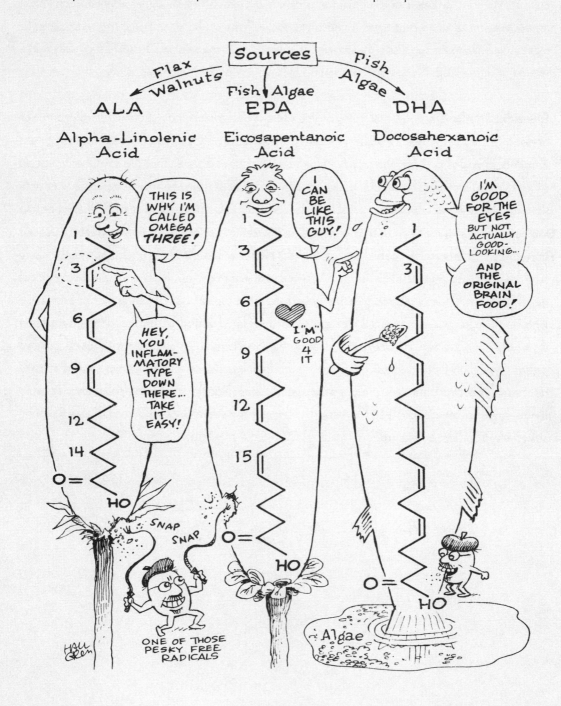

Examine Your Eats. The foods we eat also influence the delicate hormonal balance that controls our moods and emotions. So it's worth experimenting with different foods (peanut butter cups don't count) to see if small adjustments can help. Sometimes, though, those neurochemical imbalances make deep dips—and it's hard to recover from them. Plus, resist the temptation to treat your anxiety or depression with overeating; looking in the mirror afterward may only make you more depressed. Nuts, fruits, and vegetables may help raise serotonin levels.

Consider Meds. We know that many moms-to-be like to avoid medications altogether for fear of dousing their babies with any pharmaceuticals whatsoever. While there's been conflicting data on antidepressant medications and adverse effects, it does appear that a class of antidepressants called selective serotonin reuptake inhibitors, or SSRIs, frequently have fewer side effects than the disease itself. Examples of SSRIs include Zoloft (sertraline) and Prozac (fluoxetine). In fact, most human studies show that SSRIs have not led to an increase in birth defects. Because hormones and other chemicals do cross the placental barrier, it can be said that a melancholy mom may lead to a melancholy baby. If you suspect you might be depressed, get professional help right away. Talk to your ob/gyn and get a referral to a professional therapist or psychiatrist who can help you work out your issues, get to the bottom of your problems, and help determine if you need medication. Most experts believe that SSRIs need to be taken with a side dose of professional therapy to be most effective. And remember that when medications are medically necessary, avoiding them only prolongs the agony. Ultimately, the effects on pregnancy seem to be the same for those who treat depression with medication and those who don't. So we ask, why suffer when you don't have to?

YOU-Q:
The Worry and Anxiety Quiz

There's an old joke that a developmental psychologist had a child and then wrote a book about her theory of how children develop. Then the psychologist had her second child and wrote a book on individual differences in children. Then she had a third child and quit the field and took up yoga. Pregnancy is the same way: No two pregnancies are alike, even your own. So it's natural to be a bit worried, somewhat stressed, and even a bit blue when you're going through pregnancy. This test helps gauge those levels, so you know what you can do to make the most of your pregnancy.

PART I: Worry

To get started, answer the following questions on a scale of 1 to 5, 5 being you are Very Worried.

I worry . . .	Not at All Worried 1	2	3	4	Very Worried 5
1 about the pain of childbirth.					
2 about the delivery of my baby.					
3 that I will have a miscarriage.					

I worry . . .	Not at All Worried 1	2	3	4	Very Worried 5
4 that my baby will not be healthy.					
5 that my baby will have a birth defect.					
6 that pregnancy has made me gain too much weight.					
7 that pregnancy has hurt my appearance.					
8 that I will have difficulty caring for my baby.					
9 that the baby will hurt my relationship with my partner.					
10 that things I did before I got pregnant will hurt my baby now.					
11 about getting good health care for me and my baby.					
12 that I will be a bad parent.					
13 that I will not be able to afford my baby.					

Worry Score

For this test, add up all of your scores.

You should have a number from 13 to 65.

Issues

Worry is clearly a natural part of pregnancy. First, pregnancy (and particularly a first pregnancy) involves a tremendous feeling of venturing into the unknown. Humans are wired to treat unknown situations with avoidance, and worry is the emotional expression of the activity of the avoidance system. Some amount of worry is probably quite adaptive, though. Because worry is associated with avoidance behavior, it serves as a mechanism that prevents women from engaging in potentially risky behaviors that they might have engaged in prior to pregnancy. Thus, a moderate amount of worry is likely to be healthy.

Another reason why pregnant women experience worry is through misattribution processes. That is, women experience a lot of discomfort over the course of pregnancy. There's physical discomfort from body states that are changing rapidly. There's also mental discomfort from changes in hormonal balances over the course of pregnancy. Some of these discomforts have an obvious cause. For example, the baby kicks and causes pain. For others, the cause of the discomfort may be less obvious. In these cases, women may attribute their discomfort to whatever is bothering them at the moment, whether it is actually causing the issue or not. So a woman may end up worrying about finances, not so much because finances are a potential problem but because thoughts about finances are a good attribution for the current level of discomfort she is feeling.

Finally, high levels of worry are problematic. High levels of worry are associated with rumination, or repetitive thoughts about the source of worry. Rumination can help maintain the level of worry and stress, so the cycle of rumination needs to be broken. Rumination also causes attention problems, because the object of rumination displaces other thoughts. In addition, high levels of worry create chronic stress. There are important medically relevant effects of high chronic stress, including changes in eating patterns, constriction of blood flow to the fetus, and lowered immune system function. So while a moderate level of stress is helpful, high levels of chronic stress must be addressed.

PART II: Depression

Answer each of the following questions on a scale of 1 to 5; 5 being this is Very True of Me:

	Not at All True of Me 1	2	3	4	Very True of Me 5
1 I am sad all the time.					
2 I am disappointed in myself.					
3 I frequently feel like crying.					
4 I don't consider myself as worthy as I used to.					
5 I am irritable all the time.					
6 I often have thoughts of harming myself.					
7 I feel I have many bad faults.					
8 I feel that the future is hopeless.					

Depression Score

For this test, add up all of your scores.

This score should range from 8 to 40.

Issues

Depression is a potential problem during and after pregnancy. The rapid changes in hormone levels during pregnancy influence mood. Short-term and short-lived changes in mood are common during pregnancy, but a sustained period of depression should be brought to the attention of your doctor as quickly as possible.

Visualizing Where You Are

During pregnancy, depression and worry also belong right in the middle of a bell curve. Too little of them, and you probably aren't taking things seriously enough. You might end up engaging in behaviors that hurt you or the baby. Too much, and you may be suffering from a problem that requires your doctor's attention. So, just like Baby Bear in "Goldilocks and the Three Bears," you want to be just right. To figure out where you are, take your score on the worry test and approximate your level on the chart on the next page. Then take your score on the depression test and mark it on the left side. Now draw a line upward from your mark on the worry test. Draw a line to the right from your mark on the depression test. Put a big dot at the point where the lines cross. You are here—er, there!

We have labeled the regions of this depression/worry territory. There's a section in the middle, and that's about where you want to be. A moderate amount of worry and a little mood swinging are normal in pregnancy. If you're there, you don't need to feel bad or worried about the amount that you feel bad or worried.

The other regions on the graph require some attention.

If you live at the bottom left, you're just too laissez-faire. You ought to be at least a little worried about pregnancy. You need to be alert to what you are doing to maximize your health and your baby's health.

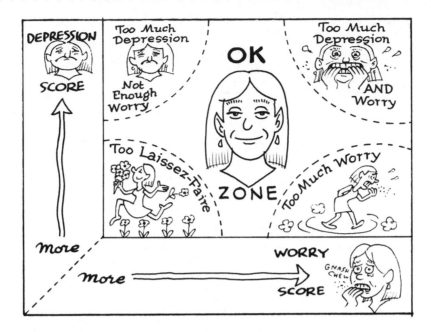

If you live at the bottom right, you are not that moody, but you are definitely worrying too much. Too much worry and anxiety during pregnancy is a problem.

If you live at the top left, then you are not that worried, but you are showing signs of depression. Depression is common during pregnancy, but it is still something to be taken seriously.

If you live at the top right, then you are experiencing both a lot of worry and some signs of serious depression. This is a matter that you should take up with your doctor immediately.

7

Let's Talk About Sex

How Hormonal Changes Can Do
Quite the Number on You and Your Body

From the moment you first learned you were pregnant, your priorities got changed faster than a leaky diaper. Suddenly, your world no longer revolved around your work, your mate, or your Thursday-night appletinis. The center of your belly became the center of your universe.

That, of course, is part of the parenthood plan. You sacrifice much of your time, your money, and your sleep for the love of raising a child. The result? Worth every one of those trade-offs.

But as you have probably surmised from our previous chapters, there's a fine line between healthy and unhealthy sacrifices. That is, it's not helpful to you, your relationships, or your children if your sacrifices come at the expense of your own health. We saw a bit of that in action in the last chapter as we explored emotional and mental issues that pregnant women face. The next two chapters are going to take the topic a step further by tackling some of the physical concerns.

This chapter addresses so-called soft health issues—those that seem not to carry much serious health risk but are important just the same in terms of how you feel about yourself and the world around you. What all of these symptoms have in common is that they are caused by fluctuating pregnancy hormone levels. (In the next chapter, we'll address the so-called hard health issues, which include more serious medical complications.)

You've already learned how much your baby grows and changes every day in your belly, and you don't need a full-length mirror to know that your body is undergoing some pretty major changes as well. Those changes occur primarily in the size, shape, and appearance of your external physique, but they also manifest themselves in the way you feel internally when it comes to such things as sex drive and the way you interact in your intimate relationship. Most of these aren't health issues per se, but they can influence your anxiety, stress, and emotional levels, which, as you learned from the last chapter, can become health issues if you let them get out of control.

The big biological player in most of these issues? Estrogen. You produce more estrogen in one pregnancy than you will in the rest of your entire nonpregnant life combined. In short, your pregnant body is going through a hormonal firestorm, and that affects not only how you look but also how you feel. Your goal here is to embrace your pregnancy and learn to celebrate the changes in your body and even in your relationships. After all, the way you handle those changes, in part, plays a role in what happens *after* pregnancy as well—in terms of both your health and your happiness.

The Estrogen Effect

As we explained in the introduction, we decided against writing a chronological account of pregnancy mainly because so many issues can span the length of the entire pregnancy and also because we believe that it makes sense to look at entire systems and their functions as they work throughout an entire pregnancy. That said, the second trimester is when you'll probably experience the most significant changes in your body. It's also, for many women, the most enjoyable part of pregnancy. In the first trimester, you may be dealing with nausea and fatigue, and in the third trimester—when the baby has grown enough to use your bladder as a stepladder—you're feeling quite uncomfortable. But the second trimester usually brings a renewed sense of well-being: You're feeling good, you've got the glow, you're doing A-OK. That, dear friend, means some dramatic pregnancy symptoms are right around the corner.

Beginning at week fourteen, the placenta is fully operational, pumping out continuously high levels of estrogen and progesterone, among other hormones. Just to put it all in perspective, a pregnant woman produces more estrogen in one day than a nonpregnant, premenopausal woman generates in three years. Wow. And that's not even mentioning progesterone, which is also revving high. The reason? Both hormones play huge roles in preparing for and supporting pregnancy.

- By increasing the number and size of blood vessels that supply the uterus, estrogen helps increase blood flow, ensuring that enough nutrients make it to your developing baby. In fact, there's a tenfold increase in blood flow to your uterus from the beginning of pregnancy until the end.

> Factoid: The uterus grows from 60 grams to 1,200 grams during pregnancy, or from about the size of a walnut to the size of a beach ball.

- While helping the uterine lining thicken to prepare for implantation, estrogen also plays a major role in increasing the overall size of the uterus. It does this by increasing the number and size of the cells, so the uterus can be stretched to accommodate a growing baby.
- Estrogen helps increase the number of white cells in the blood, thus improving immune function. This comes in handy, since pregnancy is an immune-compromised state, yet you still need to protect the fetus from infections. Increased white blood cells travel along with blood-clotting factors, the latter to decrease the chances of bleeding in the very vascular uterus and placenta (and thus of not supplying nutrients to the baby) and to decrease hemorrhaging during delivery. The downside of this partnership is that it increases the chances of blood clots forming in your legs and elsewhere. We'll discuss this at greater length in the next chapter.

One of the most wonderful ways we see estrogen working is through the so-called pregnancy glow you may be exuding. While many of us assume that you glow because you're happy, proud, and excited about the adorable baby booties you're planning to buy, it's actually a physical effect of pregnancy. Estrogen stimulates your blood vessels to gain more nitric oxide effect, which opens up your arteries and arterioles (small arteries). This increases blood flow to your baby and, as a side effect, makes your skin shine.

As you can see, these changes are largely good: The increased estrogen is designed to nurture and protect your baby. But you can also imagine that with such hormone intensity, you're bound to experience some changes that don't feel good at all.

That Lovin' Feeling: Your Sex Drive

Last chapter, we talked about how your pregnancy-related mood swings can cause you to laugh one minute and ball up in a heap of tears the next. The same applies to your bedroom moods as well. One minute, you may crave nothing more than a steamy sex session, and the next, you may feel about as sexy as clay. While your partner may think your mood changes are maddening, the truth is that it's not your fault—it's your hormones.

On one hand, much of what's happening in your body is working to boost your sex drive. As your estrogen and progesterone levels rise, they cause changes in your body that increase your libido. Estrogen increases vaginal lubrication, heightens sensitivity in your breasts and nipples, and improves blood flow to your pelvic area. The increased curves around your hips and breasts may also make you feel sexier. Add those symptoms together, and it's a righteous recipe for romance. Not having to deal with birth control can be liberating as well.

On the other hand, those hormones can conspire against you—especially in the beginning, when nausea and fatigue dictate that the bed be used for sleep, rest, and foot rubs *only*. And in the last trimester, you may feel more uncomfortable than a concrete couch, meaning that there's, oh, say, zero chance you want to have sex.

The X factor in the sex-drive equation is the relationship between your changing moods and your changing body, both of which are influenced by your changing hormone levels. The result is that how you feel about your body (and how you think your partner feels about your body) plays a part in whether or not you want to do the satin sheet salsa. Just as every woman's pregnancy is unique, so is every woman's sex drive—and yours may change from day to day or hour to hour. We should point out that because of a dramatic falloff in estrogen, it's likely your sex drive will drop dramatically immediately after birth and remain low for several months if you are breast-feeding. This makes sense be-cause a pregnancy so soon after delivery would mean that nutrients would be di-

> **Factoid:** Uterine contractions associated with orgasms are different from the contractions you'll feel during labor. If you have a normal pregnancy, orgasms—with or without intercourse—don't seem to increase the risk of premature labor or premature birth. Likewise, sex isn't likely to trigger labor even as your due date approaches.

verted to one offspring at the expense of another. And because your body needs extra time to heal after the rigors of childbirth, your lack of libido serves as a hor-monally mediated protective mechanism.

So what's a woman to do?

First of all, if you do want to have sex, go ahead. As long as your pregnancy is pro-ceeding normally, you can have sex as often as you like.★ There are uncommon cases in which you shouldn't have sex, and your doc will guide you. She may recommend that you refrain from sex if you're at risk for preterm labor, you're leaking amniotic fluid, your cervix begins to open prematurely, or you have placenta previa. (See page 52.) If your uterus is in a typical position, there's no risk of hurting the baby during intercourse because the amniotic fluid protects the baby from impact. The angle of the vagina, relative to the space in your womb, decreases the probability of

---

★ It's not uncommon for pregnant women to experience a small amount of bright red bleeding dur-ing intercourse, especially during the first trimester. The bleeding is caused by swelling of the capillar-ies in the cervix. When irritated during sex, they burst and release blood. While it's generally nothing to worry about, you should still mention it to your doc or midwife.

Sex After Birth

After you give birth and enter into the early stages of parenthood, there are plenty of things you want to do (sleep!). And there are plenty of things you may want absolutely no part of (sex!). And for good reason: With the sudden drop of estrogen after birth, you lose your libido and the lining of your vaginal canal thins out, making sex feel as if you're losing your virginity all over again. Plus, there's added pain if you've had stitches or an episiotomy (the cut made to help give more room during a vaginal delivery).

Now add in other, more subtle complications of postpregnancy libido: You may feel guilty because you haven't had sex in a long time, and he has conflicted thoughts about going back into the place where he watched his child come out. It's tricky all the way around. Most docs recommend that you wait six weeks after birth to put anything in your vagina. That includes oral sex. The goals are to allow your body to heal, avoid infections, and help with the psychological issues. When you do venture back, it's especially important that your partner realize you need plenty of foreplay—and if you're nursing, lubricants—and that you'll need birth control if you choose. Many people wrongly assume that they can't get pregnant while they're nursing.

direct contact with the growing fetus. Plus, because there's a mucous plug that blocks the cervix during pregnancy, there's virtually no chance of unintended contact between what's inside of you for nine months and what may be inside of you for only nine minutes.★ (We'll offer some suggestions for comfortable sexual positions for pregnant women in our tips at the end of the chapter.)

The loss of sex drive may not worry a woman as much as how that loss of libido might affect her relationship with her partner. It goes something like this: He wants sex, you don't. You know he wants sex, and you feel bad about not wanting it, especially since you know your sex life will be on hold for a few weeks after you deliver. So you either force yourself to have sex when you really don't want to, which is pretty disheartening, or you put him off and worry that he's going to look elsewhere.

★ Give or take.

The simplest thing you can do to help remedy this situation is to talk with your partner. Silence is the romance killer: Just explaining to him that your back hurts or you're totally zapped will do wonders toward helping him understand that there's more to sex than sex. Beyond communication, the solution to this sexual scenario really comes down to adaptation—that is, your ability to change your sexual relationship so that it's not about the sex per se but, rather, about increasing the eroticism, sensuality, and passion in your relationship. Making that kind of mutual pact with your partner will go a long way toward keeping your old bond while you're focused on creating your new one. And while you're at it, appreciate your mate for the little compromises he is willing to make for your happiness, even if the resulting sex isn't quite what you had planned.

What a Body: Is Image Everything?

Throughout your life, you've seen your share of bodily changes. You went from a stick figure to an hourglass. Maybe you've gained weight, maybe you've lost some, maybe you've hacked off your hair, or maybe you've even surgically straightened your nose or plumped up your lips. No matter what changes you've been through, the bodily changes that happen during pregnancy are about as dramatic as they come. Those changes very much influence how you feel—and can contribute to the stress levels we talked about in the previous chapter. Here's an outline of what you can expect as your body undergoes this miraculous transformation.

Body Shape

The growth around your midsection doesn't happen just because Freddy Jr. has decided to camp there for the next forty weeks. It also happens because you store extra fat during pregnancy, and most of that fat is typically deposited in the center of your body. (That fat storage decreases later in pregnancy, when Freddy needs more nutrients.)

During pregnancy, the placenta secretes a chemical called prolactin, which attaches to dopamine receptors on brain cells. Dopamine is a pleasure hormone that's associated with addictions; when you become addicted to something, it's because a feedback loop causes you to seek things that raise dopamine levels. Prolactin seems to turn on addicting elements in the brain, thus making you, for example, want to eat more food. But it seems to have a protective element as well; prolactin is likely the hormone that helps you tolerate such dramatic body changes and not have as much anxiety over them as you would under different circumstances. It stimulates your endorphin system so that you feel less pain and more able to ignore minor anxieties; it makes sense that nature makes that available in the pregnant state, eh?

One of the biggest stresses among pregnant women is worrying about whether their bodies will ever bounce back after pregnancy. That fear, of course, just adds to the cascade of other anxieties. While we're going to suggest ways to help you get your prepregnancy body back (see our training plan on page 310), it's a little trickier to manage the psychological aspect of body image. Part of the process is learning to revel in the miracle of pregnancy and to appreciate both the sexiness and the saintliness that come along with it.

Factoid: Lots of people believe that the shape of their belly reflects the gender of the baby inside. You've got a boy if you have a basketball belly (with no fat anywhere else), and you're carrying a girl if you're shaped more like a watermelon (fat all the way around, like an inner tube). The truth is that belly shape has nothing to do with the gender of your child but rather your body type, fitness, and genetics—specifically, the elasticity of your belly, as well as the length of your belly from your pubic bone to your xiphoid process (the lowest junction in the middle of your chest).

Breasts

If belly changes get all of your attention, we can guess exactly what gets his. We all know that your breasts serve a more important purpose than hypnotizing your partner, but it may help to know a little bit more about how and why they change. Simply put: As estrogen, progesterone, and fat storage increase, so does your breast

Tough as Nails

Examine one of your fingernails. How does it look? Hormones, as well as prenatal vitamins and a healthier diet, cause nails to grow a bit faster than usual during pregnancy. While some women's nails get harder, many women find that their nails get softer and break more easily. If so, protect your nails. When you're doing any kind of work that's hard on your hands, like washing dishes or gardening, wear rubber gloves with a cloth lining. It will also help to trim nails short, which you'll want to do after the baby is born anyway. If you have your nails done at a salon, avoid places where there's a strong odor or where all the manicurists are wearing masks, and remember to bring your own instruments unless you are certain that the salon sterilizes its tools. You also want to avoid places that may use a chemical called MMA, which is highly toxic. Same goes for you: Avoid polishes and removers that contain MMA or acetonitrile, and make sure to paint your nails in a well-ventilated room.

size. As the milk-producing glands get bigger during pregnancy, you can add as much as a pound of tissue and two cup sizes to your breasts.

It's very common for your breasts to get very sore early in pregnancy; in fact, it's often the way that women first realize they are pregnant. They'll also start to itch as the skin begins to stretch. At the same time, you'll notice your nipples and the surrounding areolas getting larger and darker, and more veins and bumps beginning to appear in the area. Biologically, this happens as your blood volume increases during pregnancy. Evolutionarily, this happens for a different reason. Remember what we said in chapter 4 about black-and-white toys and the ability of newborn babies to see contrast? Newborns need high contrast not just to figure out how to shake a rattle but to make sure their mouths hit their targets. Darker, more prominent nipples act like runway lights at an airport, directing the youngster to her vital source of food.

Speaking of which, that's the other big breast change you're going to experience. Unfortunately, you may feel like a 1930s faucet—leaking, leaking, leaking. A small amount of leaking of premilk (called colostrum) can start as early as the end of the second trimester; major leaking generally occurs after giving birth. You'll also de-

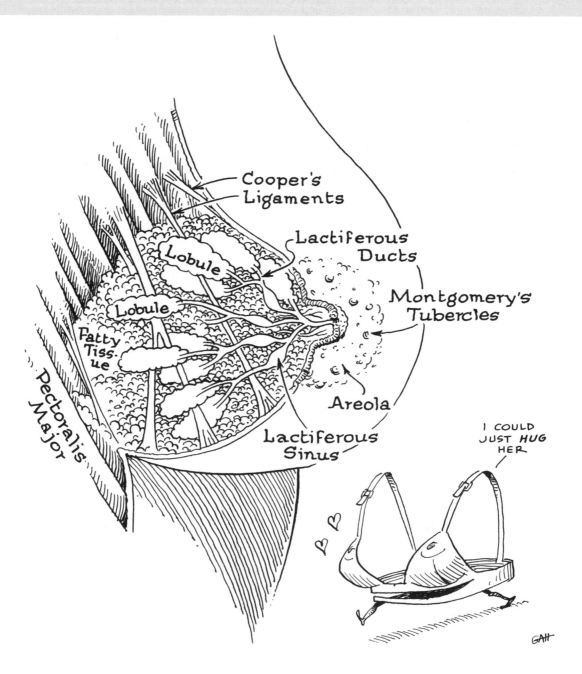

Cooper's Ligaments

Lactiferous Ducts

Montgomery's Tubercles

Lobule

Lobule

Fatty Tiss. ue

Pectoralis Major

Areola

Lactiferous Sinus

I COULD JUST *HUG* HER

velop Montgomery's tubercles: small, harmless bumps on your areolas. These bumps actually secrete a lubricant that discourages bacteria growth—a reason not to wash your nipples with soap, as we mentioned earlier. This lubricant will also help prevent your nipples from cracking during breast-feeding.

Skin

No matter whether your skin is typically dry, oily, or something in between, skin type is never static. It can change depending on your hormones, the climate, or what type of gunk you cake on your face and body. Normally, though, during pregnancy you'll notice that your skin does appear healthier—most likely due to the enhanced blood flow that gives you "the glow." But that's not always the case. Some other skin changes you may notice:

- Stretch marks: These bleeping striations appear when the dermis (a middle layer of skin) cracks and splits in order to expand. The redness will go away within a year, which helps immensely, but there's little you can do to eliminate them completely, because once those cracks happen, the damage is done. In the meantime, stay out of the sun, so that the marks don't become darker and more visible.

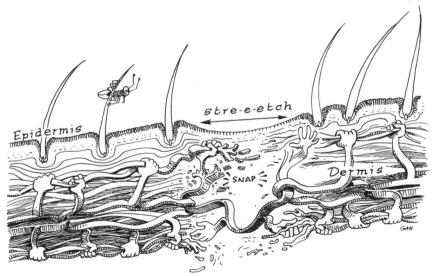

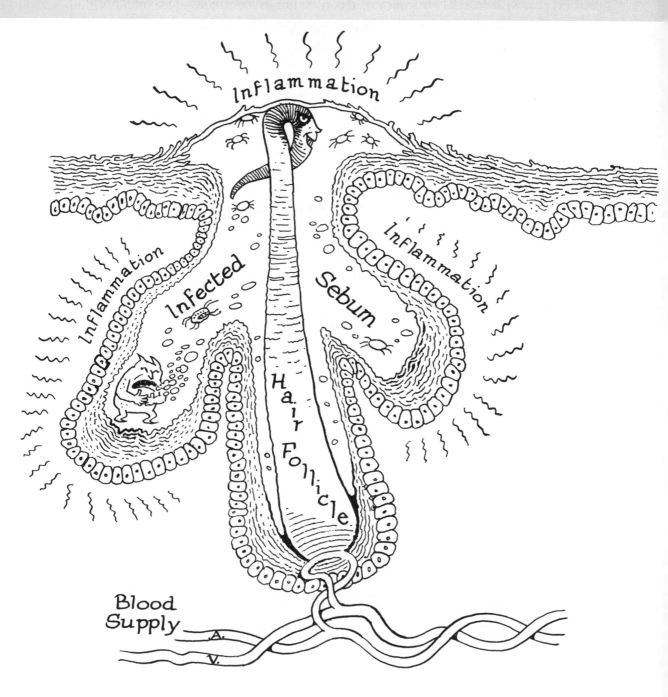

- Acne: The pores in your skin can sometimes get blocked by dirt, by built-up makeup, or by accelerated skin growth from increased estrogen. When that happens, the oil in your skin can't drain out, and bacteria start to grow, causing irritation and acne. And if a woman is prone to acne, pregnancy may worsen it all over her body, not just her face. Over-the-counter treatments such as benzoyl peroxide are generally considered safe, though we recommend waiting until after the first trimester. Check with your doc, because some acne medications like Accutane (isotretinoin) are considered extremely harmful during pregnancy.
- Darkness: Sometimes the midline of your abdomen can take on a brownish or black color called linea nigra, or you can get brown patches on your face or neck, a condition called melasma (also nicknamed the ominous "mask of pregnancy"). Both eventually fade, but if you're impatient, a steroid cream (for use after pregnancy and breast-feeding) may help clear this up. Fair-skinned women typically don't get the dark line but are more prone to red rashes.
- Genital changes: Besides the fact that your vaginal walls thicken during pregnancy and your clitoris (which is biologically like the tip of a penis) enlarges, increased blood flow to the area can lead to changes in the color of your labia. Seeing black, blue, or even purple can be a change you didn't expect, but all are perfectly normal.

Hair

Here's yet another change attributable to the master pregnancy hormone: Estrogen extends the growing phase of the hair-growth cycle, so that fewer hairs fall out than normal. Typically, we lose about one hundred hairs a day after they have finished a normal growth cycle. But in pregnancy, with that extended growth phase, hair is fuller. It's also shinier. You can thank estrogen for that too; it helps produce sebum, natural oil that comes from our hair follicles. After birth, however, expect to be cleaning a lot of hair out of your drain. When estrogen drops from your body, hair drops from your head.

Around about now, you may be wondering whether it's safe to dye your hair dur-

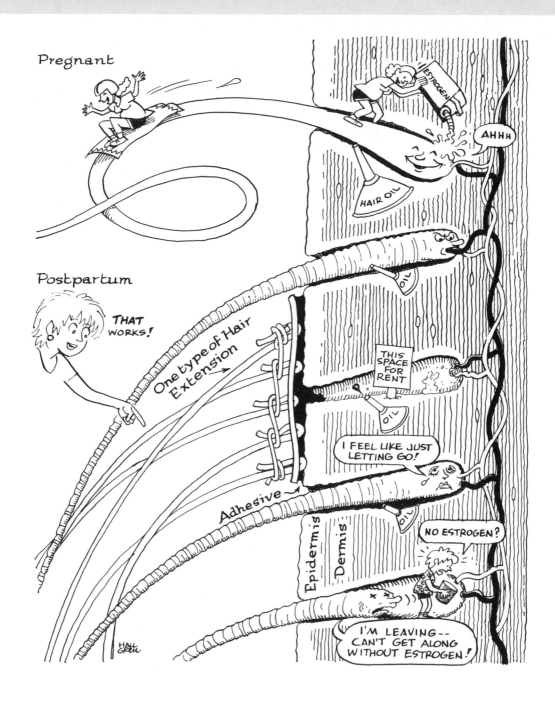

ing pregnancy, as 50 percent of mothers-to-be do. Here's our take: Hair coloring is not recognized as a danger during pregnancy; although some studies link cancer to hair dyes, the research is fairly weak. Some of the chemicals in hair dye can be absorbed through the skin via the scalp; highlighting or streaking involves less direct contact with the scalp. Temporary dyes that you apply at home are less toxic than permanent ones, but make sure that you wear gloves and use them in a well-ventilated area to avoid breathing in fumes. Another option: pure henna, a semipermanent dye that's been used for thousands of years. It's messy and has to be left on for four to eight hours, but it's safe and leaves an orange-red hue. Other colors of henna don't count because they may contain potentially risky metallic compounds.

> **Factoid:** You just learned that the hair on your head can grow thicker and fuller during pregnancy. Same is true for body hair, probably because of an increase in the male hormones called androgens. Yep, your body produces them, too. This comes in the form of more facial hair and stray hairs on your breasts, belly, and back. Most will be gone three to six months after you give birth; in the meantime, you can safely tweeze, wax, or shave as you wish. Permanent hair removal techniques are likely safe, but don't you already have enough discomfort to deal with? Plus, it's a waste of money, since the hair will fall out on its own anyway.

Hot Flashes

Pregnant woman are hot. Literally. In fact, seven out of ten women experience hot flashes or night sweats during pregnancy. This happens when intense heat spreads throughout the upper body for anywhere from thirty seconds to five minutes—typically starting in the neck and head but sometimes starting in the breast or lower. The intensity and frequency vary.

Nobody's quite sure what causes hot flashes, although we do know they can be triggered by spicy foods, hot drinks, alcohol, and stress. But some research shows that fluctuating levels of—you got it—estrogen may be at the root of them, with low blood sugar and hyperthyroidism also thought to cause the uncomfortable sensation. If you find that the hot flashes are more than just a temporary discomfort, talk to your doc about looking for a root cause, and take some of the precautions we outline below.

YOU TIPS

On the grand scale of health concerns, there's no doubt that sex drive, body image, and soft skin rank lower than anything that directly puts you or your child in harm's way. But to dismiss these softer health issues as inconsequential would be a mistake just the same. That's why we offer these tips for helping you feel the best that you possibly can.

Drum Up Your Drive. Look, there's absolutely nothing wrong if you don't want to have sex. (Men, read that again.) Perfectly fine. But the problem in some relationships is that sex is often seen as a symbol of the overall state of the relationship. Lack of sex can mean the ol' spark is gone, which can mean that a relationship is losing a bit of mojo. So what we want you to work on is not forcing yourself to increase your sex drive but to ramp up your sensuality and find other ways to physically and thus emotionally bond with your partner. (Men, read that again.) If the sex comes, fine. But if not, you've still made sure to connect on deeper levels.

For you guys out there, here are some suggestions that will go a long way toward making your partner feel good about herself and feel even better about the two of you:

- Foot rubs. Give them. Daily.
- Take a bath together. Grind up dry oats into a fine powder and sprinkle them into the tub. It can be incredibly soothing, as well as help decrease any itching she may have. For extra bonus points, light a candle and dim the lights.
- Every two weeks, take a picture of her to document how her belly has grown. Women we know report that it's an incredibly sensual activity—and one that you'll both look back on as pretty darn amazing.
- Exercise together. Focusing on each other's bodies gives you the double benefit—good for your health and for your relationship.
- Take baby classes with your partner. (See YOU Tool on page 190.)

- Flirt. Adapt your old-fashioned techniques to your new-fashioned technology. A random short text or email just to say you love her will go a long way (but nothing that will get you fired if you use a corporate device).
- Bust your tail around the house. The biggest thing you can do to help ease her anxiety is to take care of the things that you *can* do. You can't develop milk glands, but you can stock up on diapers, prepare the baby's room, go grocery shopping, cook meals (see "Pop's Pregnancy Recipes" on page 349), clean the litter box, or do anything that helps take her stress levels down a notch or two. Better yet: Do them without her having to ask.

Just Do It. If you are in the mood for sex (foot rubs worked, huh?), take comfort in the fact that you're not going to hurt your baby during intercourse. That said, we know that the standard missionary position with him on top is likely the least comfortable of all as your belly gets larger. Here are some alternative ways you can connect:

- **Two Spoons:** Lie side by side, with him behind you. The shallow penetration in this position might be more comfortable.
- **Ride High:** When the woman's on top, there's no pressure on her belly, and she can control the speed and depth of movements.

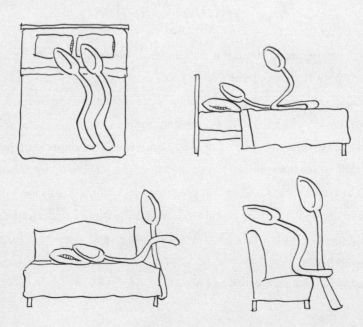

- **Comfort on the Comforter:** She lies on the edge of the bed, with her knees bent and feet on the edge of the bed. He stands at the edge.
- **Loving in the Living Room:** She kneels on a couch, with her belly facing the back of the couch and her arms on the back of the couch to support her weight. He penetrates from behind.

Get Some Support. We're not talking emotional support; we're talking about feminine support—namely, in the form of a comfortable bra. To help relieve soreness from swollen breasts and chafing from underwire bras, you want to find some pregnancy bras with these characteristics: a deep band under the cups (not wire), wide shoulder straps, soft fabric to minimize itching, and back fasteners (they offer more flexibility for adjustment than the ones that fasten in the front). You may want to sleep in a bra, especially if you're leaking, so make sure to find a comfortable one. Many women think that sports bras work especially well.

Check Them Out. Just because he may be spending an extraordinary time lingering on your blossoming bosom doesn't mean that you should skip doing the same. In fact, it is important to

A Fighting Chance

We've spent some time talking about the nice parts of relationships (Two Spoons!), but for some women, there's a much darker side. In some cases, pregnancy can trigger or escalate domestic abuse (abuse being defined as physical, sexual, and/or emotional). Not only does this put both mom and baby in direct danger, but it can also lead to problems that can adversely affect pregnancy, such as drinking, poor nutrition, depression, and so on. Given the fact that abuse tends to carry over after pregnancy and lead to a whole host of problems down the road, it's imperative that pregnant (and nonpregnant) women who are in abusive relationships seek help immediately. Contact the National Domestic Violence Hotline at 800-799-SAFE/799-7233 or www.ndvh.org; and remember to clear the memory cache and history files from your computer if you visit the website, so your partner will not be able to trace your activities online.

continue with breast self-exams during pregnancy and get any suspicious lumps checked out by a doc. Of course, what makes self-exams so tough is that your breasts are going through a heck of a lot of changes during pregnancy and may be tender to the touch. But take a deep breath and examine them anyway.

Save Your Skin. While some women get the smooth-skin glow during pregnancy, others get just the opposite: extreme breakouts. Before you try anything crazy, realize that 15 percent of people develop some type of allergic reaction to various products, including cosmetics. It's worth laying off the goop for a week just to see if your face will respond. After pregnancy and breast-feeding, you can start using a prescription Retin-A (tretinoin) cream if you plan on not being pregnant again. But take precautions: Pregnant women should never use Retin-A, which can cause severe birth defects. At the same time, use a soap without preservatives to help decrease oil and stimulate skin-building collagen. It'll take about a month for the treatment to begin working, and your skin may appear worse initially because of irritation from the medication. Add a niacin cream to help reduce the irritation. In the meantime, here's the plan for perfect skin care during pregnancy:

> Factoid: We don't know why, but malignant melanoma is the most common cancer to thrive during pregnancy—so have your partner examine your entire body for unusual moles early on and again at six and eight months. Report any suspicious spots to your doc or a dermatologist. Use the ABCDE checklist: asymmetry, border irregularity, color variety, diameter of more than 6 millimeters, and evolving (a spot that changes appearance).

- Wash your face with a gentle cleanser, one that won't burn your eyes.
- Use a moisturizer based on your skin type. Oily skin doesn't need a moisturizer. In fact, at ages younger than fifty and in any location save a desert, *most* skin doesn't need a moisturizer. Using one actually inhibits your skin's production of protective oils, even several weeks after you've discontinued it. Look for a lotion or a cream (as opposed to a gel or a liquid) that contains antioxidants in the form of vitamins A, C, and E, which will ward off toxins so that more collagen can form.

Screening for STDs

As part of your prenatal visits, you'll be screened for sexually transmitted diseases. Why? Because of the potential complications that can be passed to the fetus. Here are some of the ones that your doc or midwife may discuss with you:

Herpes: While uncommon, herpes can be potentially fatal to the fetus. C-sections reduce the risk of transmission from mom to baby.

Chlamydia: Pregnant women with untreated infections run the risk of having their babies acquire conjunctivitis and pneumonia.

Gonorrhea: If untreated in mom, infant may contract conjunctivitis and require antibiotics.

HIV: Transmission from mom to baby can happen in utero, during delivery, and during breast-feeding. If you are HIV-positive, you should pick an ob/gyn who has experience delivering other women with HIV; babies need to be treated within the first hour of delivery.

- Exfoliate your face using a washcloth and water rather than a chemical product. The mechanical removal of dead skin ensures that chemicals often used for exfoliation won't be absorbed and passed on to your baby.
- Use a sunscreen with zinc oxide and a sun protection factor (SPF) of at least 30 every day. No excuses. It's a mechanical blocker, so it isn't absorbed into the skin like many chemical sunscreens. Such blockers also work immediately, so you can put them on just as you're leaving the house.

See the Stretch. We're sorry to say that it doesn't appear that any topical treatments can eliminate stretch marks. A lot of damage takes place when that dermis tears and irritation ensues. There is some evidence, however, that daily massage may help prevent marks in the first place, so ask your mate to give regular rubs to the most common sites of stretch marks: your abdomen, thighs, and breasts. We're guessing he won't mind a bit. Use cocoa butter or vitamin E, as limited research suggests that the massage cream may help.

Hang On to Your Hair. Remember that because you're not losing much hair during pregnancy, the individual strands are going to stick around a lot longer than usual. They're no longer alive, however, so you want to treat the extra hair you are holding on to like a wet silk blouse. No excessive heating or combing, and avoid shampooing unless your hair is dirty. The fewer chemicals on your scalp, the better. Organic hair products are a wise choice if you feel you must use something.

Fix the Flash. Hot flashes may feel like the body's equivalent of lightning storms, and sometimes they can feel just as impossible to control. Since there are many possible causes, it's difficult to pinpoint a single cure that works for everyone. If you do suffer from them, try these tactics to help keep you from flashing:

- Wear breathable, layered clothing.
- Don't exercise when it's hot. Mornings and evenings are better. And if midday is the only time available, swimming is an excellent choice.
- Talk to your doc about possible medical reasons for the hot flashes, like thyroid-related issues; medications may be required to control them.
- Avoid taking herbs, which can do all kinds of things to your body that might throw your hormonal system out of balance.
- Aim to drink enough water—usually two quarts—every day to keep your urine clear enough to read through, and keep focusing on a diet that includes protein, fiber, fruits, vegetables, and grain.
- Keep a diary of your flash history, so you can try to identify (and then avoid) your common triggers.

YOU TOOL

HOW TO PICK A BIRTHING CLASS

Candles, satin, and Barry White CDs get all the attention when it comes to romance, but one of the ways you can best bond with your partner is by signing up for a childbirth class to help you prepare for pregnancy, delivery, and life beyond. Birthing classes teach you a lot about breathing techniques to prepare you for labor. (Some say it's to distract you from pain; others say it's to help you tune into and manage your pain.) While there are online classes available, we discourage you from them because two of the biggest points are to share the wonder of the birthing process with your partner and to find other moms-to-be who can serve as a support system both now and after birth. Here are some tips to help you choose a class that's right for you:

• Select a class with a philosophy that matches yours. The Lamaze method, the most popular in the United States, focuses on relaxation but also encourages mom to learn how to respond to pain, both with and without medication. The Bradley method focuses on a natural approach that involves the father as birth coach and discourages the use of medication. For more information on each, check www.lamaze.org and www.bradleybirth .com.

• Ask about what topics will be covered. Most classes will cover the gamut, including anatomy, stages of labor, reducing labor pain, medications, complications, newborn and postpartum care, and breast-feeding.

• Check the certification of the agency and ask for the credentials of the instructor. Some of the biggest certifying organizations include Lamaze International, the Bradley method, and the International Childbirth Education Association.

• Pick classes offered over a period of six weeks rather than the marathon weekend ones.

You'll remember more if you spend less time in class, even if the course is spread out over several weeks. And choose one that has five to ten couples in it. You'll learn from others.

- Keep a pregnancy diary that allows you to track your aches, discomforts, and side effects.
- Check with your insurance company to see if it will reimburse you for classes (many are free). No matter what, the investment is worthwhile.
- Practice techniques you learn in class, but don't worry if you forget, because your nurses, doula, doc, or midwife will help you when the going gets rough in the labor room.

8

Body in Motion

Tackle the Unpleasant, Uncomfortable, and Sometimes Risky Side Effects of Pregnancy

*U*ntil we live in a world where you can perform do-it-yourself human cloning in your basement, there's no debating this fact: You are now experiencing the most amazing biological event that can happen to a human, as you morph from a body of one to a body of two (or more).

As you undergo this radical change, you will experience plenty of blips, burps, and bumps along the way—some that may have long-term and serious health implications, and some that may make you feel as helpless as an umbrella in a tropical storm. As we go from a chapter in which we discussed some of the milder side effects of pregnancy to a chapter in which we'll talk about some of the more serious ones, our goal is simple: to keep you healthy and strong for your own good, as well as to best prepare you to handle the rigors of parenthood.

We hope that you forgive our somewhat laundry-list approach to this chapter, but we've organized this material to help you easily find the information that you need to address whatever issues you may be facing. While all mechanical side effects that you may experience during pregnancy have a variety of causes, there does seem to be a common link among them: a hormone called relaxin. In this chapter, we want to help you understand why these side effects might occur—and what you can do to minimize their damage.

Hormonal Hijinks: When Good Goes Bad

For the last couple of chapters, we've been pounding you with plenty of "relax" commands. Relax and you'll feel better. Relax and let pregnancy run its course. Relax and let the soft sounds of raindrops cascade over your ears and comfort your soul. Sweet, isn't it? Now, however, it's time to amp up the biological bantering and discuss a different kind of relax—namely, relaxin—a vital pregnancy hormone that also can be the source of some decidedly unrelaxing aches and pains.

Before we talk about its side effects, you first need to understand the hormone's purpose. Relaxin does just what you'd think it does: It relaxes. Most important, it relaxes the intrauterine ligaments. Why? Because if you don't increase flexibility down in your fetus's living quarters over the next forty weeks, trying to grow a baby in the uterus would be like trying to squeeze a mountain lion into a file cabinet. Not gonna fit. Your body needs flexibility so the uterus and pelvis can accommodate a baby that will grow from a couple of cells to the size of a midsized watermelon.

As you might imagine, that relaxation effect isn't limited to your uterus. Relaxin also relaxes other parts of your body, like your arteries, which have to handle your increased blood volume without sending your blood pressure through the roof. That's a good thing, right? Opening up the arteries also increases blood flow to the uterus so that more nutrients can get to the baby.

So far, it seems that relaxin is all good. What could be wrong with being more flexible, staying loose, and letting your body expand and dilate all around you? But take that argument one step further. Do you really want everything to go all loosey-goosey? Sometimes your body needs to be tight and inflexible. For instance, what happens when the muscle that prevents stomach acid from creeping back into your esophagus starts to let down its guard? You got it: Acid goes the wrong way up a one-way street, and you feel as though you're dining on Duracells.

In addition, consider the fact that two hormones that influence sex drive—estrogen and progesterone—come with side effects similar to relaxin's. Estrogen, for example, also opens up the esophageal sphincter and thus lets more acid spill back up. Progesterone contributes to loosening up the ligaments and joints throughout

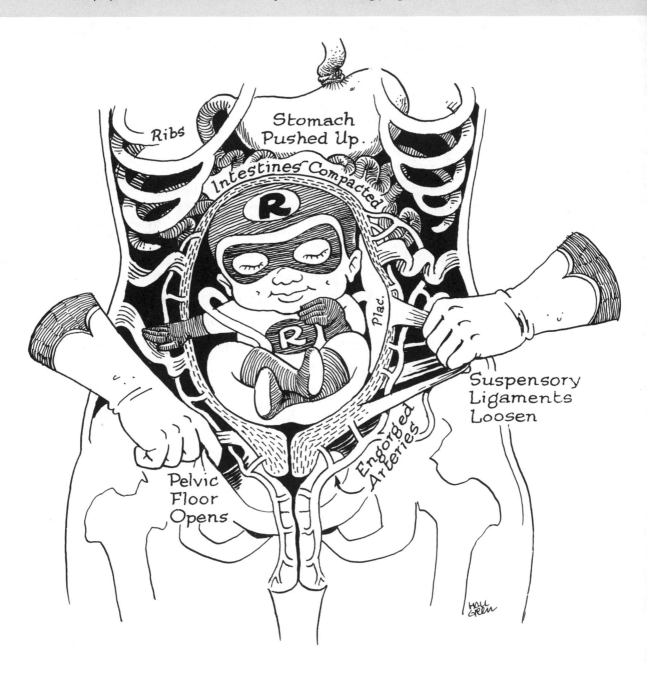

your body. It may be good for growing and delivering a baby, but it's not so good when you trip over a curb and tear the anterior cruciate ligament in your knee. That looseness partly explains why menstruating women are eight times more likely than men to suffer a torn ligament.

Hormonal and chemical changes happen for a reason, and that reason is to best protect you and your baby during gestation and delivery. But sometimes that protection comes at a price. What we're going to do throughout the rest of the chapter is help you cope with these body changes so that, just maybe, you won't have to pay full price.

> **Factoid:** Along with all the other body changes that happen during pregnancy, you can also expect your back to expand—that is, not just your cup size increases as your breasts grow, but your band size as well. Both your back and hips open out to accommodate your growing baby. That means that even if you do shed all of your baby weight, you still might not return to your prepregnancy dimensions.

GI Woes: Digestion Problems

You don't need to be a gastroenterologist to know that there's a lot going on in your tummy. Your uterus is growing, you're feeling weird, and your relationship with food is as on and off as a celebrity romance. That's all to be expected as your body figures out how to deliver nutrients to your child. At the same time, progesterone slows down the entire digestive process, which leads to a host of complaints, like constipation. In this section, we'll move through the entire digestive system—from one opening to the other—to help guide you through some of the more unpleasant symptoms you may be feeling.

Mouth/Teeth

Throughout your pregnancy, you've spent a lot of time focusing on the changes you can see: your belly, your breasts, your feet that feel like flippers. Many changes, though, happen beneath the surface. For instance, as pregnancy increases your circulation (relaxin opens up the arteries), more blood flows throughout all of your mucous membranes. Remember, that's A1 info when it comes to your sex life: Increased blood flow means increased comfort and sensitivity during sex. But such isn't the case when it comes to your airways. The increased circulation causes the lining of your nose and airways to swell. Since we're dealing with a pretty confined space when it comes to your face, that swelling restricts airflow, making you more likely to experience sinus infections, congestion, and snoring. Also, the extra blood vessels are fragile, predisposing you to nosebleeds.

What we're most concerned about here, though, is that the increased circulation also softens your gums, leading to minor bleeding when you brush or floss. That does *not* mean you should slack off on brushing and flossing, under any circumstances. One thing we certainly don't want to see is periodontal disease in pregnancy, because pregnant women with this condition are at heightened risk of gestational diabetes and are seven times more likely to have babies born too early and too small. That's not a typo: *seven* times more common. Gingivitis, an infection of the gums that can lead to periodontal disease, affects half of all pregnant women. (Swelling and excessive bleeding are the symptoms, not the cause.) Gingivitis starts when bacteria go forth and prosper between your teeth and gums. The stuck food attracts and nourishes bacteria and inflames the gums. Estrogen not only makes you more sensitive to bacteria, it magnifies the inflammation, which can irritate the inner lining of your arteries and cause them to narrow. If you're diligent about brushing and flossing and get regular cleanings from a hygienist, you can significantly decrease the risks associated with gum problems. But skip the mouthwash, as most include a chemical, triclosan, that pregnant women should not ingest.

No matter what, do not avoid going to the dentist when you're pregnant. In fact, you ought to go regularly every six months before, during, and after your pregnancy. Ideally, you should address all tooth and gum issues before you conceive, but if something crops up when you're pregnant, do not hesitate to treat it. Even dental X-rays are okay when you're pregnant, as long as you wear a lead shield to protect everything below your jaw. Gum disease is potentially more dangerous to your fetus than the radiation from an X-ray.

Breath of Fresh Air

On the surface, it would seem that asthma in mom would mean problems for baby. After all, when mom can't receive proper oxygen, it hinders baby's ability to do so too. But having asthma doesn't have to be a problem; in fact, while asthma is very common during pregnancy (both for people who have it beforehand and for those who develop it during pregnancy), you can control it with little effect, if any, on the fetus. (If you don't control it, you increase your risk of developing high blood pressure and placental issues.) There are asthma medications that are considered safe to take during pregnancy, and if you have asthma or asthmalike symptoms—lots of wheezing and coughing—you should make sure to communicate that to all of your docs, so they can help determine which medication is best for you.

Some steps you can take to help avoid asthma attacks:

- Quit smoking, and avoid secondhand smoke.
- Avoid having large meals if you're prone to developing reflux (and even if you aren't).
- Take sanitary precautions, especially around people with a cold or the flu.
- Be aware of things you're allergic to, and avoid them. Same goes for other contaminants, irritants, and things that trigger asthma symptoms for you—like a certain type of exercise, perhaps.

Heartburn

As if you haven't had enough food troubles during your pregnancy (eating too much, not eating enough, throwing up what you manage to eat), the pregnancy gods thought it would be amusing to throw in one more obstacle. Acid reflux, when acid from the stomach that helps break down food percolates up into your esophagus, is pretty darn common during pregnancy. As we alluded to earlier, relaxin and other hormones soften up the sphincter at the top of the stomach. So instead of having a steel fire door to keep acid where it belongs, the junction between the stomach and the esophagus works more like a revolving door, letting the stomach acid travel back up. Second, as your baby grows, it pushes upward and changes the angle of the junction between the stomach and esophagus. What was once a 90-degree angle becomes straight, making it even easier for the acid to shoot up.

Gas

Don't be alarmed if you occasionally slip into foghorn mode. Our guts, influenced by the neurotransmitter serotonin, all respond a bit differently to foods we eat and to bacteria that line our intestines. During pregnancy, fluctuating levels of serotonin cause the intestines to move in ways that can expel gas at less-than-predictable times. While there's nothing technically harmful about having gas, we know that it can be uncomfortable—and we also know that it's not the kind of background music you want playing at your baby shower. So you'll find our tips for relieving the gas at the end of the chapter.

Constipation and Hemorrhoids

As we move down to the final stop on the digestive tour, it's worth taking a moment to think about the wonders of the human body. Here's one of our favorites: The structure of the anus is exactly like the structure of your lips. You read that right. If you purse your lips together as if you're blowing out candles on a birthday cake, the folds in your lips look just like the veins in your anus that fill with pressure when you try to move your bowels.* And that can be hard work, due to the fact that progesterone is slowing down the speed at which your intestines move your waste downward—making constipation a common side effect of pregnancy.

Hemorrhoids are also frequent in pregnancy. The veins near the anus bulge because of the relaxing effects of pregnancy hormones on the vessel walls as well as the increase in blood flow to the area. That, combined with the heightened pelvic pressure from the expanding uterus and the straining from more difficult bowel movements, causes the blood vessels to distend and poke through the sphincter that keeps

---

* A hand mirror can confirm this if you don't believe us.

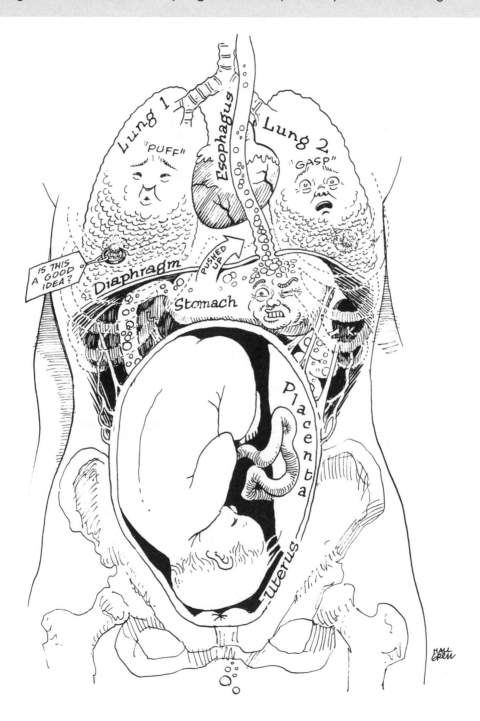

Figure 8.2 **Acid Trip** When relaxin weakens the connection between the stomach and esophagus, acid from below the diaphragm can travel up toward your mouth, causing reflux.

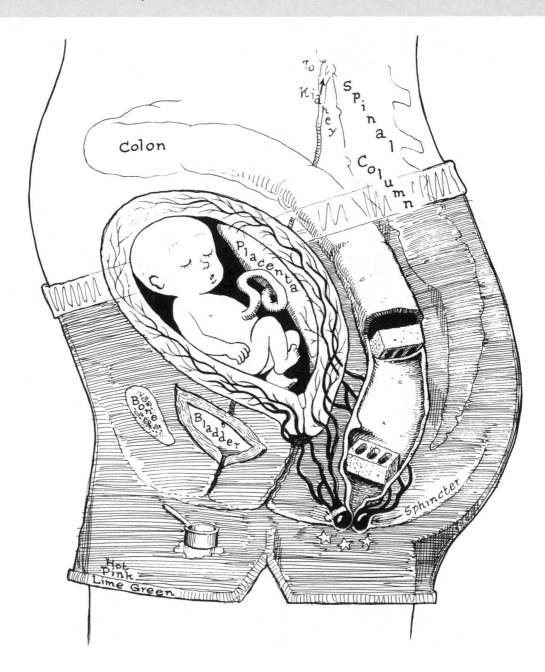

the anus closed. The result: hemorrhoids. When you're trying to move concrete-hard poop toward the exit (it's hard because it moves through the colon so slowly), those swollen hemorrhoid veins are scraped, so they bleed and can cause pain or itching. Hemorrhoids usually go away after delivery, but in the You Tips section, we do offer some remedies that can help soothe the pain.

Infections Down Under: Problems of the Vaginal and Urinary Systems

When we deal with a part of the body that plays *the* vital role in making and delivering a baby, it shouldn't come as much of a surprise that it also gets plenty of attention in the middle. While we've already covered sex-related issues when it comes to the female parts, it's also worth spending some time on vaginal and related issues that may be less pleasant.

Bladder/Urinary Infections

Normally, the pelvic floor is made up of muscles that are as tight as a drum, which keep everything in your pelvis suspended and hold all surrounding tissues in place. But when relaxin comes in to loosen everything up so the baby can fit into that space, the pelvic floor becomes less taut. That means you're more likely to leak urine out (when you cough, sneeze, or sound the foghorn), and it also means there's a greater chance of bacteria flowing back in. In addition, the acute angle between the bladder and the urethra (the tube through which urine exits) relaxes, making it easier for bacteria to enter.

Interestingly, the chemical consistency of urine changes a bit during pregnancy. For one, urine is less dense because there's more fluid in your body, making it less resistant to bacteria; dense urine acts like a roadblock to bacteria by stopping its growth. Secondly, the increased sugar in your blood needed to feed your baby sometimes leaks into your urine. Since bacteria like eating sugar about as much as foot-

Figure 8.4 **Chutes and Bladders** Once again, relaxin is the culprit. As everything gets a little looser to accommodate the baby, so do all the tubes and junctions that influence urinary flow. That relaxation makes it easier for bacteria to swim upstream and cause bladder infections.

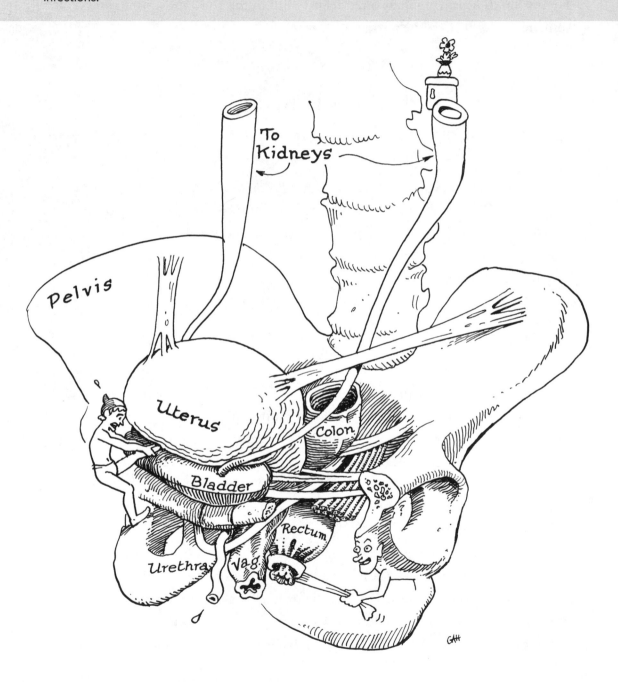

Herbal Answers

Sometimes it may be worth trying unconventional methods for some of your aches and pains. These are some alternative treatments that have been shown to be generally safe and many experts argue are effective. Discuss them with your doctor.

The Issue	A Remedy
Bleeding gums	Calendula or myrrh (add fifteen drops to 2 ounces of water and swish in your mouth)
Constipation	Chlorella (1,500 mg daily); the cracked cell wall version is absorbed better
Gas	Papaya, ginger
Hemorrhoids	Witch hazel cream
Edema	Dandelion leaf (a natural diuretic), quercetin, garlic
Varicose veins	Bilberry
Nosebleeds	Vitamins E or A and D ointment inside the nostril and a humidifier in your room.
Sinusitis	A Neti pot and N-acetylcysteine (500 mg) for two weeks.
Excess saliva	Mints, chewing gum, crackers, or lemons (and don't be afraid to carry around a spit cup).

ball players love buffets, your urine becomes a ripe place for bacteria to grow. About 15 percent of pregnant women experience urinary tract infections (UTIs), which can be safely treated with medication (the antibiotic nitrofurantoin is a common treatment) and by drinking 100 percent cranberry juice (its acidic nature helps).

Yeast Infections

Right this very minute, you have tiny organisms called yeast living on your skin and inside your vagina. Because your vagina is an acidic environment, the fungus typically does not grow mighty, and you generally aren't even aware those little buggers are hanging around down there. But—there's always a but—things can change when that acidic environment changes. In a nonpregnant state, antibiotics can change the vagina's pH balance (between acidity and alkalinity) by decreasing the population of the protective lactobacillus bacteria, making you more susceptible to yeast infections. Three-quarters of women will have one at some point. In pregnancy, the increased amount of sugar in the vaginal secretions, which can also become less acidic, makes it easy for yeast to flourish.

You know you have a yeast infection because the fungus comes along with its four best friends: redness, discharge (usually white and cottage cheesy), itching, and irritation. Though yeast infections are uncomfortable, they're not considered a serious health threat. Antifungal medications can help; topical medication can be messy, so talk to your doc about oral treatments for use after the first trimester.

Bacterial Vaginosis

If your vagina smells like ammonia, it's a good bet that you have a vaginal infection called bacterial vaginosis, which is caused by an overgrowth of flora in the vagina and affects 15 percent to 20 percent of pregnant women. Along with the odor, you'll also likely have a milky discharge and some irritation. Unlike with a yeast infection, which doesn't affect the baby at all, there does seem to be a link between bacterial vaginosis, which commonly occurs in the first trimester, and premature labor, as well as infection of the amniotic fluid, placenta, and newborn. During the first trimester, all you can use is topical treatments. Since they generally aren't very effective and have serious side effects, docs usually wait until the second or third trimester to give oral medication. We also advise women to add probiotics to their diet every day to help keep the vagina, as well as the intestines, healthy. We prefer the spore form of probiotics found in pills or frozen yogurt rather than the live culture in yogurt. That's because the latter generally doesn't survive your stomach acid all that well. Only 600,000 to 1 million of every 2 billion bacteria survive compared to 600 million of every 2 billion of the spore form.

Muscle Mania:
Problems of the Musculoskeletal System

Pregnancy is a forty-week workout. You're carrying an increasingly heavy load over all kinds of terrain in all kinds of environments without a break. While your work will be paid off with the ultimate reward, that doesn't mean your muscles and ligaments aren't being taxed along the way. These are some of the bigger musculoskeletal issues that you may face.

Back Pain

Not that we want to equate your baby with a box being delivered from your favorite store, but in a way, pregnancy must feel a lot like you're working the twenty-four-hour shift at UPS. You're carrying a big load, and your back takes the brunt of the pressure—especially as the weight of the baby and the increased size of your breasts want to pull you forward, putting more pressure on your spine. Now add in the fact that many pregnant women stop exercising, which means they especially stop doing the core abdominal exercises that help make their internal girdle strong and supportive. And don't forget that all of your tendons and soft tissues are more lax because of Relaxin and Co. Finally, as you may have noted, your belly moves from flat to convex during pregnancy, which increases the curve of your back, shifts your center of gravity, and causes your sense of balance to change. After you've done the math, you can see what the answer is: a perfect storm of back trouble. Your back isn't engineered to be as strong and supportive as it should be under the best of circumstances—remember, we were made to crawl—and pregnancy additionally stresses the system.

Because the odds are stacked against your spine, we recommend resistance training exercises that focus on your core to help maintain some of that internal strength in your abdominal and lower back muscles that support your back. The earlier you start, the better. Also, keeping an eye on your posture automatically builds the core muscles, even when you want to curl up on a couch like a kitty.

You should also be aware of a type of back pain that's common in pregnancy called sciatica. This happens when your baby presses on your sciatic nerve, which runs all the way from your spine to your lower legs. Sciatic pain feels more like knives than the dull, throbbing pains that come with muscular strains. There's no real cure for sciatica, but some of our tips can help quiet the pain.

Joint Issues

Relaxin helps soften the connective tissues of the body—relaxing the pelvic joints, ripening the cervix, and preparing your body to deliver. The side effect of these critically important changes is that loose ligaments make it a lot more difficult to exercise, because they make you much more prone to sprains. Remember, while ligaments need some flexibility to assist in joint movement, they also need some stability to help keep your joints in their proper places.

If you're not careful, there's the potential for a vicious cycle here: You find it difficult to exercise because of joint pain or because you injured a joint during exercise, so you stop exercising. You stop exercising, and you lose strength in your supportive core muscles. You lose that support, and your body feels about as strong as a cotton ball. So you hurt, you ache, you slow down, and you definitely don't exercise. That's why it's critical to maintain your fitness during pregnancy—safely and effectively. Our workout on page 310 will help you do so.

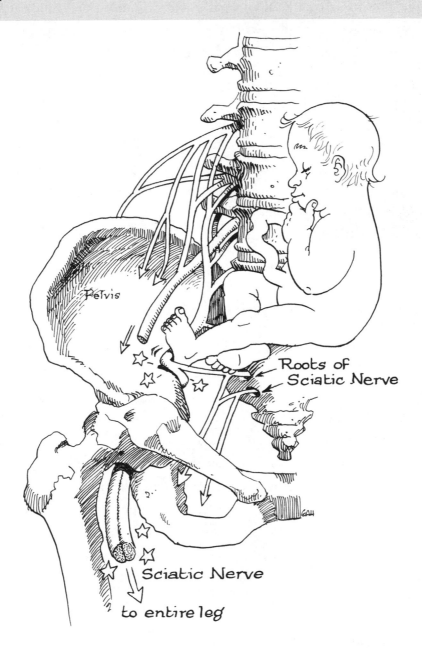

Pelvis

Roots of
Sciatic Nerve

Sciatic Nerve

to entire leg

Carpal Tunnel Syndrome

Bet you didn't expect to be reading about carpal tunnel syndrome here,* but if you think about the major biological changes going on during pregnancy, it shouldn't come as a surprise. You're flooded with hormones that help the uterus grow (including chemicals that resemble growth hormone), but your body doesn't have an off-on switch that allows you to pick and choose which parts of your body respond to them. As your uterus grows, so do a lot of other tissues. In most parts of your body, that's not a huge problem. But think about your wrists and forearms. In such a narrow area, the tissues swell and compress the nerves. That's when you feel the shooting, paralyzing pains. Surgery isn't necessary in most pregnancy-related carpal tunnel cases, and splinting your forearms usually helps control the pain, though it may mean you have to lay off the daily mommy blogging for a while. After pregnancy, the condition goes away within a few weeks in at least two-thirds of women.

Faulty Flow:
Problems of the Circulatory System

Here's a circulatory fact that'll win you big bucks on your next *Jeopardy!* appearance: Uterine veins dilate up to 60—repeat: six-zero—times larger than normal during pregnancy. If you've paid attention at all during your reading, you know exactly how and why this happens. Relaxin helps relax the artery beds, and estrogen causes the cells lining your arteries to secrete nitric oxide to open them up. This dilation ensures that blood runs freely to and from your uterus, to supply nutrients, drain waste, and create the perfect little darling who will soon be trying to eat Tupperware containers. All of that arterial blood comes back to your heart by flowing into dilated veins. Because blood pressure is lower in veins than in arteries and the walls of the veins are already loosened, there is a chance that blood can pool or stagnate in the presence

---

* And not in some future book called *YOU: At the Office.* (Hey, that's not a bad idea!)

of elevated estrogen levels, putting you at risk for clots. Sleeping on your left side can help keep things flowing smoothly.

In addition, fibrinogen, which estrogen increases, works like cement between bricks to clot blood and slow down or shut off blood flow. In the grand scheme, you need this slowdown mechanism to prevent you from hemorrhaging during pregnancy and delivery. But as you can guess, this quick-fix mechanism means you have an increased tendency to clot during pregnancy. Some specific circulatory problems:

DVT

One of the most worrisome potential complications of pregnancy is deep vein thrombosis, when clots form in the large veins of the legs and pelvis. DVT is the leading cause of maternal death in the developed world.

Why does this happen? You have a lot of blood in your veins during pregnancy, and relaxin relaxes those veins. When the pressure of the uterus reduces the flow of blood back up to the heart from the legs, blood pools and becomes stagnant. Because of the increased presence of fibrinogen and other clotting factors, that blood is more likely to clot. You can help reduce the risk of lower-leg clots by wearing compression stockings to force blood back up and elevating your legs above your heart.

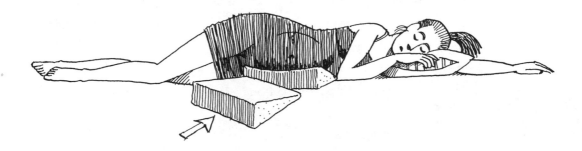

On the Side

More Problems, More Solutions

Foot Issues	Sad to say, you may have to retire your shoe collection after pregnancy. The combination of the relaxing of your soft tissues and the extra weight you're carrying can cause your feet to grow one-half to one full shoe size. During pregnancy, you're also more prone to developing plantar fasciitis, an inflammation of the tissues at the bottom of your feet that is particularly painful when you step out of bed in the morning or stand up after being seated for a long time. Wear low-heeled, cushioned shoes (shoe or heel inserts can help relieve some of the pressure) instead of walking with bare feet, to keep from aggravating the inflammation even further, and try massage and gentle stretches. Here's how to do the stretch: While sitting in a chair, place your foot over your knee. Pull your toes toward you while keeping your heel firm. Do this first thing in the morning and three or four times during the day.
Vision Problems	There's some evidence to suggest that estrogen may cause physiological and vascular changes in your eyes, leading to dry eyes and vision changes. Your tears normally come from the upper outside of your eye, where they are secreted, and travel across your eyeball to drain into your nose. That course of tears across your eye keeps your entire eye lubricated. When estrogen spikes during pregnancy and swelling changes occur, your eyeball bulges outward, changing the course of your tears. They now flow down the less resistant path from the upper outside of your eye straight down to the lower outer edge—that means you need a Kleenex and your eyes become dry. Often, these changes resolve after pregnancy—especially the vision changes—so don't run out and buy expensive new glasses. If you wear contacts, you may want to switch to your prescription glasses. There's some fear that changes in the eye during pregnancy can mean that contacts you previously wore may not fit properly, drying the eye out and potentially leading to some corneal damage.

Headaches	With links between hormone levels and migraines, it's no surprise that you may experience terrible headaches during pregnancy. (Or the opposite: Many women enjoy a remission from migraines, especially during the second and third trimesters.) If you have migraines, be aggressive about looking for triggers such as caffeine and chocolate, so you can eliminate them. If headaches persist, seek help from an expert in headaches to reduce the severity and frequency of these very stressful events. Medication may be warranted; there are several options that are safe in pregnancy.

When traveling long distances by car or air, it's a good idea to stop or get up every hour or so and stretch or stroll to keep the blood circulating in your legs. If you're at risk for DVT (you have a prior history of DVT or clotting, have had two or more miscarriages or stillbirths, or there's a family history), you can be tested for thrombophilia, a genetic condition that predisposes you to clotting. If you test positive, your doc can prescribe heparin injections to decrease the risk of clotting.

Edema

Weight gain during pregnancy doesn't just do a number on your wardrobe, it also changes the way fluids move throughout your body. The additional weight (and gravity) actually slows down the circulation of both blood and other fluids. The result: You retain fluids in your legs, your hands, even your face, and feel as if you're blowing up like the *Willy Wonka* blueberry girl. The fix: Elevate your legs when you're sitting or lying down, and watch your salt intake. Also, sitting in a tub or swimming may help you deflate. Though there's little data behind it, anecdotal evidence suggests that drinking water—as counterintuitive as it may seem—might help reduce swelling.

Top 10 Things You Need to Know About Preterm Contractions and Cramping

10. You can experience contractions even in the first trimester as your body adjusts to the pregnancy. Some causes: The stretching of the ligaments around the uterus can cause cramps, as can constipation and gas pains. If it's accompanied by spotting, bleeding, and abdominal pain, you need to see a doc to rule out an ectopic pregnancy.

9. In the second and third trimesters, if cramping comes along with diarrhea and back pain, it could be a sign of preterm labor.

8. Preterm contractions are different from Braxton Hicks contractions—random contractions that happen in the second and third trimesters.

7. Dehydration can cause contractions. Drink plenty of fluids.

6. Some women cramp after amniocentesis. Some docs prescribe a glass of wine afterward to soothe the cramps. We don't recommend that. We recommend number 5.

5. Good contraction and cramping soothers: a warm bath, an empty bladder, and rhythmic breathing.

4. Another contraction causer, just FYI: sex and orgasms. Nothing to worry about.

3. You can perform a self-test to see if your contractions are really contractions: Lie down and place a hand on your uterus. If your entire uterus is hard during the cramping, it's probably a contraction. If it's hard in one place and soft in others, it may just be the baby moving around.

2. You may be in preterm labor if contractions come every ten minutes rather than intermittently.

1. There's never any harm in calling the doc to report cramping or contractions, so she can walk you through any accompanying symptoms to try to determine what's happening.

Hypertension/Preeclampsia

As many as 10 percent of pregnant women suffer from a condition called preeclampsia, characterized by high blood pressure and the presence of protein in their urine. Preeclampsia usually starts in the second trimester. You may experience symptoms such as swelling, sudden weight gain, headaches, changes in vision, and upper abdominal pain.

Or you may have no symptoms at all; your provider may pick it up during a routine prenatal visit. Women under age twenty and over age forty are at increased risk, as are women who have a vitamin D deficiency, high blood pressure, diabetes, migraines, obesity, or a family history of preeclampsia, or who have had a urinary tract infection or periodontal disease during pregnancy.

The cause? It's not known, but a tantalizing clue lies in the observation that the longer you've been in a sexual relationship with your partner and the more children you've had together, the less likely you are to develop preeclampsia. This has led to the theory that preeclampsia is mom's immune reaction to foreign proteins from dad in the placenta, which causes inflammation of the linings of mom's blood vessels. The result: elevated blood pressure, damage to the kidneys and liver, as well as placental abruption or intrauterine growth restriction. Preeclampsia may also put you at risk of heart disease later in life.

While the only real cure for preeclampsia is delivery, if you're diagnosed with the condition and the baby's lungs are not yet mature, you may be placed on bed rest. This helps get blood to your uterus and gives your child more time to get the nutrients needed for organ development before birth. Corticosteroids may be used to accelerate the fetus's lung maturity while anticipating a possible early delivery, and you'll most likely be given medications to help normalize your blood pressure.

> **Factoid:** Feeling short of breath during pregnancy doesn't mean that you're literally unfit for motherhood. It's normal. Your lungs are processing about 40 percent more air than they do when you're not pregnant and, as the baby grows and takes up more space in your body, decreasing in size. So you may find yourself huffing and puffing even when you do nothing more than walk from one room to another. If the breathlessness persists at rest, you should call your doctor and be evaluated.

YOU TIPS

The "no pain, no gain" mantra may help to sell gym memberships, but it doesn't help during pregnancy. Just because you're going through a natural biological process that comes with a fair share of nuisances doesn't mean that you have to accept them as they come. No doubt, your body is enduring a tough climate and weathering many different types of storms. You can fight your way through some of them, but you might as well try to avoid others altogether. These tips will give you the tools you need to take your discomfort level down a few notches.

Ease the Heart Ache. To keep acid from migrating back up your esophagus, prop your head up while you're sleeping. That may mean using extra pillows, sleeping in a recliner, or elevating the head of your bed by slipping bricks under the two legs at the headboard. You also want to avoid wearing tight clothing, which can squeeze acid up, and eating within two hours of going to bed.

Get to the Bottom of Things. You can soften that cementlike feeling of constipation by drinking a little more fluid such as prune juice or water, eating a little more fiber, and even using glycerine suppositories. Assuming that your kidneys are working fine, try 200 milligrams of magnesium twice a day, in either pill or capsule form.

To help ease the pain of hemorrhoids, try soaking in a warm sitz bath with Epsom salts or magnesium. A sitz bath is one in which you sit in a tub and soak just your bottom and hips. The aquatic environment will soothe some of the burning associated with the hemorrhoids. You can also try topical arnica gel or cortisone cream, but tell your doc if you do. If the hemorrhoids still bother you after delivery (most resolve themselves by then), you can have them clipped in an office procedure that usually doesn't even require anesthesia.

Quiet the Storm. The last thing you need during pregnancy is to feel like you're the conductor of a twelve-piece trombone section, so follow these guidelines for silencing your Sousa.

- Make sure not to gulp your food, so that you don't swallow air, which leads to increased gas production. Chewing gum or sucking on candies can cause the same effect as swallowing, especially sugar-free candies and gums that contain sorbitol. Excessive consumption of these may have a laxative effective, increasing the chance that your invisible issues can quickly turn into visible ones.
- Antigas medications like simethicone are safe and worth trying. They work by pulling all the gas bubbles together. Put a couple drops of Beano into your food (especially beans; thus the name) to help reduce gas.
- Steer clear of foods that cause gas before "public events" where you want to avoid drawing the wrong kind of attention to yourself. These include beans, cabbage, cauliflower, broccoli, asparagus, onions, and Brussels sprouts, as well as milk and milk products, high-fiber grains such as bran, and fruits such as apples, pears, and peaches. These are great and beneficial foods, but not in the four to eight hours prior to an important meeting or outing. Same goes for sodas and fruit drinks.

Take Two for Your Teeth. On your to-do list, you may rank taking care of your teeth at about the same priority level as clipping hedges. But that would be a mistake. Make sure you have an oral fixation for at least a few minutes a day to help prevent infections that could spread to your child.

- Visit your dentist at least once during pregnancy (and make sure to get regular prenatal care) to reduce the risk of infections. Even better, visit your dentist twice in the year before you are likely to get pregnant. Remember, since 50 percent of pregnancies are unexpected, this may simply mean visiting your dentist regularly. We hope you do.
- Brush at least twice a day for two minutes and floss once a day.
- Avoid sugary foods; they feed the bacteria and cause a big old plaque buildup. Instead eat foods that help maintain healthy gums and teeth, including those with lots of calcium, vitamin B12, and vitamin C.

- Rinse your mouth out with water to help counteract any unpleasant taste you may be experiencing from nausea or morning sickness.

Tighten Up. To help counteract all the sagging that's going on in your pelvic floor, you want to practice Kegel exercises. First, find the muscles that you would use to stop urine flow. Now squeeze and hold for five seconds, then release for five seconds. Do ten repetitions three times a day. The beauty of Kegels is that nobody needs to know you're doing them. The exercises will not only help strengthen muscles to help combat pregnancy-related urinary leakage but also help tighten the entire structure for lifelong pelvic health.

Stay Fresh. Yeast infections can be as annoying as they are itchy, so that's why you should take precautions to keep them from developing (though they are quite common). These tips will help.

- Avoid tight-fitting or synthetic-fiber clothes; wear cotton panties instead. You should also avoid panty hose. The tightness increases the likelihood that the area will become a breeding ground for the bacteria.
- Use a blow-dryer on a low, cool setting to dry your genital area after a shower or after sweating (and change out of wet clothes immediately). Bacteria like things wet. Spurn them by giving them a Sahara-like setting.
- Wipe from front to back to prevent bacteria from your rectum from making the journey from the back of the bus to the front.

Get Your Back Back. Of all the pains in your life (in-laws don't count), back pain can be the most confusing. It's hard to pinpoint the cause and even harder to figure out how to fix it. You can take many different paths in the course of preventing and treating back pain. Some ideas:

- If you're slumped over a computer or curled up on a recliner, it may feel okay at the time. But poor posture is simply an invitation for life-stopping back pain. No matter where you are, think about lifting your head up and back, as if a string were pulling the top of your head toward the ceiling. As you lift up, you relieve some of the tension in your spine.

- Stay active and exercise. Women who exercise regularly have the body strength and tone to help support their backs—and thus manage back pain—during pregnancy. In addition, we want you to focus on core exercises that help develop your internal muscular system. (See our exercises on page 310.)

(See our exercises on page 310.)

> **Factoid:** Even though it may be uncomfortable, wear a seat belt. The pressure of a seat belt on impact is ten times less than the pressure of a steering wheel. Whether you're the driver or the passenger, put the lap portion across your hip bone below your belly, and put the shoulder strap between your breasts and across the side of your belly.

- If you're craving some more passive comfort, you can try massage. It can help loosen up tight muscles that have become strained from the stress of carrying around all that extra weight.
- Sleep on your side with a pillow in between your legs.
- Use good form even when you aren't pregnant. That means squatting down to pick things up (rather than bending at the waist), sitting in chairs with good back support, and putting one foot on a stool if you're standing for long periods (to reduce some of the pressure on your lower back).
- Belly braces that fit like a girdle help your posture by elevating the uterus. They're available at maternity clothing stores or online.
- Massage in an over-the-counter ointment called Tiger Balm, which may relieve some muscular pain.

Fiber Up. Fiber, along with plenty of water, can lessen your constipation and may even decrease your risk of preeclampsia. Some research suggests that eating 25 grams of fiber a day, including 100 percent whole grains, can reduce the risk of preeclampsia by up to 70 percent. More studies are needed to substantiate these findings.

Part 4

YOU

Bringing Baby into the World

9

Special Delivery

Find Your Way Through the Adventure
That Is Labor and Birth

That sure came quick, didn't it? Just a few pages ago, we were talking about such things as how to stop your head from pounding with stress, as well as the most comfortable positions for having sex. Now you're ready for the big transition: when your baby travels from the warm, comfy quarters of what might as well be goose down amniotic fluid to life on the outside.

Now's also when reality hits you with sledgehammer like force.

How . . .

Is . . .

This . . .

Baby . . .

Going . . .

To . . .

Get . . .

OUT . . .

Of . . .

Me?

Time to get in touch with your inner Elastigirl; the incredible adventure of labor and delivery is about to begin.

Naturally, your mind swirls with questions. You wonder about such things as how long you'll be in labor, whether you'll be able to manage the pain, and if your hubby has properly charged the camera battery. (See page 233 for good photo-taking tips.) As you prepare to leap into the unknown, we want to give you a few pep-talk pointers to help guide you through the process:

- If you take only two pieces of advice along with you as you go into labor, let them be these: One, stay flexible and remember that labor can be unpredictable. And two, keep in mind that the ultimate goal is a healthy mom and a healthy baby; there's no extra credit for doing it according to a preconceived plan if there turns out to be a better way.
- There are a handful of things you can control during labor and delivery—such as who accompanies you, how you are monitored, whether or not you move around, and your choice of pain management. The rest you need to leave up to your doctor or midwife. It's not about telling your doctor what to do but about finding a doc before 2:41 a.m. who has similar beliefs, goals, and strategies as you. Remember, you originally chose this person because he or she shares your priorities, beliefs, and goals regarding childbirth; now you have to trust that he or she will get the job done right.

When it comes to labor and delivery, you want to be an active participant in the health care team that will make your labor go as smoothly and safely as possible, whether you decide to do a traditional hospital delivery or choose an alternative method, like a home birth. If you stay reasonably calm and pay attention to the fundamentals, chances are heavily in your favor that everything will work out just fine.

Because there are so many ifs, ands, and buts in the delivery process, we figured it would be best to approach this chapter a little bit differently from the rest. We're going to help you envision the various pathways you might take to reach your ultimate goal: holding your newborn baby. So think of it as the first of many, many, many* board games you're going to be playing over the next decade.

★ Many, many, many, many, many, many, many . . .

Just follow the rules of such classics as Candy Land or Chutes & Ladders: moving forward and backward as various situations dictate (though sometimes your laboring body may feel as if it's playing Twister). Follow the arrows, answer the questions, and move toward your final destination: The Promised Land of Parenthood.

This game of life isn't a trivial pursuit, and it's surely one that can boggle your mind—especially if you don't have a clue about how the whole operation works. But believe us, you don't have the monopoly on anxiety; every mom feels like she's manning her own biological battleship and worries about the risk and trouble that might lie ahead.

So let's get started. Ready? Yeah, baby.

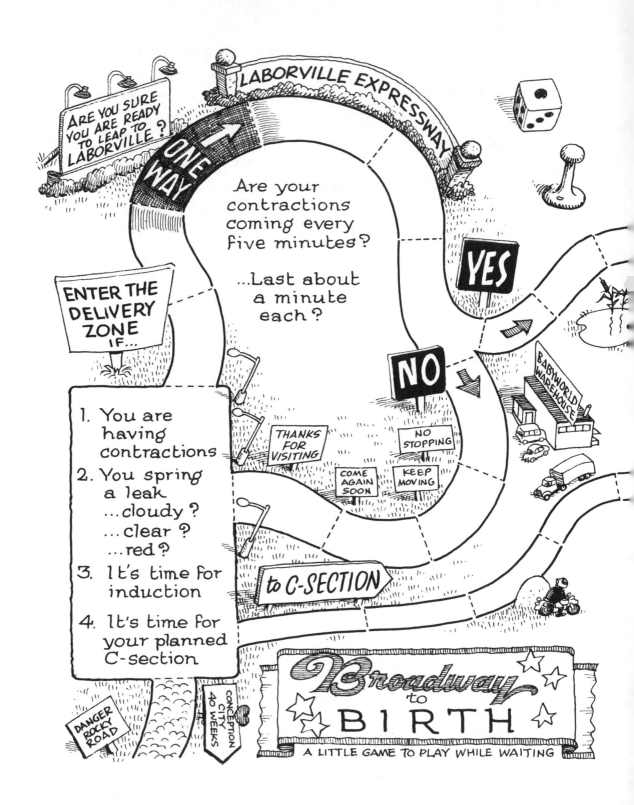

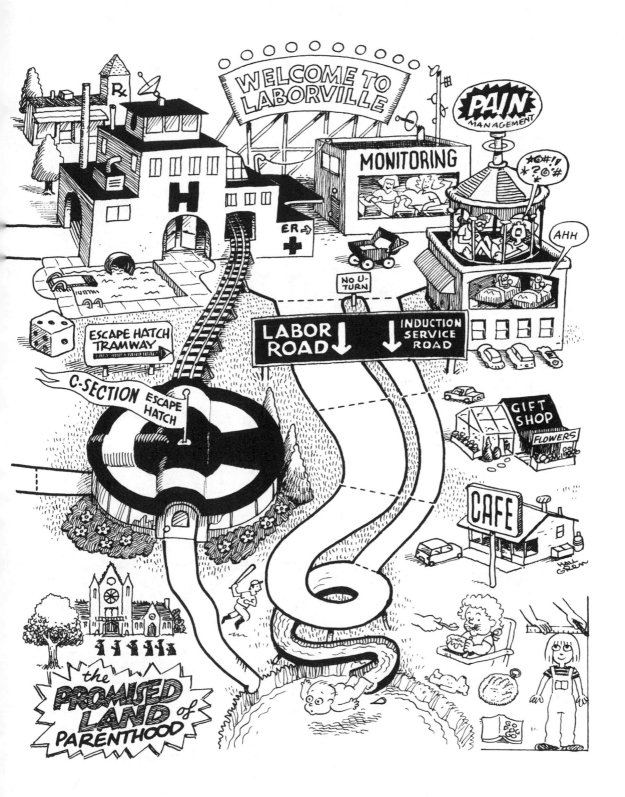

Broadway to Birth

Welcome to the end of pregnancy. You may be a few hours or a few days away, but in either case, you're about to drop the "to-be" from your mom-to-be title. Your overnight bag is packed, and boy,★ are you ready. But is your baby? Ask yourself the following questions to see which path you need to take.

START HERE

Are you past forty weeks? — YES → **Move to the ISLAND of INDUCTION page 240**

NO

Do you have a planned C-Section? — YES → **Move to the ESCAPE HATCH page 241**

NO

Did you spring a leak? — YES → **Is it clear fluid, and did you previously test negative for group B strep?**

YES

NO

NO

You should call your provider, but it doesn't necessarily mean you're in active labor. All it means is that your water broke—that is, you're leaking amniotic fluid. (Important: no sex or baths after water breaks.) If nothing happens within twenty-four hours, your provider may want to induce labor. If so, *move to the ISLAND OF INDUCTION* (page 240). Typically, a doc will instruct you to stay at home. *Move ahead one space.*

If it's yellow, green, or bloody fluid, your provider will likely tell you to go to the hospital. That's because there may be meconium (fetal stool; yes, they make it while inside the womb) in your amniotic fluid, signaling that the child may be in distress. In this case, you would *advance to LABORVILLE* (page 228). But at some point prior to going into labor, you may also pass blood-tinged, thick mucus. Think of it as a cork in a bottle of wine. Docs call this the bloody show; it looks a lot like phlegm. This doesn't necessarily mean that you're in active labor; in fact, it can occur up to a week before labor begins. A bloody show is generally a positive sign that your cervix is dilating and does not require you to call your doctor. If you tested positive for group B strep, there is a higher chance that this bacterium can find its way into and infect the uterus now that the water is broken, since the sterile sac has been compromised. *Move ahead one space.*

★ Or girl.

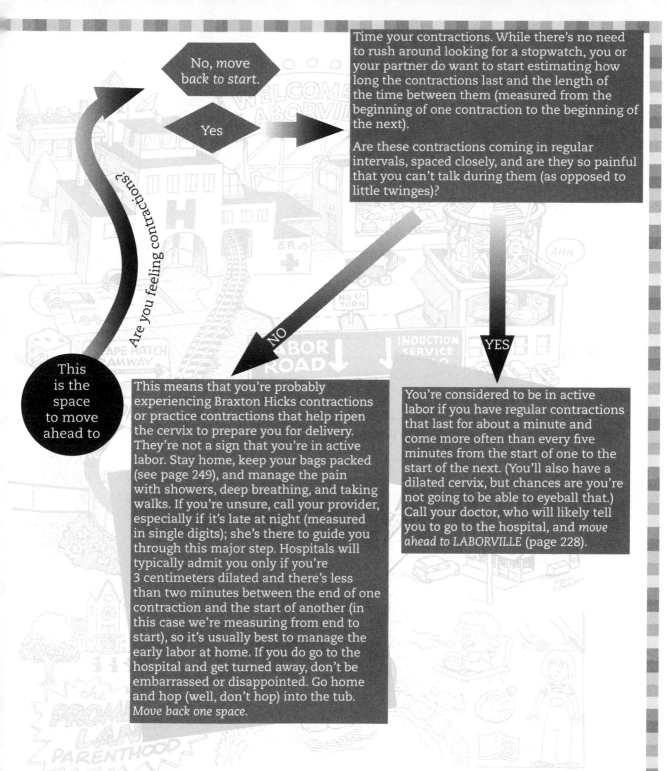

No, *move back to start*.

Yes

Time your contractions. While there's no need to rush around looking for a stopwatch, you or your partner do want to start estimating how long the contractions last and the length of the time between them (measured from the beginning of one contraction to the beginning of the next).

Are these contractions coming in regular intervals, spaced closely, and are they so painful that you can't talk during them (as opposed to little twinges)?

Are you feeling contractions?

This is the space to move ahead to

NO

YES

This means that you're probably experiencing Braxton Hicks contractions or practice contractions that help ripen the cervix to prepare you for delivery. They're not a sign that you're in active labor. Stay home, keep your bags packed (see page 249), and manage the pain with showers, deep breathing, and taking walks. If you're unsure, call your provider, especially if it's late at night (measured in single digits); she's there to guide you through this major step. Hospitals will typically admit you only if you're 3 centimeters dilated and there's less than two minutes between the end of one contraction and the start of another (in this case we're measuring from end to start), so it's usually best to manage the early labor at home. If you do go to the hospital and get turned away, don't be embarrassed or disappointed. Go home and hop (well, don't hop) into the tub. *Move back one space.*

You're considered to be in active labor if you have regular contractions that last for about a minute and come more often than every five minutes from the start of one to the start of the next. (You'll also have a dilated cervix, but chances are you're not going to be able to eyeball that.) Call your doctor, who will likely tell you to go to the hospital, and *move ahead to LABORVILLE* (page 228).

Laborville

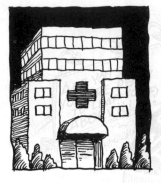

At this point, you can see the finish line, but the marathon of pregnancy isn't quite over yet. If you go to the hospital, the triage team will give you a quick assessment to determine whether you're ready to be admitted. (We realize that not all of you will be having hospital deliveries, although 99 percent of deliveries are in a hospital or birthing center and 90 percent are assisted by doctors. If you're not in the majority, *please pull the HOME DELIVERY option card*.)

They'll check your blood pressure and temperature, take blood and urine tests, and strap monitors to your belly so the medical staff can monitor both your baby's heart rate and the frequency of your contractions. Then either the nurse or the on-call physician or midwife will check your cervix and determine whether or not to admit you. If you're not admitted because you haven't dilated yet, they may send you home; if this occurs, do not pass go, do not collect your tax deduction, and *please return to BROADWAY TO BIRTH*.

If you're very uncomfortable with the contractions and your cervix is not dilated, or you live far from the hospital, they may invite you to walk the floor, and they'll assess you every two hours to determine whether you're in active labor.

After you've been admitted, an IV may be inserted. If you're planning natural childbirth, you can negotiate to have only the Hep-Lock inserted and not be attached to the IV tubing or bag, which frees you up to walk around and change positions more easily. The Hep-Lock is a plastic tube put into your vein and capped off until ready for use; a tiny bit of heparin used to be put into the tube to keep it open, hence the term Hep-Lock. (You should have it there in case of emergency.) You'll also be hooked up to two monitors: one to measure the timing and strength of your uterine contractions, the other to measure your fetus's heart rate. If there are any concerns about the heart rate, your provider will assess you and your baby closely and may decide you need to *move ahead to the ESCAPE HATCH,* page 241). If you're planning to walk around, ask about intermittent monitoring, so that you don't have to be strapped to a machine the whole time. (From the hospital's point of view, the path of least resistance is to have you in bed, so if you don't want to have your movement restricted, you often have to advocate for yourself or have your doula or a family member do it for you.) Sometimes you will be asked to stay in bed no matter what you had planned, and your baby may thank you.

Besides assessing fetal heart rate and contraction frequency, your provider will also perform an external exam to estimate fetal size and position; these give her clues as to what to expect as your labor progresses. By this time, contractions are coming as frequently as Seattle rain, and your pain levels may be rising so fast that you're about to throw concrete blocks at the next person who asks if he or she can help. While it's of little comfort now, try to remember this: Pain usually signals that your body is continuing to make oxytocin, the hormone necessary for labor to progress normally. *Move to THE HOUSE OF PAIN* (page 230).

Home Delivery
OPTION CARD

More and more women are deciding that the most comfortable place to have a baby isn't the place that houses hundreds of other patients and tasty cafeteria mystery meat. It's in their very own homes. In this case, your primary caregiver will be a midwife. Her job is to monitor your labor, help with pain management, advise you on birthing positions, and assist with the final delivery and postpartum care. If a complication occurs, a midwife will also decide if and when it is necessary to transfer you to the hospital. Home birth is a viable choice for low-risk moms, and the rate of complications appears to be about the same when comparing home and hospital births among low-risk cases. Home births are still very uncommon (about 1 percent in the United States), but they're a reasonable option for many.

Any woman considering a home birth must be:

- Healthy (free of hypertension, preeclampsia, gestational diabetes, premature labor, congenital heart problems, infection, and so on) and less than thirty-five years of age.
- Eating a sound prenatal diet.
- A nonsmoker (both you and your partner).
- Able to take an active role in giving birth.
- Willing to cope with the pain and hard work of labor.
- Laboring within thirty minutes of a hospital (including at time of peak traffic; your baby may want to come during rush hour).
- Living where midwives are permitted to practice outside a hospital.
- Able to cover expenses if your insurance is limited to hospital births.
- Also important to note: Many states require an ob/gyn backup for home births. That's because even low-risk moms can have last-minute complications that can be disastrous for the baby. In cases where the baby needs to be intubated or resuscitated, thirty minutes is twenty-nine minutes too far away from doctor, anesthesia, and nursing support.

The House of Pain

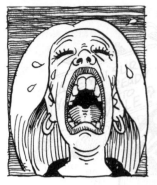

Some women know in advance that they will want pain medication during labor; others plan for a natural childbirth. But even if you intend to have natural childbirth, the fact of the matter is that you don't know how much pain the delivery will cause or how your body will respond to pain until you experience it, so it's good to learn what medical and nonmedical options for relief are available.

Before we get into specific remedies, it may comfort you to recall that delivering a baby is exactly what your body is designed to do—and it will do so instinctively. If you're wondering why our offspring don't slip out of us effortlessly and painlessly like puppies, it's because we have bigger brains and can walk on two legs. Good evolutionary trade-offs, for sure.

It's smart to think about your pain management options ahead of time and to know what your hospital offers and what kind of discussion you can have with your anesthesiologist. Here's a brief summary:

Breathing techniques have long been endorsed to help pain management. While there's no data to suggest that they are more effective than distraction, they may work for some. (Incidentally, we do endorse breathing, no matter what technique you choose.) See more details on childbirth classes in chapter 8.

Perhaps the most common way to relieve pain is the simplest: **Change your position.** Sitting on a birthing ball, for instance, gets you upright and seems to relieve some of the pressure. Also try walking, rocking on all fours, squatting, leaning over the bed, and hanging on to your partner.

Alternative therapies like acupuncture and aromatherapy (massaging scented oils on your body) are commonly used and may be reasonable options. Another that seems to be effective is: hypnotherapy, but you have to have proper training, so it takes some preparation.

Water therapy is the nouveau pain relief technique. Soaking in a tub of warm water seems to help relax the uterus and alleviate pain. Newer hospitals often have tubs. If yours doesn't, you can rent one. But check with your hospital first before rolling up with a U-Haul. See more info on page 233.

Some have also found that **injections of sterile water** relieve pain. The injections are given in four spots above the crease of the buttocks, and while the injection is kind of painful, it may work to relieve overall pain by redirecting some of your pain from the nerves that are associated with labor.

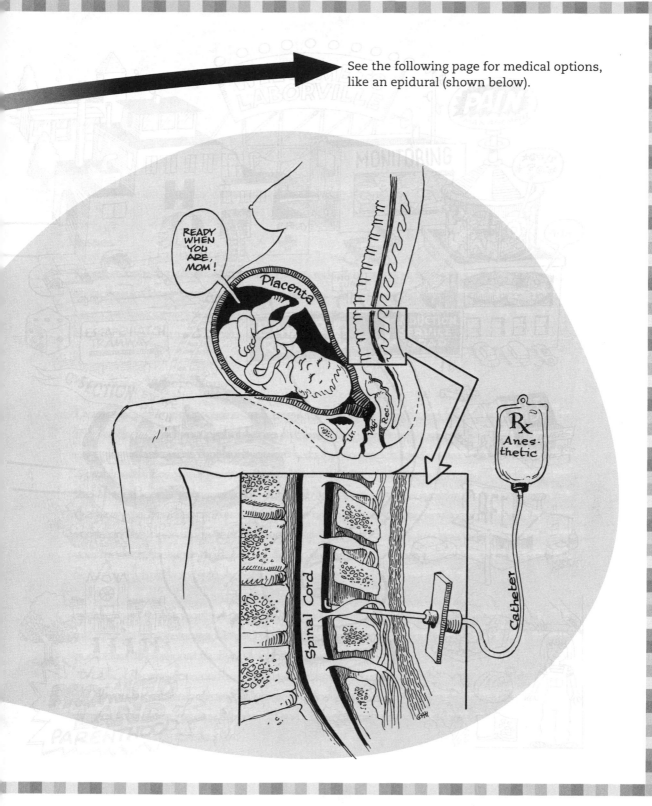

See the following page for medical options, like an epidural (shown below).

Here are your medical options.

A walking epidural (which can be patient controlled, by the way) gives a low dose of anesthesia that allows you to move around (and sometimes even walk) without all the pain. The upside is that your motor nerves are not blocked if it works as it should, and the nerves that help you balance are usually spared from numbness too; we wouldn't want you falling down. The downside is that not all pain nerves may be blocked.

A patient-controlled epidural is almost standard practice these days. A press of the button allows you to deliver the dose of medication you need to help control the pain. It gives you some degree of control in a situation where you might not have much, which works not only medically but psychologically as well, to improve your delivery experience. An epidural delivers a very small amount of medication into the spinal space shown on page 231. Note that epidurals aren't always 100 percent effective and can have side effects such as itchiness, backaches, headaches, and hypotension.

A spinal epidural (really a spinal block and an epidural delivered to you within one needle) can be given to women who are very far along in the labor process (up to 9 centimeters or even fully dilated, depending on the hospital). Within two breaths, you can get relief.

Narcotics (opiates) can also be given to relieve pain. There is some link between opiates and respiratory distress in newborns, but a delivery team in the hospital can take care of any issues. (It's why narcotics aren't recommended for home births.) They're not a great choice, because they can make you—and even the baby—woozy, but their upside is that they generally help take the edge off the pain. They're typically used if it's too late for an epidural; also, narcotics can be given with any doctor's prescription, while an epidural needs the skills of an anesthesiologist.

Nitrous oxide (N_2O, aka laughing gas) is almost nonexistent in the United States when it comes to delivery but is almost universally available in Canada and in England—underscoring the fact that cultural differences can influence medical decisions. N_2O is virtually risk free and is thought to be a great adjunct to other pain remedies by helping you get through some of the really difficult contractions. You can ask for it but may not get it, as many hospitals have a bias against nitrous oxide. That fear was originally based largely on the hypothesis that it could cause oversedation and create DNA replication difficulties in your newborn; those fears are now considered unfounded. Other fears that N_2O contaminates the environment of others have been overcome with clever gas-scavenging devices.

Move ahead to EXIT STRATEGY.

Factoid: More and more women are deciding to have underwater deliveries. The tub needs to be big enough to hold two or three people in two or three feet of water. When the baby comes out, the midwife or doc cuts the cord while the baby is still underwater—and then the baby gasps for his first breath when he's removed from the tub. Though it's not all that common, the moms who go the aqua route say they love it. Soaking in warm water seems to help relax the uterus and alleviate pain. Humans, indeed, may have come from the water to the land and then returned to the water, only to come back—perhaps why we can be born underwater. (Other mammals can't do this, apart from whales and manatees.) Just plan for it ahead of time. More and more hospitals and birthing centers have tubs, but if yours doesn't or you're planning to deliver at home, you can rent one. (See the website of a company called Tubs to Go, at www.aquadoula .com.)

Factoid: Worried that the fire-breathing dragon tattoo on your lower back will interfere with an epidural? Don't be. Though there's a lot of concern these days about inked-up moms getting a needle of another kind, there's no research to suggest that there's any risk involved.

Father Figures

During labor, dads can feel as useless as toothless cobras. While partners can't erase the pain of delivery, they can do a whole lot of good in other ways. Some options to turn a helpless feeling into a helpful one:

- Massage your partner.
- Communicate with loved ones in the waiting room and in other parts of the world; have the laptop and camera charged and ready to go.
- Be in charge of the suitcase to bring to the hospital (see page 249), making sure that everything's in there.
- Promise to do whatever she you wants you to do, whether it's being silent, singing and dancing, or offering up your jaw for her to punch straight on.
- Take great pictures in the delivery room. Some good shots: the big clock in the delivery room at the time of birth, the scale when the baby is being weighed, the room number where the baby was born, the doctor/nurses/midwife, and even the placenta. (Some will say it's gross, but it was your baby's lifeline.) And, oh yeah, maybe one or two of the baby.

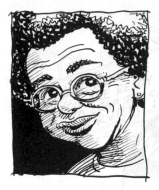

Exit Strategy

Your doc or midwife will consider two things to make sure that you're ready for the final push(es): dilation and effacement. You have to be dilated 10 centimeters for there to be enough of an opening for the baby to get through. And your cervix also has to change its shape; normally, it feels like a nose, but during labor it stretches and thins out, like an inflated balloon. When the cervix has fully thinned out, you are 100 percent effaced and good to go.

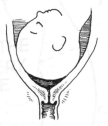

Ripening

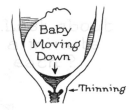

Baby Moving Down

←Thinning

Effacement

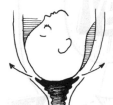

Dilation

Pushing can take anywhere from a few minutes to a few hours. At this point, you may want to experiment with different body positions. Lying flat on your back is actually not the best position for delivery because it collapses the diameter of your pelvis a half inch to an inch, making it feel as if you're pushing uphill. Here are some options that are used frequently in both home and hospital deliveries. They work to ease the baby's way out by freeing your hips and keeping them higher than your knees, as well as by increasing the diameter of your pelvis. This allows pressure from the baby's head to be applied evenly to your cervix, which helps it open. Incidentally, you can use a balance ball with any of these positions.

- Kneeling or sitting: Lets gravity help you.
- Hands and knees: Allows you to move and rock your hips to help ease pain during contractions.
- Squatting: Works best if you've practiced daily squatting before delivery. Some Navajo women grab a strong rope that's hung from the ceiling to decrease the pressure on their legs when they squat; don't do this with a home delivery unless you have a specially constructed ceiling and have practiced squatting and hanging before. (See page 326.) Your knees aren't higher than your hips in this case.

If Your Child Is Breech

If your child is in breech position during labor, your doc will consider a couple of different factors to determine whether the baby can be delivered vaginally or will require a C-section. These factors include whether you've had a full-term live vaginal birth previously, the size of the pelvis versus the size of the baby, and the baby's position. (There are variations of breech, like one foot up and one foot down, or the umbilical cord in front of the baby.) If the doc determines that everything is in optimal position and there's enough room, she may decide that it's okay to try a vaginal delivery. However, the breech position does increase the chance of both episiotomy and the use of forceps. If not, or if the baby is in distress, she will likely recommend a C-section.

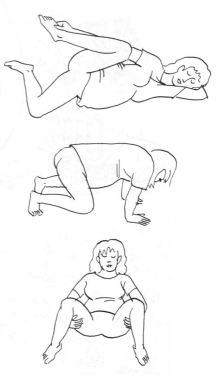

- Standing: Lets you open your legs wide while you hold on to something to help you balance at the peak of contractions.
- Left lateral position with one leg up that relieves compression of the major vein known as the vena cava.

Now, as with every process, unforeseen events can sometimes arise at various points during delivery. If so, *move to DESTINATION DETOUR* (page 238). If you and your doctor have determined at any point before or during delivery that you're going to need a C-section, *move ahead to ESCAPE HATCH* (page 241). This is almost always the case for multiples or breeches who are not in the head-down position.

In a typical vaginal delivery, a baby goes through phases that sound like the instructions to perform a backflip with a half twist: engagement, descent, flexion, rotation internally, extension, and rotation again externally once the head clears your pelvic floor. But there are no instructions at all; your

Baby's First Breath

In the midst of everything that's going on, you may not have noticed one of the most beautiful parts about the delivery process: your baby's transition from living underwater to living in air. Nine months of work culminates in the cutting of the cord (the first of many times you'll do that). Before the first breath can happen, blood has to move from the heart to the lungs, which up until this point were like rigid sponges that allowed nothing to get through. A substance called surfactant (like soap film) prevents the lungs from collapsing so the air sacs can fill with air. The first breath, which typically happens within forty seconds of the cord being cut, sometimes needs to be prompted through a little rubbing or jostling of the baby—not the stereotypical spanking. With premature infants, steroids can be given before or even after birth to stimulate surfactant secretion to help keep their lungs open after they are born—a process known as accelerating the maturity of the lungs.

child just naturally performs this routine to transition from womb to world. Degree of difficulty? Depends on a lot of factors, including the size and shape of baby and of mom's pelvis. Here's how it usually works:

- When the pelvis is large enough for your baby, he moves into the pelvis. In most cases he starts out sunny-side up—with his face looking to mother's pubic hair line. As he progresses through the pelvis during labor (called the descent), the baby has to undergo a series of motions to make sure he is ready for the launch and twists from sunny-side up to facing down toward mom's buttocks.
- He flexes his head (moves it forward onto his chest) to fit the shape of the pelvis. That's called flexion.
- He rotates his head (called internal rotation) around the joints of the pubic bones. This allows the widest part of his body to fit through the widest part of mom. Here's when we say the baby is engaged.
- Finally, he lengthens and rotates his head (external rotation) so that he can maneuver the rest of his body around those joints and show his head. This allows the ob/gyn or midwife to go in for the assist while mom pushes for the final dismount.

As the time of the birth nears, you're going to feel as though you need to have an intense and urgent bowel movement. But you need to resist the urge to push your baby right out with all your might, as you would with such a bowel movement. That's because a huge push could cause a painful tear. Instead follow the instructions of your doc, nurse, or midwife, breathing in short, quick breaths to avoid the overwhelming urge to push and pushing slowly when instructed to do so. They will give you specific instructions and guidance during this time. You (or your partner) may ask your provider for a hand mirror to help you focus your pushing efforts.

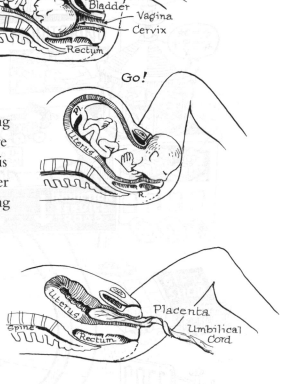

Sometimes your contractions may slow down during this stage, and your provider may suggest trying different positions to help. If your labor stalls, even at this late stage, she may recommend administering oxytocin intravenously to make the contractions become more regular again. Just before delivery, you may feel very hot and may vomit, as your body is trying to expel the fetus. As the head emerges, you will feel a burning sensation around the opening of your vagina. That's called the ring of fire and is caused by the maximum stretching of the tissues and nerves of the perineum (that's the space between the rectum and vaginal opening). Usually your doctor or midwife will massage this area to help it stretch or give you a local anesthetic in anticipation of performing an episiotomy to help the delivery along.

A perfect 10! Applause! Cheers! Tears!

Move ahead to THE PROMISED LAND OF PARENTHOOD (page 244).

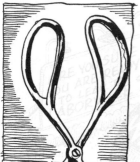

Destination Detour

Sometimes labor doesn't progress; it stalls or stops (the equivalent of having to lose a turn) or takes other twists. These are some of the potential roadblocks and ways that your provider will help you past them:

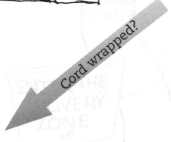

Cord wrapped?

Shoulders stuck?

Descent of head stalled?

As the baby's head emerges, it is very common for the umbilical cord to be wrapped around the baby's neck. Your provider will check to see where the cord is. If it is wrapped around your baby's neck, your provider will try to reach in and untangle the cord. If she can't, the cord will need to be cut, and your baby will be delivered quickly.

Sometimes, after the head is delivered, a shoulder can get stuck on the way out. While it commonly happens when the child is large and the pelvic floor doesn't stretch as it should to accommodate the broad shoulders of a big baby, it may occur in other instances, as with a fast delivery. If this occurs, your provider will immediately avail herself of several options: Commonly, she will push your knees to your shoulders to change the angle of the birth canal or put pressure on the area around the top of the pubic hairline above the bone to help push and guide the baby's shoulder to deliver. Alternatively, if she can fit a hand in the vagina, she can reach the infant's arm and guide his shoulder out; the rest of the infant will be delivered with ease. If not, she may instruct you to *move ahead to ESCAPE HATCH* (page 241).

For any number of reasons, labor may stall. As long as it isn't because the baby is too large to fit and just due to exhaustion in the mom from pushing, alternative techniques may be tried. For example, as long as the head has descended low enough, a vacuum or forceps may be applied to the head to help mom during her pushing. As long as they are applied correctly, they are both safe. With the vacuum, a small swelling may be formed on the baby's scalp in the shape of the vacuum cup. This usually resolves in 24 hours after the child is born.

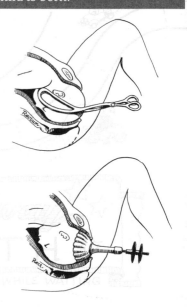

Episiotomy

An episiotomy is performed when a very large baby is anticipated, if he gets stuck, or if a change in his heart rate signals that he may be in distress and needs to be delivered quickly. If it appears that delivery may cause damage to the top of the vaginal area, the doc may decide to perform an episiotomy to relieve the pressure and prevent a painful tear.

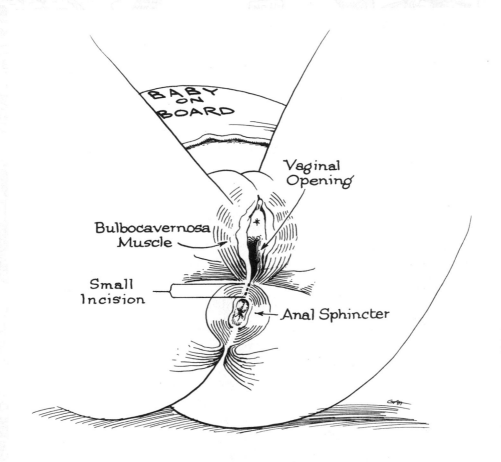

Vaginal Opening

Bulbocavernosa Muscle

Small Incision

Anal Sphincter

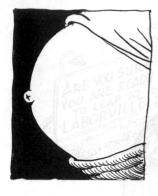

Island of Induction

Docs may choose to induce your labor for many reasons. Maybe your water broke and it contained some fetal waste (meconium), or your baby is showing signs that it needs to be delivered faster. Maybe you're suffering from preeclampsia, chronic high blood pressure, or diabetes. Maybe your baby is getting too large. Or maybe you're more than a week past your due date. Docs generally don't let pregnancies go on indefinitely because after forty weeks the placenta begins to lose its ability to deliver oxygen to the growing fetus. Once the determination is made that your baby is going to be better off outside rather than inside, your doctor will suggest a procedure to start your labor called induction.

Some moms even request an induction for scheduling purposes—say, an out-of-town mother-in-law has planned a visit to help. These so-called social inductions are very controversial, and the mom must be very near her due date for docs even to consider it. Induced labor is associated with an increased rate of C-sections, possibly due to the conditions that prompted the induction, so your doctor will carefully consider the well-being of both you and your baby before scheduling a procedure that may increase your risks.

To induce labor, your doc will check the dilation and effacement of your cervix. At that point, she may apply a prostaglandin gel, which will soften and ripen the cervix to prepare it for labor. It may take a day or so for the cervix to get ready. The doc may also give you intravenous oxytocin to start contractions. Oxytocin speeds up labor, and it makes your contractions feel especially, well, brutal—more like being hit by an eighteen-wheeler than the steady rhythm of ocean waves. So most women whose labors are induced opt to receive pain reduction therapy early in the process. Good choice, in our opinion. Another option: a doc may do what's called stripping the membrane. If your cervix is open, she may sweep her finger across the baby's head. That may be enough to disturb the connection between the baby's sac and your membrane—thus stimulating prostaglandin to get things moving.

Move back to EXIT STRATEGY (page 234) or move ahead to ESCAPE HATCH (page 241).

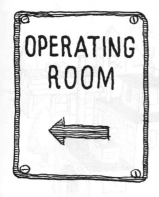

OPERATING ROOM

Escape Hatch

One of the biggest challenges in the labor and delivery process is deciding if and when it's time to stop the natural delivery and perform a cesarean section. C-section rates vary by hospital from 8 percent of all deliveries to up to 50 percent, indicating that there's no set standard. Decisions are often dictated by hospital norms and traditions, as well as the experience of the obstetrician or midwife involved, in addition to your health and your baby's.

Whether or not to perform a C-section can be a tricky call. A doc needs to determine whether there's some kind of problem that's stopping the child from making it down the birth canal or whether the child is in such distress that he needs to be pulled from mom pronto—judgment calls that need to be made under pressure. Sometimes a doctor knows ahead of time if a C-section is likely; factors include being an older mother, having diabetes, having a larger-than-average baby, having multiples, having placenta problems, and having a breech baby. Of course, a C-section comes with its share of risks for mom, such as infection, difficulty breast-feeding, and a negligible future risk of small bowel obstructions from scarring.

> **Factoid:** One of the several benefits of vaginal delivery is that your child's gut is colonized from flora in your vagina. A child delivered by C-section doesn't have the honor of traveling through that vault, so he's not exposed to the same bacteria and is often colonized by hospital bacteria. The good news is that you can make it up with breast-feeding, because then he ingests beneficial bacteria and immunoglobulins from around your nipple.

Also, the child's breathing can be compromised briefly after a C-section because a vaginal delivery tends to squeeze fluid out of the baby's lungs. But those risks also come with benefits, the most important of which is a decreased risk of fetal death or disability—because the medical team can get a distressed baby out and give him the medical attention he needs.

As you know, there's not a whole lot you can do if you and your birthing team decide on a C-section. It's their job to do all the dirty work: give you a spinal/epidural-block anesthetic; sterilize your skin; make the incision above the pubic hairline; and peel the bladder off the lower part of the cervix so the baby can be delivered through an incision low in the uterus. A low incision is the key to having a VBAC (vaginal birth after C-section—should you decide to have another child). If the incision is high in the uterus, where the muscle

You Want to Do What?

While some women fear C-sections the way spiders fear shoe soles, some women choose to have C-sections. Why? A woman may choose to have a C-section if there's a family history of damage to the pelvic floor during vaginal birth or because she's already been through a traumatic vaginal delivery. Some women who have suffered prior sexual abuse or trauma often don't want anything in the birth canal. (But anecdotally, some previously abused women report that vaginal birth, along with therapy, can actually make the natural birthing process healing.) If you're thinking about having an elective C-section, your doc should:

- clarify your request and obtain your consent;
- check other medical problems related to your health and history;
- check the number of children you'd like to have;
- correctly determine the gestational age of your baby at the time of the delivery;
- confirm that the hospital bill will be covered by insurance.

contracts, it is more likely to burst during the next pregnancy, so your doctor would recommend planned cesareans for subsequent pregnancies.

Prior C-sections do increase the risk of subsequent C-sections, as there is an heightened risk of the placenta not being in the right place during the next pregnancy. In addition, the same risk factors that prompted a cesarean the first time may still be present the next time around, so women and their docs are more comfortable taking this route. For these reasons, the incidence of recurrent C-sections is 92 percent; the U.S. Centers for Disease Control and Prevention (CDC) would like to reduce the rate to under 63 percent. In fact, about two-thirds of women who have repeat C-sections could have VBACs, but most elect not to. If you are interested in having a VBAC, discuss this with your doctor. More things to consider:

- Generally all ob/gyns will make sure that you are provided with compression stockings before the surgery. Because your legs won't be moving, any pooling of blood will leave you at increased risk for developing a clot in your leg veins.
- It's okay—and encouraged—to have your support person sitting next to your head in the operating room behind the curtain, talking to you and encouraging you

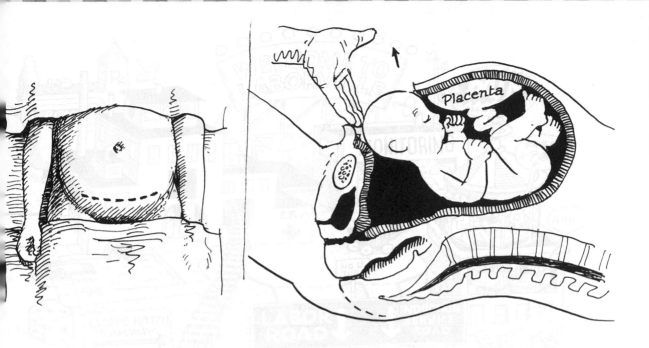

throughout the procedure. The anesthesiologist or nurse anesthetist will also be with you at the head of the bed.

- Immediately after, the delivery team will keep the baby warm and check its lungs while your doc fixes you up, so it may be a few moments before you're able to bond with your baby. As long as all is well with your baby, many nurses will encourage your support person to take this chance to bond with the baby and hold it at your side until your surgery is over.

Advance to THE PROMISED LAND OF PARENTHOOD (page 244).

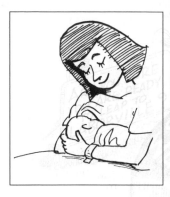

The Promised Land of Parenthood!

You did it! Your job as a caregiver is over in one sense and just beginning in another. Enjoy one of the most amazing thrills you'll ever experience. While you're doing that (and breathing a wee bit easier), the delivery team will be up and about, attending to all kinds of immediate tasks for both you and your baby. Sometimes, if an urgent issue arises, you may suddenly see a host of other professionals or equipment appear in the room. Rest assured, this is why you paid them, so they will do what is right for you and your baby as the need arises.

Once delivery of the infant is complete, your provider will cut the umbilical cord and get the baby's blood type. *Go to SAVE THE BLOOD option card* (page 246). The team then checks your baby to make sure that he is breathing and moving well, and they help wipe

First, the delivery team will help you deliver the placenta by applying pressure to your abdomen. They'll inspect it when it comes out to make sure it's all there (more on what docs look for in a placenta on page 55). If a piece is missing, they'll do an ultrasound to locate the missing tissue, and plans will be made to remove it. Ideally, this should occur within the first fifteen minutes after labor, since your cervix is still dilated and you may still be enjoying the effects of anesthesia. However, they may wait longer if necessary. If the missing fragments can't be removed at the bedside, you may have to undergo a procedure called a D&C to get them out.

TO YOU

Hepatitis B
OPTION CARD

Most hospitals give hepatitis B vaccines to newborns. Here's where we deviate from the norm. We don't think it's necessary to expose your child to a vaccine at birth if you're not in a high-risk group. In fact, none of the authors of the book had his or her kids vaccinated for hep B at birth. This can be delayed until as late as age two and a half if there is no risk involved (see page 399). Discuss this with your pediatrician before delivery.

the baby off so that his body temperature does not drop, because babies can't regulate their temperature well. The birthing team will then let you hold your baby and will encourage skin-to-skin contact. A newborn will move toward the breast when placed on mom's abdomen—a useful instinctive maneuver, as the infant's suckling stimulates mom to release oxytocin, which helps the uterus contract so that the placenta can detach and be delivered. Most of the time, you will receive a dose of oxytocin, either through your IV or as an injection into muscle tissue, to help restore uterine tone and decrease the amount of blood lost after delivery. (If you don't want oxytocin, you may be asked to stimulate your nipples, which also releases oxytocin.)

What else are they doing?

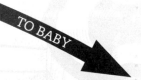

At one minute and again at five minutes after delivery, nurses will give your child an Apgar score to assess whether your baby may be at risk and need further close monitoring soon after birth. On a scale of 0 to 10 (10 being the best), the test measures appearance, pulse, grimace, activity, and respiration, with a max of 2 points for each category. Don't worry: Few babies get a perfect 10. That's because lots of babies lose points for having a bluish tint to their extremities. See the full test below.

In an initial pediatric pit stop, the nurses will give your baby a quick once-over. It's perfectly okay to ask that they delay this for a bit so you can bond with your baby, but since nurses are so used to routines and delivery floors are busy places, sometimes they may not be able to grant a delay. Here they'll:

- Put antibiotic ointment in his eyes to protect against chlamydia, a common bacterial infection that the baby might have been exposed to on the way out.
- Prick his heel to get a blood sample to determine his blood type and check for an enzyme deficiency (called phenylketonuria, or PKU) that can cause mental retardation.
- Give him a shot of vitamin K to help prevent bleeding, because the baby can't make vitamin K yet.

Pull the HEPATITIS B option card.

The Apgar Score

	Score of 0	Score of 1	Score of 2
Skin color (appearance)	Blue all over	Blue at extremities, body pink	Body and extremities pink
Reflex irritability (grimace)	No response to stimulation	Cries when stimulated	Sneezes/coughs/ pulls away when stimulated
Pulse rate	None	Less than 100	More than 100
Muscle tone (activity)	None	Some flexion	Active movement
Respiration	None	Weak or irregular	Strong

Save the Blood

OPTION CARD

Well before delivery, you'll be asked whether you would like to bank some of your baby's cord blood for stem cells. If you are not asked, ask your doc yourself. We recommend that you save the blood. That's because cord blood can be used to help treat nearly fifty different conditions. In fact, there's a 1-in-2,700 chance that your child will need that blood by age twenty-one and an even greater chance that somebody in the family will be able to use it. You'll need to prepare ahead of time if this is something you want done during the delivery. Private cord blood banking costs up to $2,000 to process the specimen, then about $100 a year for maintenance. The public option is free, but as with a regular blood bank, your specimen can be used to help someone else; if your child needs the specimen, you cannot get your sample back.

YOU TIPS

Granted, when it comes to this point in the pregnancy process, you're not in total control of the situation. Nature, your birthing team, and possibly modern medicine all play pretty big roles in the ultimate biological transition. That doesn't mean you don't have any choices, however. So here's what you can do to help yourself through the delivery process:

Be Flexible. It's okay to come up with a birthing plan on how you envision your pregnancy will proceed. But since labor and delivery are unpredictable, there are actually only a few things you have any degree of control over (pain management, your mobility, monitoring, and the people around you). And, according to Murphy's Law, the more you plan, the more unpredictable your labor will be. Rather than drawing up a detailed birth plan, we believe it's much better to prepare for all the options, understand how the process works, and talk to key players on your delivery team. If you've picked a team that has the same philosophy as you, you'll be comfortable no matter what twists and turns occur.

> **Factoid:** There's no need to limit fluids during labor, though hospitals do like to restrict them because vomiting during labor in certain positions is very common, and anesthesiologists fear aspiration, or inhaling vomit into the lungs. Laboring women do better when they're hydrated. Please, though, no red Kool-Aid or Hawaiian Punch. Hospital staff prefer you to stick to clear fluids. By the way, obstetrical anesthesiologists consider pregnant women to always have a full stomach; that's because it takes longer for them to empty their stomachs. So orders of not eating during labor are, as one OB colleague says, plain ol' common sense.

The No-Embarrassment Zone

Two questions you may be afraid to ask:

Do I need to shave before labor?

While pubic hair serves some functions (it helps prevent chafing, for one), the amount of pubic hair you have for delivery doesn't matter. So do whatever you're comfortable with: trim it, wax it, or just leave it alone.

What if I push out something other than the baby?

With all the pushing that's going on, it's not surprising that about half of all women have a bowel movement during labor. While we surely understand why you'd be self-conscious about it, delivery teams are used to it; it's perfectly normal, so don't think another thing about it. One way to help minimize the chances that you will: a high-fiber diet with plenty of water will help keep your intestines clean.

It is a sign that you are making an excellent pushing effort if your bladder spontaneously empties as you push, so don't worry about this. If the team predicts that it will need forceps or a vacuum or if the baby is large, they may want to use a catheter to drain your bladder and give themselves some more space to work.

Speed the Process. If you're experiencing a high level of discomfort but the baby has decided that she wants to camp out in your belly for a while longer, you can try to move things along. While there are not superstrong data, it does appear that breast stimulation brings on labor for some women. Other options that could help: downing some castor oil, rubbing evening primrose oil on your belly, or just plain and simple walking. Sex, by the way, has not been shown to work, but there's no harm in trying.

Create the Ideal Atmosphere. Just because you're going to be staying in the hospital for only a couple of days doesn't mean that you can't give your room a personal touch. With just a few

Pack Your Bags for the Hospital

Items for Labor: two tennis balls (for partner to massage your lower back); aromatherapy (if permitted by hospital); fully charged camera; music (if allowed).

Items for Hospital Stay: cell phone and charger; laptop for sending instant birth announcement/photos or Skyping/ichatting with faraway friends and relatives (check hospital's internet policy first); phone numbers for health insurance company and pediatrician (both should be informed right away about birth); nail file for baby; extra socks, flip-flops, change of clothes (still maternity, we're afraid); toiletries.

Items for Departure: car seat, going-home outfit for baby.

The Reason for Stillbirths

A stillbirth is a miscarriage that takes place after twenty weeks. Most stillbirths are related to some preexisting condition that compromised the placenta in some way. While many moms feel very guilty, thinking that it was something that they did, the fact is that 99 percent of stillbirths are not due to anything the mom could have done differently. We would urge you to try to exchange your feelings of guilt for those of grief. Typically, an autopsy will be performed to help determine the cause, and docs will usually focus on uncovering the cause in the hope of preventing it for the next pregnancy. Should you find yourself in this position, the nursing staff and your doc or midwife will help you and your partner through this unsettling time. They will give you the option of gathering mementos such as pictures, so you can grieve in your own way. And of course, hospitals do offer grief counseling services and chaplains to help you through this traumatic period.

Factoid: In some cases, you may be given magnesium through an IV to help prevent seizures associated with preterm labor and preeclampsia; side effects include muscle weakness and fatigue. It is perfectly safe when given in a controlled environment by your medical team, but as always, be a smart patient and question everything put into you or your IV, including the names and dosages of all medications.

Factoid: Probiotics for mom have a double benefit. When taken regularly, they decrease the weight gain that mom experiences and reduce the risk of infant diarrhea. We like the spore forms, as they survive better to populate your intestine with friendly bacteria.

items, you can create an environment that will help relax you. For instance, bring your favorite music to play, your favorite blanket, a comfy pillow, and photos of a beloved pet, family member, or another child. (Those will come in handy when you're asked to pick a focal point during the tough spots of delivery and when your other children visit.) And don't be shy about changing the mood of the room by adjusting the temperature, dimming the lights, or even using scented oils, creams, or lotions.

Take a Tour. Ask the hospital for a tour of the facilities a few weeks beforehand. This will give you the opportunity to check everything out, ask questions, and inquire about the availability of birthing balls or tubs. Plus, just seeing the place where you'll deliver will help ease your mind—after all, part of the fear of the process is the fear of the unknown.

10

And in the Beginning . . .

Challenges—and Rewards—of the First Month After Delivery

We all know what a honeymoon period is. For bosses, employees, lovers, or presidents, the honeymoon period is that blissful time when you can learn the ropes and get used to your new gig before reality sets in and the bleep hits the fan.

But when it comes to parenthood, as warm and wonderful an experience as it is, the bleep hits the fan (and the diaper and the onesie and the receiving blanket) pretty much the moment you bring bubby home. Though you're basking in the glow of that beautiful baby of yours and how you've never, *ever* felt anything like the soul-gripping joy of being a parent, babies allow no time for you to learn the ropes. Reality hits you hard. And often. They need to eat, you need to sleep; your nipples are sore and your brain is numb; they get diaper rash and they get gas—morning, noon, night, and seventeen times in between. Ain't no hammocks on this honeymoon, mama.

Add in the fact that everyone and their mother (not to mention yours and his) want to tell you what to do, how to do it, and when to do it, and you've got your own personal board of parental advisers, whether you like it or not. In this chapter, we're going to help you filter the advice by detailing the top eight issues and stresses that you will likely face in the first month of parenting and giving you the information that you need to make decisions that work best for the health and happiness of you and your baby, as well as the rest of your family.

1. Feeding Your Child

A Primer on Breast-Feeding and Formula

Above all, we believe that breast-feeding is the best way to feed your child, although we realize that it's not an option for some people; more on that in a moment. Simply, your body knows exactly what your baby needs, and it concocts the perfect cocktail of nutrients in the form of your breast milk. Breast milk contains protein, healthy fat, sugar, vitamins, and minerals that have huge effects on the health and development of your child. Not only that, it actually changes composition as your baby grows, adapting to his growing needs. Breast milk protects against infection, allergies, asthma, sudden infant death syndrome (SIDS), and a raft of other diseases as well. And that's not even mentioning the benefits that breast-feeding has for you: It burns something on the order of 500 calories a day, helps to contract the uterus after delivery, and has protective effects on your bones and against certain cancers. Bottom line: Breast milk is the ultimate nectar to the newborn.

During pregnancy, estrogen and prolactin cause the milk glands and ducts in your breasts to increase in size. If you recall figure 7.1 on page 178, the glands are where milk is produced; the ducts are the tubes that transport milk from the glands to the mini sprinkler nozzle in the form of the twenty or so small holes at the tip of your nipple. At the very end of your pregnancy, your breasts prime the pump by making a yellow, creamy substance called colostrum, which contains proteins, vitamins, minerals, and infection-fighting antibodies.

A few days after giving birth, colostrum turns to milk, and you'll experience the phenomenon known as engorgement. All of a sudden, you'll wake up and see Dolly Parton staring back at you from your bathroom mirror. For a couple of days, your breasts will be bigger than you ever imagined, and you will produce so much milk that your newborn may actually choke and sputter trying to swallow it all. This too shall pass, as your hormones equilibrate and your milk production scales down to meet the needs of your baby. In the meantime, you can ease the pain of your swollen breasts by manually expressing some of the excess milk and massaging your breasts in a hot shower. If you're set up to pump already, you can easily put away a few extra bottles. You'll probably experience a lot of leakage until your milk production gets under control. In addition to wearing a bra with nursing pads, you may need to sleep on a bath towel so as not to soak your bed.

Early on, you'll be feeding your beautiful babe every two to four hours, but it can be hard to know whether or not you're feeding the right amount, because unless you sport see-through breasts, you can't see how much is coming out of you or how much is going into your baby. If your little one is gaining weight appropriately and soiling diapers often, you are most likely giving him the amount he needs. To know if your baby is latching on well enough to get milk, the trick is to listen for a change in sounds when your baby is feeding. You should hear a transition from short, quick sucks to long, slow, deep gulps—during which you can hear swallowing and see his jaw moving up and down. When that transition occurs, you will often feel a tingly sensation in your breasts. This is known as the "let-down reflex" and it means that your milk is flowing freely to your baby.

Factoid: If you have nipple rings, we suggest taking them out during your pregnancy to help prepare your body better for breast feeding. Because scar tissue can form around the piercing, it can make it difficult for your baby to feed. (By the way, there's no danger in navel rings during pregnancy, but as your tummy grows, your navel will flatten out, making it more difficult for a ring to stay in place.)

Apart from a sharp pain deep in your breast when your baby first latches on (it usually goes away within the first few weeks), breast-feeding should not be painful. If it is, check to make sure that your baby is properly latched on: His mouth should be wide open, covering most of the areola. If he's not latched on, stick your finger inside his mouth, breaking the suction, and try again. It is important to note that babies should feed from both breasts at each feeding (burping in between). Also know that babies nurse at different speeds: Some spend five minutes on each breast, others as much as twenty.

In the beginning, breast-feeding can be very hard. While it's the most natural experience in the world, it does take work and practice to get the two of you in sync (our dance metaphor holds true even after delivery). Here are some other tips that can help you maximize your breast-feeding experience:

Make the Proper Hold. Holding your baby to your breast isn't like lugging groceries to the car. The best way to make sure that he's feeding well and comfortably is to employ one of these four positions:

- the cradle hold (the classic position)
- the cross-cradle hold (gives more control over his head)
- the football hold (good for nursing twins)
- the side-lying hold (especially good for women who have had a C-section because it takes any pressure off the incision, as well as for nighttime feedings)

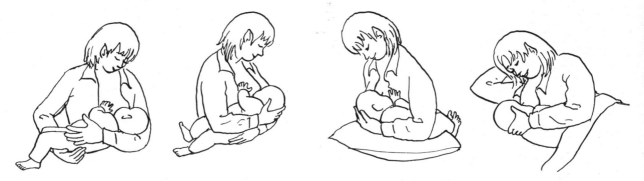

Cradle Hold   Cross-cradle Hold   Football Hold   Side-Lying

Note in all the figures the position of your arms and hands. Besides making sure that he gains easy access, your other goal is to support his head and back during the feeding. The major key to successful breast-feeding for both you and the little one is relaxation on your part. Any anxiety or stiffness you exhibit is immediately picked up by your baby, and then the act becomes a struggle. (Please tell any dads that the Heisman hold doesn't count.)

Watch What You Eat. It doesn't take a biochemist to know that pumping your own body full of spicy nachos grandes doesn't exactly make for the best-formulated breast milk. To make sure that your baby is getting the right nutrients, you have to do the same. Keep taking your prenatal vitamin and see to it that you get these nutrients, which have been deemed especially beneficial for improving the quality of breast milk:

- Protein: two or three servings a day of organically fed poultry, seafood (non-bottom-feeders and small fish; think wild—including canned—salmon, trout, mahimahi, sea bass, flounder), lean meat, eggs, low-fat dairy, and soy.
- Calcium: 1,300 mg a day (from low-fat dairy products, calcium-fortified orange juice, soy milk, tofu, broccoli). Consume no more than 600 mg in any two-hour period throughout the day, because that's the maximum your body can absorb at a time, either from food or from your calcium citrate and magnesium supplement. You *have* been taking that, haven't you?
- Iron: 20 mg a day (from poultry, seafood, dried beans and fruit, egg yolks). Your multivitamin often includes more than that.
- DHA: 600 mg a day (an algae source, available in most drugstores, is ideal, since it avoids any toxin concerns and is very palatable in pill form).
- Vitamin C: 800 mg a day (from citrus fruits, red peppers, broccoli).

Above all, aim to have a healthy, balanced diet and drink plenty of fluids. It's best to eat five or six smaller meals throughout the day rather than have three larger ones. Avoid spicy or gas-inducing foods, as well as caffeinated beverages and alcohol. Remember that you are eating for, at most, 1.2, not two. (When you're pregnant, it's 1.1, but you burn more calories when you breast-feed, so you need some additional nutrients.)

Manage the Trouble. If your child is having a hard time latching on, it could be caused by a number of reasons. For one thing, he may not be fully awake and stimulated. You can help keep him alert by removing his clothes, which will wake him up real fast. For another, he'll have trouble if you have inverted nipples, when not enough of the nipple is exposed for your baby to latch onto. You can use plastic devices found in pharmacies that fit into your bra to help stretch the skin around the areola, which

How to . . . Choose a Name

Picking a name for your child is about as personal as it gets. You may decide on a name based on your family history, your religious traditions, what sounds good, what doesn't sound good, the name of your favorite country music star, or even your favorite doc on TV. So we're not here to tell you what name to choose (Oz or Ozzie), because you already know how important it is; it's your baby's first form of personalized branding, after all.

We're not surprised that Archibald Leach changed his name to Cary Grant, Demetria Guynes changed hers to Demi Moore, and Marion Michael Morrison changed his to John Wayne. What your name says, says a lot about you.* As you're sifting through baby name websites and arguing with your mother about what sounds better, you might want to keep in mind some of the guidelines that many people like to use when naming their children:

- Don't name your child anything that you yourself wouldn't want to be named.
- Consider future implications for names that can cause confusion or teasing; for example, gender-neutral names, unique spellings of names, names that cause puns (Chris Cross), or rhyming names. And by all means, think about what his initials might spell (Andrew Steven Smith).
- If you and your partner disagree, try to find a common ground. One way: Each of you makes a separate list of five to ten names, you exchange the lists, and you each pick three from your partner's list that you could be happy with. Then work from that list of six.

Not sure what to name your child? Take a look at our Name Game on www.realage.com and doctoroz.com (although be warned, almost every name chosen on the latter site has an Oz in it). Here we'll ask you a series of questions about you and your family name to come up with some options that sound good and best represent the values you want to instill in your child.

* Linguists who study names think that how we react to a given name comes down to four factors: phonology (how the name sounds, like Coca-Cola); orthography (how it's spelled, like Kool-Aid or Mr. T); morphology (how a name is formed and changed through prefixes, roots, and suffixes, like J-Lo); and semantics (the underlying meaning of a name, like Coolio).

How to . . . Choose a Stroller

Picking your kid's first set of wheels isn't as nerve-racking as handing over the keys in sixteen or seventeen years for the real set, but there are still certain things to consider:

- Consider your lifestyle. If you live in the country or suburbs, get a newborn car seat with a stroller attachment. That way you'll have fewer worries about waking him when you move from car to stroller. If you live in the city or do a lot of errands by foot, a carriage that can be positioned to lie flat with a large basket underneath might be your best bet.
- Jogging strollers and umbrella strollers are no-no's for newborns, because they don't offer any back support.
- Above all, you're going to make a decision based on personal preference, so you should make sure to give it a good once-over and weigh a number of factors, such as how heavy it is, how the restraint straps fit, whether it has a removable seat that you can clean, the handle height (and whether it's adjustable), and whether or not you'll be having more than one child in a stroller at any given time.
- If you're going to get around using an on-the-body carrier, the baby needs to be seven days and seven pounds before you use it.
- There is some research to suggest that rear-facing strollers are better for a baby's brain development than forward-facing ones. That's not surprising. The rear-facing ones allow better interaction between caregiver and child, while forward-facing ones expose kids to more white noise (like traffic, wind, and garbles) and make it more difficult for them to hear the sweet nothings that you or your caregiver whispers to them.

causes the nipple to poke out. If you do have inverted nipples, it's best to start using these helping devices in the third trimester. Also, you'll want to be on the lookout for white spots that may develop on your baby's tongue. That's called thrush, a type of yeast infection that may be hindering him from eating well.

Relax and Get Comfortable. It's often hard to get a proper letdown if you're stressed, distracted, or breast-feeding on the go. And without a proper letdown, your baby will not get enough to eat and will be hungry again in no time. Try to set aside quiet time to nurse your baby. Sit in a comfortable chair with good back and arm support, and set yourself up with everything you need ahead of time: a glass of water, a book or magazine, the telephone within reach. If you have other children, see that their needs have been met so that they won't bother you (too much). After you and your newborn have gotten the hang of breast-feeding, your body will respond automatically to the baby's stimulation of your nipples, and you'll be able to multitask (not that we want you to do so).

Burp Right. You should burp your baby before moving him from one breast to the other, and then after he finishes. Hold him so that his head is over your shoulder, and rub or pat his back gently. The key to a successful burp: Provide a little counterpressure under his stomach with your collarbone. The gentle pushing against his belly, not the back pat, is what really does it—although patting does dislodge bubbles.

Supply and Demand. As your baby grows, he'll need more nutrition, and your body will automatically produce more and richer milk to satisfy him. If you notice that he still seems hungry after a feeding or the time between feedings is not stretching out, you may not be producing as much milk as you could or he wants. The best remedies for this are sleep and plenty of fluids. If you can't catch enough z's, at least try to relax and put your feet up as much as possible; now is not the time to start training for a marathon or even doing your usual amount of running around. Also, avoid antihistamines, diuretics, and other medications that dehydrate you. Fenugreek, an herb found in tea form, is said to help increase milk production.

Salve Your Wounds. Here's something you can rub on your nipples if you're cracking or bleeding: cow udder cream. Really. The lanolin helps heal the area and seal in moisture. Just make sure to wipe it off before feeding. If you don't live near a tractor supply store, regular old lanolin, which you can get at any pharmacy, will do the trick; it just has a slightly stronger smell than the udder cream.

Pump It. There comes a time when many moms decide they need to pump milk so they'll have it on hand for babysitters, partners, or helpful grandparents who want to help refresh you by giving you a night out or a full night of sleep. And there are times you may want to pump and dump if you consume spicy foods or a glass of wine. If you're pumping only occasionally, a hand pump will do. If you're going to be pumping regularly, it's worthwhile to rent a powerful hospital-grade pump.

The best time to pump an extra bottle is shortly after your baby's first feeding of the day, as most women have plentiful milk in the morning. Even though the actual pumping is initially an uncomfortable experience (no way around that), know these guidelines: You can store breast milk at room temperature for four to eight hours; in an insulated cooler for a day; in the fridge for about a week (mark the date you pumped on any bottles you store); and in the freezer for up to three months. We recommend you use glass storage bottles, especially when freezing, because plastic ones may leach the endocrine disruptor bisphenol-A. Also, do not store milk in plastic bottle-insert bags, as they are porous and will increase the chance of your milk going rancid.

Don't Worry About Shapes and Sizes: Breast size has no influence whatsoever on milk production. Even if you're small, that doesn't mean your child will be malnourished. The amount of milk depends more on how healthy you are and how many nutrients and fluids you get. What can be a problem is if you have a breast implant and it starts to leak. An even bigger issue: If you've had a breast reduction, your milk ducts may have been severed, and you may be unable to breast-feed. Talk with your breast surgeon if you're not sure.

Know the Myths. With all the info that's swirling around about nursing, it can be hard to know the difference between medical facts and something that the neighbor down the block told you. Some common myths and their realities:

Myth	Fact
Nursing makes your breasts sag.	Aging does, especially if you do not periodically hang upside down or do pectoral exercises.

(continued on next page)

Myth	Fact
If you didn't breast-feed in your first pregnancy, you can't in your subsequent ones.	BS (bad science). Indeed you can. New baby, new milk production process.
Once you commit to breast-feeding, you have to do it for all feedings.	You can absolutely combine breast-feeding with using formula. Your body adjusts its milk production based on demand. Low demand equals low supply. High demand, and it rises to the occasion. Many women who return to work and don't want to pump nurse their babies in the mornings and evenings and provide formula for daytime feedings.
Breast-feeding equals birth control.	We recommend you use barrier methods. While the prolactin hormone that stimulates milk production will prevent the release of eggs, one in fifty women will get pregnant while breast-feeding exclusively if not using other protection—and that doesn't count those who are combining breast-feeding with formula or solid food. If you take birth control pills containing estrogen, you have to stop breast-feeding. The minipill has no estrogen and provides a safe method of birth control while breast-feeding.

Pump and Dump. Many medications pass poorly into breast milk, so they're safe to take while nursing. But there may be times when you want to pump your milk and dump it, and feed your child previously stored milk or formula, either because you need to take a short course of a drug that is contraindicated for breast-feeding (such as a radioactive dye for a medical imaging procedure) or because you've enjoyed a night on the town that included alcohol. Basically, if you feel the effects of alcohol, then it's still in your bloodstream and your milk supply; when you no longer feel the effects, it's safe to nurse again. That said, the occasional drink in your breast milk is not a cause for concern. Contrary to popular belief, by the way, Guinness stout—or any other form of alcohol—has not been proven to stimulate milk production.

Understand Your Options. There are reasons why doctors, nurses, and midwives push breast-feeding as the preferred feeding option, the first being those health benefits, but we also recognize that there are many reasons why it might not be realistic. Some women have jobs that prevent them from nursing or pumping as frequently as they need to; some women are on medications or have conditions or infections that don't mix well with breast-feeding; some mothers of multiples feel that the process is too overwhelming; and some babies have medical conditions that require close monitoring of fluid intake. You also should not breast-feed if you have a serious infection, smoke, or are doing illicit drugs. In these cases, go to formula. Our recommendations: Choose a formula made from cow's milk rather than soy protein, because cow's milk is most similar to human milk. And read the label to find one with the highest concentration of vegetarian DHA. How much formula to give? Generally, add 3 ounces to your baby's age in months per feeding. So a one-month-old would get 4 ounces per feeding, a two-month old would get 5 ounces, and so on. When he hits about 32 ounces during a twenty-four-hour period, it's probably time to try a little solid food.

2. Get Some Zzzzzz's

Managing Sleep Deprivation

Gone are the days when you can sleep in—or sleep through the night. If you're lucky, it'll be only about ten to twelve weeks before your baby starts to sleep through the night, and by "through the night," we mean six to eight hours of uninterrupted sleep without needing to be fed. Until then, while it's not an ideal situation, your body can handle it; in a way, the multiple midnight bathroom runs you had in the third trimester helped prepare you for this. Certainly a lot of your sleep quality and length depends on how you decide to feed; if you decide to pump or use formula, your partner can help relieve some of the nighttime responsibilities. In any case, because your sleep is entwined with your baby's, your goal is to create the best possible sleeping environment for your child, which ultimately will help you too.

In the beginning, your baby will be in a constant sleep-eat cycle. Nevertheless, it's important to give him clues about when it's night and when it's day, even when he's sleeping. Healthy sleep training is like muscle building: You've got to teach his body what to do through your actions and through routines. When he naps during the day, go about your business, keep lights on, and don't go crazy dampening background noise. At night, even when you're feeding, provide as little stimulation as possible: no music, dim lights (use red; those wavelengths are not perceived by your or your baby's brains as daylight), no books, no talking, no tickling. Essentially, make nighttime feedings as boring as possible, so that he is encouraged to go back to sleep rather than to seek entertainment. Ultimately, sleep is really a habit, and if you can teach your child the difference between night and day—and when it's okay to be aroused and when it's not—you're setting yourself up for good sleep experiences.

Some other things to consider:

The Equipment: Safety-approved crib with a firm, tight-fitting mattress (see page 348), bassinet, or cosleeper.

The Routine: Help induce sleep by giving a warm bath early in the evening, followed by a massage (see page 132), stories and/or lullabies, and a regular bedtime. Routines count for babies, and once the little one gets into a pattern, it will become easy. Try to discourage bad habits for the same reason.

The Trick: The more you can teach your baby to soothe himself, the better off you'll be. So try to stay away from crutches, like rocking your baby to sleep or giving him a pacifier. Otherwise he'll learn that he can't fall asleep unless he's rocked, or he'll cry if the pacifier falls out during the night. Instead leave a small blanket in the crib, which can help comfort without being a crutch. Try to put him to sleep when he's still awake so it becomes expected—and habit.

The Challenges: Figuring out how to deal with nighttime crying is a biggie. At first, the crying will, of course, be your signal that your baby is hungry. But other times, it may be simply to get your attention. If he's been fed and the cry isn't a so-called sick cry, you'll establish better sleeping habits if you allow him to soothe himself on his own. Yes, we know, it's easier said than done—but well worth the effort.

Another big decision is whether you want to allow your child to sleep with you. For some moms, it's not an option, because they're up all night worrying about rolling on top of their children. Overall, sleeping together seems to be a cultural phenomenon. It's more common in tribal cultures and cultures that stress conformity and less common in cultures that stress independence. While babies may wake up more often if they're in your bed or in the same room with you (they can smell you), it's also easier to nurse them frequently if you don't have to get up and go into another room. Be aware that if you or your partner are taking sedatives, have been drinking, or are extremely overweight, you should

Factoid: The labor and delivery room isn't where you're going to document all the ins and outs of what happened during your delivery. But in your first postpartum visit to your provider, you want to get all the facts straight, so you have the info for future pregnancies. Find out such things as what kind of tear you had, if a vacuum was used, reasons why the decision was made for a C-section, any medications you were given, and so on. Knowing what happened during your last pregnancy and delivery will help prepare you for your next.

Factoid: Some parents bundle their babies so much that they end up looking as if they live in the Klondike. The general rule for how to dress your kid: the same number of layers of clothing as you're wearing plus one layer. And keep the baby's head covered, since that's where most of the heat escapes from.

not put the baby in your bed, because you can crush him while you're sleeping. And remember that whatever path you choose, you're establishing a habit, so, again, consider your desired outcome and reverse-engineer.

The Naps: A baby's sleep is in phase with circadian rhythms, so he'll often be sleepy at nine in the morning and two in the afternoon. Those are usually ideal times for naps. Also, just because a baby skips a nap doesn't mean he's going to go down easier or sleep better at night. He needs sleep (that's the time when the brain grows), so don't skimp on naps. The signs of sleep deprivation are nearly invisible at this age, so it's important to establish good routines early on.

3. What's Wrong with Him?

When to Call the Doc

When you have a baby, a lot of tough stuff comes with the territory: the lack of sleep, the constant running around, having to watch rerun after rerun of *The Wiggles.* One of the toughest: listening to your baby cry.

First things first: Many babies cry an hour or two a day; after all, crying is their only verbal means of communicating. While it may test your nerves, it's totally normal, and very soon into motherhood, you'll learn to distinguish among a hungry cry, a tired cry, a my-diaper-is-fully-loaded cry, and the dreaded something-is-not-right cry.

Colic—a condition in which an otherwise healthy child is crying, fussy, and irritable for more than three hours a day and more than three days in any given week—is fairly common. It's benign and usually goes away within the first three or four months. Of course, just because it isn't harming your baby doesn't mitigate the fact that caring for a colicky infant can be extremely upsetting—even traumatic—for you. Here are some measures you can try to help soothe a fussy infant.

- *Stay cool.* Babies pick up on cues from their parents. If you're temperamental because he's temperamental, he's only going to get more temperamental, and so on.

What's That Cry?

Just as a bird-watcher can distinguish the tweets of an oriole, chickadee, and a yellow-headed caracara, it won't take long before you can ID your baby's cry. But to help you early on, here are some tip-offs about what he wants when he's fussing.

If He's Also . . .	It Could Be . . .
Squirming.	He has a dirty diaper.
Turning his head to the side or putting his fist to his mouth.	He's hungry.
Pulling his legs up to his chest and has a tense body.	He has gas. Burp him.
Sweating and has red ears.	He's too warm. Check his temp and loosen his clothing.
Getting goose bumps or has some purplish tones to his hands and feet.	He's cold. Go get a blanket or a hat and socks.
Flailing his arms and legs, or turning from the light.	He's overstimulated, so take him out of his current environment to a quieter one.
Blinking and yawning, as well as kicking.	He's tired.
Squirming, looking around.	He just needs a cuddle.

- *Stretch him.* Flex your baby at the knees and hips to see if you can relieve some gas. Sometimes discomfort is related to digestive issues.
- *Move it.* Many babies with colic are soothed simply by getting up and going. Put him in a stroller or baby carrier and take a walk, go for a drive, or strap him into one of those vibrating seats.
- *Change your diet.* If you're breast-feeding, you can try to relieve

some discomfort by eliminating dairy, onions, garlic, spicy food, chocolate, caffeine, and cauliflower from your diet.

Whatever you do, do *not* shake your baby to get him to stop crying; this can permanently damage his delicate brain. If you feel yourself reaching your limit of frustration and exhaustion dealing with a colicky baby, enlist a support person—partner, friend, neighbor, relative, sitter—to give you a break.

In addition to crying, there are other signs and symptoms you should be attuned to that may indicate a medical problem:

The Signs	The Significance	The Action
The baby is having fewer than six wet or three soiled diapers a day for more than two days (or no stool for forty-eight hours if breast feeding). If he's on formula, he'll be more constipated and make around one stool every two days.	It may mean that he's not getting enough nutrients.	The pediatrician will look for signs of dehydration, such as a depressed fontanel (the space between bones in the middle of the scalp), and may suggest ways to supplement his fluid intake and nutrition.
The baby's stool is white or bloody.	If the baby's stool is white, something is wrong with his liver as it's trying to metabolize food. If the baby's stool is bloody, it can be caused by a number of things, such as a small anal tear, allergens, or even ingesting blood from mom's cracked nipple, which more commonly causes bloody spit-up.	In the case of white stool, the doc will check to see if the path between the liver and intestines is functioning normally. If the stool is bloody, it still needs to be checked out.

Call the Doc

Always trust your intuition. Better to call the doc and be told it's nothing to worry about than the other way around. Some signs when you should absolutely call the doc:

- Baby is hard to wake up, or too tired to eat, or appears weak.
- There's blood or mucus in the stool.
- He has an unusual rash.
- His eyes are red and swollen or have a yellow, sticky discharge.
- Seek immediate help if:
  - He's having difficulty breathing. (You can see his ribs sticking out when he pulls the muscles in with each breath.)
  - His lips or mouth are blue and he's breathing faster than fifty-five breaths per minute (normal is twenty to forty), or if he doesn't breathe for fifteen to twenty seconds.

The baby has a fever over 100 degrees F.	Babies have a primitive immune response, so their barriers to the outside world aren't as well developed, especially in the lungs and intestines. The fever is an indication of some kind of immune reaction to an outside invader.	A doc will check for infections of major organs, especially the brain.
The baby has turned blue in some parts of his body.	Blood is not being properly distributed throughout the body. React fast on this one unless the area pinks up on rubbing.	The doc will check to make sure that the heart and lungs are working correctly, for heart anomalies are the most common birth defects.

(continued on next page)

The Signs	The Significance	The Action
The baby has a tremor or is shaking.	If it's short in duration, it could be the Moro reflex we talked about on page 128. If the shaking lasts longer than a few seconds and is unrelated to his having been startled in some way, it could indicate some brain malfunction.	A doc will evaluate the child's brain to make sure there's no seizure disorder.
Projectile vomiting.	The pathway from his stomach to his intestines is blocked, preventing the stomach from emptying.	A doc will check for pyloric stenosis, a condition that requires immediate surgery to prevent dehydration and malnutrition.
His skin or eyes are yellow or yellowish.	He's not clearing bile (produced in the liver) from his system correctly, which is a sign of jaundice.	Depending on the severity, he may prescribed to sit under ultraviolet (UV) light. Because jaundice is so common, there's probably a good biological reason for it to happen. It turns out that bilirubin, which causes the yellow color, is a powerful antioxidant that helps the baby cope with the three times higher oxygen content in the transition from womb to breathing after birth. But don't avoid treatment if the bilirubin level is very high, as this can damage brain cells.

There's a lump in the skin near where the belly button protrudes.	The umbilical artery that connected mom and child passes through the abdominal wall. After the cord has healed, a gap may remain through which the digestive organs may protrude, causing pain and creating an umbilical hernia.	These usually close by themselves within a few years, but a doc should check it out to make sure that the intestines aren't trapped.
He's spitting up.	All kids spit up. It's a form of reflux, as the sphincter at the bottom of the esophagus doesn't always work, allowing the stomach contents to flow back up.	To check the severity, measure out 3 or 4 ounces of milk and splash it on a towel or diaper. If that looks to be the amount he's spitting up, or if his spitting up is accompanied by crying, his reflux may be more severe. Antacids and other medications can help, but do not try them without seeing your doctor.

4. What's the Matter with You?

Take Care of Your Own Health Too

Granted, we understand that right about now, all of your attention and affection are directed toward that cute little swaddled-up bubbity-boo of yours. But you can't be so focused on him that you forget about you. In this postpartum state, your body and mind are in recovery mode, leaving you vulnerable to some medical issues. If you're experiencing the following symptoms, you need to call your doc for follow-up:

The Signs	The Significance	The Action
You have a headache that just won't go away.	It might be elevated blood pressure.	Your doc will check your BP and might offer temporary medications.
You're bleeding enough to soak one large pad every hour, you have numerous large clots that are lemon sized or larger, or your vagina smells foul.	You might have an infection or a retained piece of placenta attached to your uterus.	Antibiotics will clear up the infection, but you'll also undergo an ultrasound and physical exam to see if part of the placenta is still in you or if the uterus is not healing properly. In that case, you may need a D&C to remove the remaining placenta.
You have difficulty holding your stool until you get to the bathroom, and it's not diarrhea.	You could have a torn anal muscle, sustained during the rigors of labor and delivery.	Your doc may refer you to a colorectal surgeon to repair the area.
You have swelling and pain in the back of one or both legs, or shortness of breath.	It could mean a change in blood pressure, and/or the formation of a blood clot in your leg.	Your doc will probably perform an ultrasound to see whether you have a clot. If so, you'll likely be put on blood thinners and monitored closely.
Milk is not coming in after you've already had significant milk production.	You might not be feeding the infant often enough, which is causing a decrease in your milk supply.	You may be referred to a lactation consultant, who will walk you through ways to stimulate milk production, like pumping after feedings, feeding more often, improving your nutrition and fluid intake, or reducing your physical activity.

Your breasts are painful, swollen, or red.	You may have an infection or engorgement of the breasts.	If you have an infection like mastitis, which is normally caused when bacteria from the baby's mouth infect the breast, you may need antibiotics. Hot showers, compresses, and massage can help soothe the pain. Cool cabbage leaves (steamed, then poked with a fork) placed under your bra can also help relieve pain from engorgement.
You're not feeling quite like a mother should. You're feeling overwhelmed, you're crying all the time, or you're having trouble bonding with your baby.	You may have some form of postpartum blues or clinical depression. See below.	A doc will help determine the severity and may prescribe therapy and sometimes antidepressants.

5. How's Your Mood?

Cope with the Neurological and Hormonal Changes That Occur After Birth

Laugh. Cry. Throw a stroller at him the next time he leaves the toilet seat up. Your moods are swinging, and they're swinging hard. It's no wonder; not only are you adjusting to a major life change, but you're sleep deprived and have hormones swirling around in your blood like bumper cars—stop, start, go, fast, slow, brake, aaaah! Perhaps nowhere do these hormonal changes manifest themselves more clearly than when it comes to your moods.

Up to 50 percent of all women suffer some kind of blues after giving birth. They may feel anxious, have crying spells, lose their appetite, or have trouble sleeping. The trick is to figure out how serious your mood changes are and what you need to do about them. Here's how docs differentiate among the various levels of severity:

Baby Blues: The above symptoms last up to about two weeks after birth. They usually don't require treatment; often, finding a sympathetic ear or someone to care for the baby at night so you can get some rest can be enough to get you over the hump.

Postpartum Depression: PPD is classified as having similar symptoms to those of the baby blues, but they can begin any time within the first year and last indefinitely if not treated. They usually set in after the first few weeks, not immediately, like baby blues, although they can start right away. And they often are severe enough that they hinder a mom's ability to function. Of course, this means you need to see your doc. Some women also get "scary thoughts" in which they think they might harm the baby or themselves—accidentally or on purpose. Even though they know for certain that these thoughts are illogical and they would never act on them, they can be so terrifying that they are afraid to even mention them. In severe cases, they may be so frightened that they avoid handling their babies.

Factoid: Don't think that postpartum depression is limited to women. Many men experience it, too. After all, their lives have changed as well, and they often have more trouble articulating what's going on emotionally. Encourage your partner to talk about his feelings or get together with other new fathers. Turns out that depression in dads, even prenatal depression, correlates with behavioral problems in kids as they get older.

It's sometimes hard to have perspective on your moods when you're caught up in them, and it may be a friend or relative who first notices the change. Don't be defensive. PPD is very common and very treatable. Playing the martyr will only exacerbate the problem, preventing you from experiencing the joys of motherhood and preventing your baby from the benefits of having an engaged, happy mom. Call your doc as soon as you or a significant other suspects that postpartum depression is a problem. You heard right: If you even think a problem exists, sharing the concerns with a professional is wise.

Counseling is the first-line defense to help get you back on track, and medications might be carefully added as well. You're especially at risk if you've suffered from any form of depression previously, have a family history of depression, or have recently undergone a major life change other than pregnancy. Some women who know they're at risk often ask their docs for an antidepressant just in case before symptoms set in.

> **Factoid:** Postpartum night sweats are likely caused by shifting hormones. They're common and not serious but can be alarming if you don't know they're coming.

Postpartum Psychosis: This elevated level of threat involves symptoms similar to those of PPD but also includes delusions, hallucinations, and confusion. You might also think that you want to hurt the baby or yourself, and you may not recognize those thoughts as illogical, so the risk of suicide or infanticide is greater than in PPD. Women suffering postpartum psychosis need treatment immediately. Medication and often hospitalization are the typical courses of treatment.

Above all, it's important to note that feeling a little off your game is totally normal—and even expected. But you and your partner need to be aware of the signs and clues to when the baby blues turn a deeper, darker shade.

6. To Cut or Not to Cut?

Is Circumcision the Right Choice?

Early in a baby's life, there are some things that you absolutely have to cut, like the umbilical cord and his fingernails. And there are some things you don't have to cut if you don't want to; his hair, for instance. Also falling into the latter category: foreskin.

There's been a lot of debate around watercoolers and in medical journals about what the right course of action is. Here's what we can tell you. Looking at the research, there does seem to be some evidence that circumcision reduces certain infections, including HIV and other STDs (and reduces transmission of STDs to partners many years hence). But there are no strong data to show that it absolutely must or must not be done; it's an elective procedure, after all. Most parents make the decision based on religious and cultural customs, as well as the simple "what pop looks like" or "what he'll look like in the locker room" arguments.

No matter what you decide, know that a local anesthetic is applied, and because of a baby's immature brain development, it appears that he doesn't process pain the same way as we do—so it's not as if circumcision will leave him with a lasting cross-your-legs feeling.

7. Family Affairs

Keep Your Relationships Going Strong

Oh yeah, just about forgot, didn't you? That you had a pet, other kids, neighbors, and some guy sitting his lazy butt on the couch who picks his nails and snores too loudly. Newborns have that way about them; they make you forget there's a whole other world that still would very much like your attention. Being the amazing woman that you are, however, you will try to balance all of these other people, pets, and plants that don't want you to forget about them. In chapter 7 we provided some suggestions for ways to manage your relationship with your partner; here are some additional ideas for helping your other children (and your pets) manage the family newbie:

Siblings
- *Get Them Involved Early.* Talk to them about what's happening (that is, if they don't notice your growing belly); discuss potential names you're thinking of; even consider a sibling class, which teaches them how to interact with their new brother or sister.

- *Exchange Gifts.* Have the older siblings pick out (or help pick out) an appropriate welcome gift, and then make sure to get a little something for the baby to give to the older ones. It starts the spreading of goodwill.

- *Give Jobs.* Older siblings may want to help a little *too* much sometimes, to the point that it actually slows you down. So give them jobs that can both help you and make them feel involved, like running to get the diapers or talking to the baby while he's getting changed. If your older kids don't want to be involved, don't force them; they're carving out their own space, and the bonding may take a little more time.

- *Be Patient.* Oftentimes, your older children will regress a bit after you bring home a newborn; for example, by going back to pacifiers or taking a U-turn on toilet training. It's a natural reaction, and one that you shouldn't get too upset about. Remember, the older child has gone from a situation in which he was the focus of your world to one in which he has to share your attention, and sometimes it's hard for us to fathom how that truly feels.

- *Provide Special Treats for Siblings.* Arrange special playdates, visits with relatives, or outings (circus, baseball game).

- *Spend Time with the Older Ones.* Leave the baby with a friend, relative, or sitter for a couple of hours and spend one-on-one time with your older children. This assignment is a good challenge for dad too.

Factoid: Many cultures practice what's called "kangaroo care": that is, skin-to-skin contact between parent and newborn. Early on, this method was found to increase the survival rates for low-birth-weight infants. It's now being used as an adjunct to help treat preemies, but you can also use the method to improve the parent-child relationship. It usually involves skin-to-skin contact (his front to your chest) for two to three hours a day, and it's been linked to calmer babies, improved breathing, fewer infections, and better sleep synchronization between mom and child.

Pets

- *Prep the Smell.* Have a friend or partner bring something home from the hospital with the baby's smell on it, like a receiving blanket, and give it to your pet before you return.
- *Introduce the Stranger.* Start carrying a baby doll around the house when you're pregnant; let the pup sniff it and gauge his reaction, so you know what kind of training and limits you need to set.
- *Do the Once-Over.* Make sure that your pet is up to date with all shots and health checks, and get him used to having his nails trimmed, since the only thing in the house with newborns that ought to have long nails is the tool-box in the garage. As you gradually introduce your baby to your pet, reward your pet for good behavior around the baby. Keep plenty of treats handy.

8. Get Your Body Back

How to Manage the War Wounds of Pregnancy

Nine months. Nine beautiful months. Nine months in which your body has been kicked, torn, stretched, jiggled, and put through the gauntlet of all gauntlets. Mighty nice work, you think. *Now give me my body back!!* As much as you enjoyed the pregnancy journey, you're ready to fit back into your old clothes and eliminate the aches that arose during delivery. Some guidelines for making the transition:

Weight and Waist: You see A-list moms who can fit into their skinny jeans mere hours after pregnancy, and you think that you should be able to drop baby weight just like that. But those cases are extremely rare. The smarter approach is the patient approach. Remember that it took you nine months to add the weight, and a realistic goal is for you to take nine months to drop it. Breast-feeding will speed it up, until the very end—most women hang on to the last few pounds until they wean. The key here is, of course, to make sure that you have sound nutrition (see page 286). You can also follow our workout rou-

What's That on Your Leg?

The Vein	The Treatment
Thin, red spider vein.	Laser treatment can remove.
Thick blue vein.	A hypertonic saline solution (one with a high salt content relative to your body's normal salt content) burns the walls of the vein so that it permanently closes.
Big, bulging blue vein.	True varicose veins need to be stripped surgically.

tines starting on page 310. Any good weight-loss program isn't just about the tools but also about your expectations and attitude. Be realistic, make smart choices, and you will once again see the inside of your skinny jeans. One other note: No jogging while carrying an infant; you want to avoid any shaking of her delicate brain.

Wounds: If you have a C-section scar or episiotomy tear, wash the wound briefly with warm water as often as you desire, but keep the wound dry otherwise. Change any dressings as often as they get moist. If you still feel excessive pain after a week to ten days, you should contact your doctor to make sure there are no complications. Also, for episiotomy tears (or if you have hemorrhoids), try soaking in a sitz bath: a bath in which only your hips and buttocks are in the water, with added Epsom salts. This allows more blood to get to the infected area, which should improve healing. You will be given a squirt bottle (known as a peri bottle) to rinse the area after going to the bathroom; you can also use ice packs or witch-hazel pads to soothe the affected tissues. We recommend taking stool softeners to make sure there's little stretching of the area when you're trying to go to the bathroom. (Pressing a towel on the tear during a bowel movement can help relieve some pain by providing counterpressure.)

Abs: No doubt, your belly has been through quite the delivery workout. The only problem is that this workout did more damage than good to your abdominal muscles. The prospect of trying to eliminate your postpregnancy pooch and recover a flat stomach can be daunting. Some women suffer from a condition called diastasis recti, in which the abdominal muscles separate during pregnancy, leading to said pooch. To tell if you have this problem, see if you can gently push your fingers through a gap in your stomach muscles. You can help tighten your abdominal wall by doing some of the exercises we outline in our exercise plan on page 310. But remember, the secret to a flat stomach doesn't center simply around core strength, but also around eating right and avoiding the simple carbohydrates that set up shop on your hips or waist unless you are running marathons to burn the sugar.

Factoid: A baby's first stool is often thick and tarlike because blood from the placenta gets in there and is passed along, but it will soon soften up. Before you can leave the hospital, docs will wait for that first stool—it's a sign that the junctions in the GI tract are working. In some babies, the junction between the anus and the intestines isn't functioning properly, a condition called Hirschsprung's disease.

Dark Spots and Belly Lines: The linea nigra is the dark, vertical line that often appears between the belly button and the pubic area during pregnancy. Hormones, which are also responsible for your darkened areolas, a new crop of freckles, and an impressive variety of other skin anomalies (like the mask of pregnancy★), are behind this weird little stripe. It will usually fade over a few months, but spending time in the sun can permanently tan it. Eating foods containing folic acid might help fade any skin discolorations, so try some leafy green veggies.

★ The mask of pregnancy allows women to retain folic acid by blocking sun, which changes the nature of this critical vitamin.

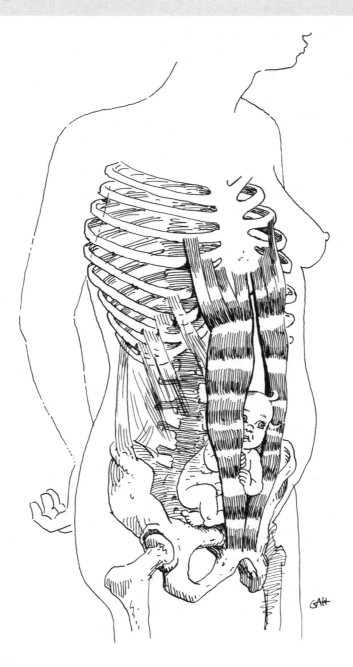

Figure 10.1 **Stomach Turning** Abdominal muscles can get separated during pregnancy (it's called diastasis recti), which can give the appearance of a stomach pooch. Certain abdominal exercises (see page 310) can help rectify the recti.

How to . . . Change a Diaper

No rest for the weary. A baby's first food means a baby's first poop, which means a parent's first diaper change. Use this step-by-step guide to make the first of, oh, seven million changes that you'll be making over the next few years.

- Lay your baby flat and lift his ankles. For boys, put a wipe over the penis to avoid a spray.
- Slide the diaper underneath so that the top of the diaper is even with his belly button.
- Bring the front of the diaper between his legs.
- Unfasten the tabs on the side, point his penis down, and close up.
- Make sure it's snug. Diaper leaks can ruin your day—or at least your carpet.

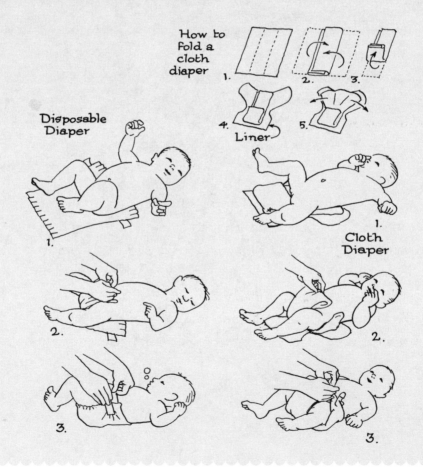

How to Fold a cloth diaper
1. 2. 3. 4. Liner 5.

Disposable Diaper
1.
2.
3.

Cloth Diaper
1.
2.
3.

How to . . . Give the First Bath

Considering that a wet baby feels as slippery as a freshly hooked fish, the first bath can be a little intimidating. Aim to bathe him every two or three days (you can give sponge baths in between), and don't give the first bath until the umbilical cord has fallen off. Use a mild soap, washcloth, and baby shampoo. Use a sink with foam padding or a special infant tub lined with a soft towel (no real tubs until he can sit up himself). Fill it with a few inches of warm water and make sure that it's not too hot. Wipe your baby's face and eyes with water and move down the body, adding soap if you like. Save the diaper area for second to last, and finish up with a warm-water shampoo, using fresh water and a nonstinging shampoo. Washing his hair last will keep him from being cold throughout the entire scrubbing.

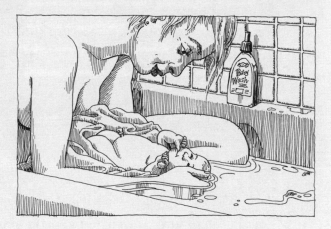

Hair: During pregnancy, with your estrogen at a high level, your hair goes through a strong growing period, but when your estrogen level drops after delivery, your hair will drop into your shower drain. This can start within a few weeks or months and will level off within a year. You can't stop the process, but you can try to minimize the damage by doing scalp massages to increase blood flow to the scalp and stimulate hair follicles, and by avoiding harsh brushes that can tear hair. If the hair loss seems excessive (you're losing clumps more than six months after delivery or developing bald spots), you might want your doc to check your thyroid levels, since thyroid hormone deficiency can be associated with excessive hair loss.

11

Your Pregnancy Plan

Use This Checklist to Arrive at
Life's Most Amazing Destination

We don't care if you've traveled to the top of Everest, to the bottom of the ocean, or to any city, coastline, or monument in any of the 195 countries around the world. We think you'll agree that the most amazing journey of your life is the one that you're taking right now. The coolest part about this trip? The destination is like no other, and it's all yours. When you reach the Promised Land of Parenthood, you'll discover that it's filled with laughter, tears, love, challenges, burps, insomnia, exhaustion, first words, tooth fairies, violin lessons, baseball catches, report cards, Legos, Barbies, driver's ed, and all of the ups, downs, and upside downs that parenthood has to offer.

First things first: You gotta get there, and this is what our plan is all about. In this forty-week flight of pregnancy, you serve as the pilot of a plane (your body) that's carrying one, two, or more VIP passengers. Of course, there are copilots (your partner and/or your doula) and air traffic controllers (your doc or midwife) who will help you arrive safely and sanely. But as you know, the main responsibility for guiding this jet★ falls into your lap (or what used to be a lap). This plan contains everything you need to know—from choosing the best fuel to performing physical inspections—to

★ Note we did not use the phrase "jumbo jet."

have a great takeoff, a smooth ride, and the perfect landing. We'll show you how to weather the storms of stress, and we'll even try to help you put some parts of your life on autopilot so that you can sit back and enjoy all there is to see during this amazing flight.

Before you accuse us of a literary flight delay by beating this metaphor into the tarmac, the comparison does make perfect sense in a very important way: As is the case with flying, the most vulnerable times during a pregnancy are at takeoff (right around conception) and landing (at delivery). Throughout the book, we've given you the background and biology about the way your body works so that you can understand why that's so—and how the things that you do very much influence those beginning and end points. Here you'll find a cheat sheet containing our best advice to help get you to the gate safely and happily. Because after the flight is over and you introduce your very special passenger to the world, that's when the real journey begins.

Please fasten your seat belt and enjoy your flight.

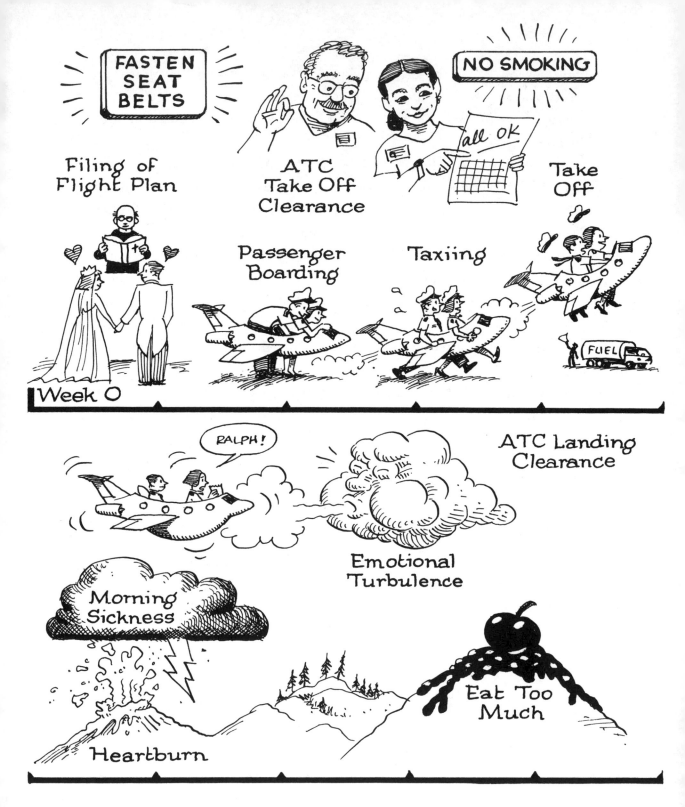

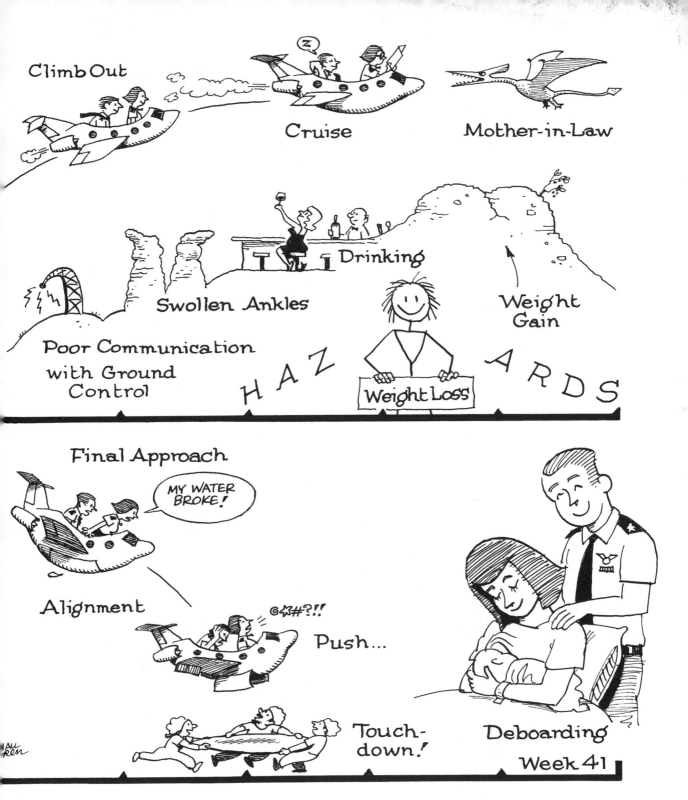

Fuel Levels: Nutrition

If you've read this book (and even if you skipped ahead to this point while sipping on your favorite bookstore-bought beverage), you surely know that the greatest way you can influence the health of your child is through the foods you choose to eat and the ones you choose not to eat. Your nutrition directly influences your child's, as the placenta supplies all the nutrients he needs. The tricky part about pregnancy is that either end of the extreme isn't good. Eat too much or the wrong kind of food, and you run the risk of developing health problems for both you and your child. Eat too little, perhaps because of extreme pregnancy-related nausea, and you might not be supplying your child enough nutrients to develop properly.

While there's certainly an ideal fuel plan, which includes healthy foods, prenatal vitamins, calcium, DHA, and other nutrients, the most important thing to remember is that there's plenty of wiggle room. Forty weeks is a mighty long time, and if on some days you stray from the ideal, that's perfectly normal—and perfectly okay. Your body and your baby are pretty darn resilient. The key is for you to think about your fuel plan over the long run, making as much of an effort as you can to provide the highest-quality fuel that you can.

See more details in chapters 3 and You Tool 5.

Good Fuel

- Fruits
- Leafy green vegetables
- Cruciferous vegetables—broccoli, cauliflower, arugula, cabbage, and Brussels sprouts—help detoxify your liver so that it can metabolize chemicals from the outside world as well as all your raging hormones
- Fish (non-bottom-feeders, especially salmon and trout)
- Lean poultry (skinned and nonfried)
- Lean meat (meat that has less than 4 grams saturated fat per serving; anything with *loin* in the name usually works)
- Legumes

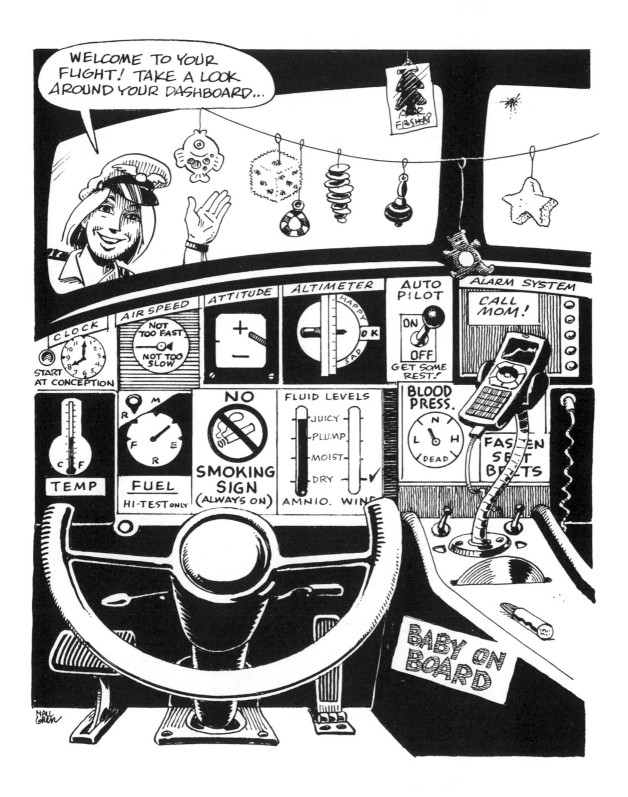

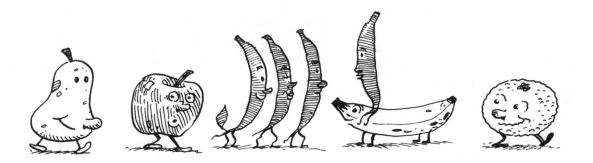

- Beans (with Beano to reduce to accompanying gas cramps)
- Nuts (especially walnuts, which have much higher omega-3 fatty acids content than other nuts)
- Cereal grains
- Low-fat yogurt and pasteurized cheese
- Soy products (tofu, tempeh, edamame)
- Oats
- Whole grain wheat products
- Foods that contain flavonols, like broccoli, radishes, onions, tomatoes
- Organic skim milk (watch calorie counts on alternative milks such as rice milk. You may choose to limit soy milk to one to two glasses daily because of phytoestrogens; there's concern that they cause feminization of the brain and other organs, including sex organs)

Bad Fuel
- Saturated fats (from four-legged animals and palm and coconut oil) and trans fats (anything "partially hydrogenated")
- Simple sugars
- Syrups
- High-fructose corn syrup
- Refined bleached flour or non–100 percent whole grains
- Soda, carbonated drinks
- Bottom-feeding fish such as shark, swordfish, tuna (higher risk of mercury)

- Any foods that have any potential safety issues, like undercooked meats and eggs, and foods where there's any question about refrigeration
- Alcohol
- More than 200 g caffeine (one cup of regular coffee or two cups of black tea) per day

Optimum Daily Fuel Levels
- Nine or more servings (fistfuls) of fruits and vegetables
- Three or more servings of whole grain and other grain products
- Three or more servings of lean protein in the form of poultry, fish, lean meat, eggs, nuts, beans, lentils, and soy
- Five or more grams of fat in the form of omega-3s (like walnuts, flax, or avocados); five grams of omega-9s (olive oil), and five grams of omega-6s (corn and nut oils)

Nausea-Fighting Fuel Plan
Crackers upon waking

Chicken broth

Iced drinks

Cold foods (weaker smell than hot foods, which can trigger queasiness)

Brown rice

Peanut butter (either by the spoonful or on crackers or whole wheat bread with honey and/or banana)★

Baked potato with salsa and/or low-fat sour cream or shredded mozzarella

Hummus and baby carrots

High-fiber cereal with skim milk or low-fat milk

Hot cereal

Yogurt

★ In healthy peanut butter, the oil will separate out from the peanuts. Or try a real nut butter like walnut or almond. Some commercial peanut butter is usually made from the worst nuts, which cannot be sold on their own.

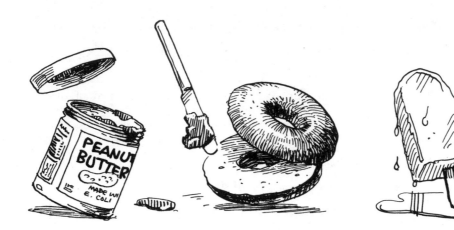

Egg salad	Marinated, baked tofu
Sliced turkey	Pasta with tomato sauce
Bagel and cream cheese	Almonds, walnuts
Rice cakes	Frozen blueberries
Canned soups (low sodium)	Frozen fruit pops

Optimum Vitamin Levels

Vitamins	**Optimum for Pregnant Women**
A	More than 7,500 IU twice a day is too much; watch for extra vitamin A in other fortified products, like protein bars, breakfast bars, and meal-replacement products.
B1 (thiamin)	25 mg
B2 (riboflavin)	25 mg
B3 (niacin)	At least 30 mg
B5 (pantothenic acid)	At least 30 mg
B6 (pyridoxine)	3 mg twice a day
B9 (folic acid)	400 mcg
B12	400 mcg twice a day
Biotin	300 mcg
C	400 mg twice a day. Remember, it's water soluble, so you need two doses over the day.

| D | 600 IU twice a day |
| E | 200 IU twice a day (or, preferably, 200 IU of mixed tocopherols) |

Minerals

Calcium	600 mg three times a day when pregnant; twice a day prior to pregnancy
Iron	15 or 20 mg twice a day while pregnant, and once a day afterwards
Magnesium	200 mg three times a day; twice a day prior to pregnancy
Selenium	100 mcg twice a day
Potassium	Four fruit servings plus a normal diet should do it
Zinc	10 mg twice a day

Additional vitaminlike substances you should get daily:

Lycopene	10 tablespoons (400 mcg) of tomato sauce a week should do it.
Lutein	A leafy green vegetable a day (40 mcg) should do it.
Quercetin	Hefty portions of onion, garlic, celery, or lemon juice in addition to the above at least once a day should do it.
DHA omega-3	A minimum of 200 mg to 300 mg per day through fish, fortified foods, or supplements. More and more prenatal vitamins are including this important nutrient, but double-check to see if your vitamin does. If it doesn't, please discuss with your doctor whether you should get DHA supplements—either standard or especially targeted to pregnant women. Recent research indicates that more DHA omega-3 may be even better; we like 600 mg to 900 mg a day.

Red-Light Toxins: Avoid

- Tobacco.
- Hot dogs, lunch meats, and saturated fats. They contain nitrates and methylates, which unwind DNA that's not supposed to be unwound.
- Alcohol.
- Marijuana.
- Radon. Splurge for a $10 kit and leave it in the basement overnight to check if your house is leaking this dangerous gas from the soil.
- Lead.
- Turpentine, toluene, and paint thinner
- Hard plastic bottles that contain bisphenol-A. (Look for the number 2 or 4, but not 3, 6, 7, 8, or 9 inside the triangle on the bottom of the bottle.) A 1 is acceptable, but it's not reusable.

Note: You can check the Environmental Working Group website (www.foodnews .org) for items that are high on the pesticide content list. And if you want to go more natural and organic, visit the website of Green and Chic (www.greenandchic.com) for products that are environmentally friendly.

Physical Inspection: Your Body

Look out the window of the airport terminal before your flight, and you'll see the captain checking her plane to make sure that everything is in good condition before takeoff. You too should be aware of the physical status of your own body, and you should perform regular checks before and throughout your pregnancy. Get your teeth checked and immunizations updated three months prior to the time you might want to get pregnant, and start the right vitamins at least three months in advance as well. Keeping your body strong through regular physical activity provides the best environment for your child, not to mention that it is preparing you for the physical and mental rigors of caring for a newborn.

See our complete pregnancy workout on page 310.

- We recommend resistance training three times a week. It will help keep your muscles strong, so you can better withstand the demands of pregnancy, as well as those of parenthood. Focus on moves that will keep your core (the muscles in your trunk area) strong. You'll also get more benefits if you do exercises that challenge your balance and make you work one arm or leg at a time. See our program starting on page 310 and our pregnancy videos (named after this book), which include specific workouts for each trimester as well as routines to prepare your muscles for the marathon of childbirth and to regain your fitness and shape after delivery.

- Walk, walk, walk. There may be times when you're tired, whupped, and feel as if you've been run over by a gaggle of baby carriages. The last thing you want to do is exercise, and that's totally understandable. But most times, you should be able to manage a walk. Aim for thirty minutes a day to help keep your energy level up and maintain a moderate level of fitness.

- If your back or knees or any other part of your body is feeling especially achy, we recommend swimming or water aerobics. In fact, we recommend them even if you don't feel achy. Take advantage of your increased buoyancy; water not only provides a good environment for your baby but will help you maintain your fitness in a safe and virtually injury-free environment.

- Tighten up your pelvic area. We recommend doing the exercises on page 326 daily. They help strengthen your entire pelvic floor, which will help you withstand the demands of labor and help you bounce back after pregnancy.

- Monitor your weight gain (and thus your risk of weight-related troubles). Don't sweat over daily numbers, because there's too much daily fluctuation when you're carrying. Instead weigh yourself weekly and track your progress over each trimester. Major differences, both up and down, warrant discussion with your doc or midwife. See page 68 for guidelines on optimal weight gain based on your prepregnancy size.

Turbulence: Stress Levels

We all prefer flights where there's absolutely no turbulence: no bumps, no seat belt tightening, no jitters. In most cases, the problem isn't the turbulence, it's the fear of the unknown—the thought that something bad is going to happen, when it's simply just a bit of a rough patch. Pregnancy works the same way: Stressors are just rough patches, and the best way to avoid stress is to prepare for the expected challenges and minimize the unexpected. Here are some preventive measures that you can take, trimester by trimester, to keep your stress to a minimum.

See more details on the biology of stress, anxiety, and depression in chapter 6.

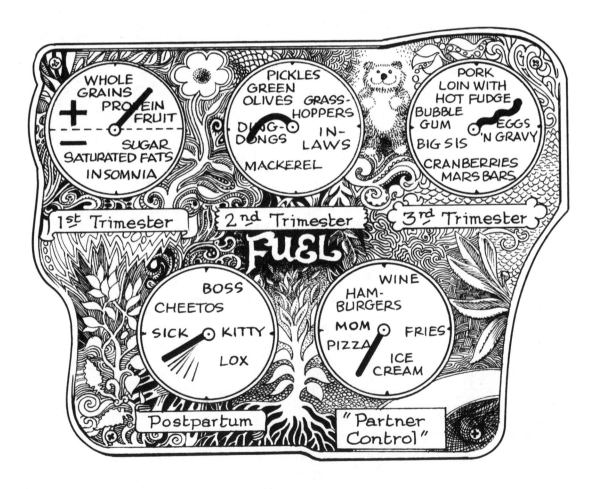

Preconception and First Trimester

- Choose a doctor or midwife whose values and reputation match what you are looking for (see page 335). Ask acquaintances for recommendations, or call the labor and delivery floor and ask nurses or staff whom they would see if they were having a baby.

- Have appropriate prenatal screening tests recommended by your provider (more details below).

- Discuss the impact of any meds you may be taking (blood pressure, antidepressants, and so on) and whether you need to switch to an alternative in order to minimize the impact on your pregnancy .

- Contact your health insurance company and know the scope and details of your plan's benefits.

- Aim for at least seven hours of sleep nightly: record your favorite late-night TV shows, watch them in the early evening, and get to bed early; catch a nap during the day.

- Enlist your partner to help with housework and pet care (especially with the cat litter, even though if you thoroughly cleanse your hands after changing the litter box, you have no increased risk of contracting toxoplasmosis), or treat yourself to some household help if you can afford it.

- Take up a relaxing, low- or nonimpact exercise such as prenatal yoga, swimming, or walking.

- Tell one person at work that you are expecting, so she can cover for you when you need to go for a checkup or escape to the ladies' room for a nap.

- If you will need to move before baby is born, start looking now and try to move before the third trimester.

Second Trimester

- Meet with HR at work to discuss maternity leave policy and formulate a plan.
- Seek out at least one support person you can confide in who has been through pregnancy before: mother, sister, friend.
- Seek support from other pregnant women, either online (at www.realage.com/youhavingababy; or the website Pregnancy and Children, developed by the nonprofit agency Adoption Services, at www.pregnancyandchildren .com) or in person. Prenatal exercise classes are a great place to meet other moms-to-be, as is your local Y or even your doc's or midwife's practice.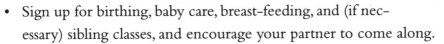
- Sign up for birthing, baby care, breast-feeding, and (if necessary) sibling classes, and encourage your partner to come along.
- Spend time with your partner. Go on dates or just relax together. Remember to keep romance in your relationship; it's a sure way to stay connected during a distracting time.
- Treat yourself to a prenatal massage by an experienced masseur.
- Listen to music that brings joy or calm to your life.
- If you have long-standing issues with your mother, try to deal with them, either by yourself or with the support of a professional.

Third Trimester

- Tour the hospital.
- Get the nursery ready: Buy supplies and decorate, but have your partner paint and lay the carpet.
- Interview doulas if you will be using one.

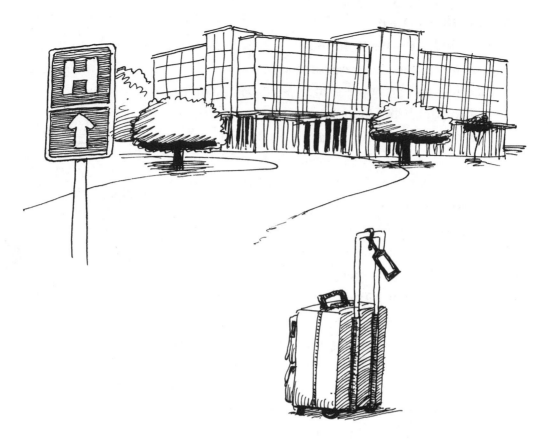

- Choose a pediatrician. (See page 339.)
- Plan for assistance immediately postpartum (doula, baby nurse, nanny, grandma) and for care of other siblings and pets while you are at the hospital.
- If you will be using day care, reserve a spot even if you don't plan to return to work for several months.
- Practice good sleep hygiene.
- Prepare your baby supplies (see page 345).
- Pack your bag for the hospital.
- Prepare meals for the freezer or get a good supply of take-out menus (meals are a great baby shower gift!).
- Discuss baby names with your partner or use our baby naming program at www.realage.com.

Copilot To-Do List

- Deal with the wheels: If you drive a pickup or subcompact, you should upgrade to a four-door car, since newborns can't ride in the front seat. Also, make sure that you have a safety-approved infant car seat prior to your baby's arrival.
- If you haven't already, contact a lawyer and write wills and health proxies; also, if appropriate, establish trusts.
- If you do not already carry life insurance, consider purchasing a policy.
- Help out around the house as much as possible: cooking, cleaning, laundry, child care, pet care.
- Be a sympathetic listener.
- Discuss with your partner what role she wants you to play at delivery (see page 233) and which special items she may want during labor (photos, candles, music).

Postpartum

- Sleep (or at least rest) when the baby sleeps.
- Delegate or ignore all nonessential tasks.
- If you don't regularly rely on housekeeping help, invest in a weekly house cleaner for the first few weeks (another great shower gift!).
- Monitor your moods.
- Enlist breast-feeding support, if necessary. Lactation consultants are often available at hospitals and birthing clinics; others make house calls. Info is also available through La Leche League International (www.llli.org).
- Limit visitors—ideally, to those who are helping you.
- Get out of the house and go for a stroll—with or without baby.
- Join a new-moms group (check your local Y) or mommy-and-me exercise group (such as Strollercize).

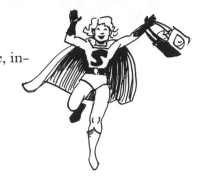

- If you plan to return to work and use in-home child care, interview nannies.
- Ask for help; don't try to be Supermom.
- Relax, trust your instincts, and enjoy being a mom!

Air Traffic Control: The Role of Docs and Midwives

It's pretty amazing how hundreds of flights go into and out of airports every day, taking off and landing at intervals that seem like mere seconds. Pilots can't do it alone; they need the help, guidance, and expertise of air traffic controllers, who can see the big picture of what's happening in the skies all around them. Your traffic controllers (docs, nurses, midwives, and other supporters) are there to do the same thing: to help guide you, to help steer you in a different direction if need be, and to keep the big picture in mind. We want you to understand what they do and that it is perfectly, absolutely, undeniably A-OK for you to call if and when you need their guidance.

Ideally, you should have a preconceptual (yup, you heard that right) visit with your provider to make sure that you are in optimal health before becoming pregnant. But don't worry if you discover that you are pregnant before having a chance to meet with your doctor or midwife; these conversations and tests will occur during your first prenatal visit. Most women's first prenatal visit occurs between six and eight weeks after the first day of their last menstrual period. As long as your pregnancy is considered low risk and is progressing normally, you will visit your doctor monthly for the first twenty-eight weeks, then every two weeks until thirty-six weeks, and weekly thereafter. If you go beyond forty weeks, your doctor will want to see you once or twice a week until you give birth.

To help find a doctor or midwife, see page 335.

To help find a doctor or midwife, see page 335.

Note: Weight, blood pressure, and urine samples are taken at all visits.

Preconceptual Visit or First Prenatal Visit

- Health history.
- Immunization history. Ideally, you should be up to date at least three months prior to pregnancy so that you do not contract immunization-preventable infections while you are carrying. Being immunized will also help you pass healthy antibodies to your child during breast-feeding.
- Partner's health history.
- Health history of close family members and direct blood relatives: father, mother, sisters, brothers, grandparents.
- Discussion of any medical problems you may have and medications you may be taking.
- Conversation about drug, alcohol, and/or tobacco use.
- Assessment of risks for exposure to communicable diseases through sexual practices, work, travel, or changing the cat litter.
- Physical exam, including weight and blood pressure.
- Pelvic exam and Pap smear to check for cervical cancer and other infections.
- Urine sample to test for infection, protein content, and sugar.
- Blood sample for blood type, Rh status, anemia, syphilis, hepatitis B, immunity to rubella (German measles), immunity to chicken pox (if you can't remember having had it), and HIV. The last test is optional but recommended and is mandatory for pregnant women in certain states, as the risk of transmission can be decreased by altering regular obstetrical practices.
- Depending on your ethnic background and medical history, a blood sample may be taken to assess risk for genetic disorders such as cystic fibrosis, sickle-cell disease, thalassemia, Tay-Sachs, and diseases common to those of certain patterns of ancestry.
- A tuberculosis skin test may be offered if it hasn't been done in recent years or if you have a history that suggests exposure to the TB bacteria.
- A prescription for prenatal vitamins with folic acid and a DHA supplement.

First Prenatal Visit

- A test to confirm pregnancy (may be urine or blood).
- Determination of due date based on the first day of your last menstrual period. If you are uncertain, an early ultrasound may be done to confirm the dates of your pregnancy.
- Discussion of nutritional, exercise, and sexual guidelines; appropriate weight gain; common symptoms of pregnancy and those that require immediate attention—both emotional and physical.
- Glucose challenge test if you're at high risk for diabetes (family history, obesity), you have a prior incidence of gestational diabetes, or you previously had a very large baby.
- Your provider may perform an ultrasound to refine your due date and look for a fetal heartbeat.

Second-Trimester Visits

- Beginning with your twelve-week visit, your provider will listen for your fetus's heartbeat.
- Your provider will check your hands, feet, and face for swelling; if at risk, you'll undergo a workup for preeclampsia.
- Beginning at your twenty-week visit, your provider will measure your abdomen to check the fetus's growth.

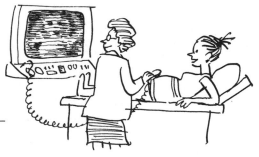

- Between eighteen and twenty weeks, a sonogram is commonly done to see whether your baby's health and growth are progressing normally.
- Between twenty-four and twenty-eight weeks, every pregnant woman receives a glucose screening test for gestational diabetes.
- Your provider may check your blood once more for anemia.
- Blood test for Rh antibodies if you are Rh-negative and your partner is Rh-positive or unknown; if antibodies are not detected, you will be given an injection of Rh immune globulin at twenty-eight weeks.

- In addition, your provider will ask questions to ensure that you are staying in good mental and physical health as your pregnancy progresses. For instance, you'll be asked about fetal movement and the pattern that is developing, so that you can learn to monitor this important health tool.

Third-Trimester Visits
- Your provider will continue to monitor the fetal heartbeat at every visit and document your perception of consistent fetal movement.
- Continue to monitor the growth of the fetus by belly measurement.
- Check for swelling of your hands, feet, and face.
- Check the fetus's position. If it's not in head-down position near the time of delivery, your provider will offer you options.
- Check the adequacy of your pelvis for vaginal delivery and the condition of your cervix.
- If your glucose screening test showed high blood sugar, you will be administered a glucose challenge test.
- Between thirty-five and thirty-seven weeks, as part of a pelvic exam, you will be screened for the presence of group B streptococcus in your vagina.
- If you were anemic early in your pregnancy or didn't have your blood checked in the second trimester, you may have your blood tested again for anemia.
- If you are at high risk for sexually transmitted diseases, you will be re-tested.
- If you had placenta previa or low-lying placenta earlier in your pregnancy, you will have another ultrasound to determine the location of the placenta, and the delivery mode will be planned as necessary.
- If your pregnancy is high risk or you experience certain problems, you may have a biophysical profile or nonstress test to help with decisions about the timing of your delivery.
- If you go past your due date, your provider will conduct an ultrasound to check the amount of amniotic fluid and may also order a nonstress test or biophysical profile to determine the baby's condition. These tests may be

given once or twice a week until you either go into labor naturally or are induced.

Prenatal Tests

In every pregnancy, there is a chance of having a baby with a birth defect or a genetic condition. You and your doctor will discuss which screening and/or diagnostic tests are appropriate for you, depending on your risk factors.

Screening Tests

Screening tests are not designed to diagnose a genetic syndrome but to provide a more accurate risk estimate for certain conditions, such as Down syndrome. There's no test (as of now) available during pregnancy that will rule out all possible genetic diseases and guarantee a healthy baby (see box on the carrier test). If you have any concerns regarding diseases that run in your family, it may be worthwhile to meet with a genetic counselor to discuss the risks for your baby and appropriate testing options during pregnancy.

Common screening tests include:

- First-trimester screening. Typically consists of blood work and an ultrasound to measure the thickness of the skin at the back of the fetus's neck (called nuchal translucency), which indicates if there's a risk that the fetus has Down syndrome.
- Maternal serum screening, sometimes called a quadruple check, which is performed in the second trimester.
- Combined test using components of the first two.
- Screening for a group of common birth defects, called open neural tube defects, can be performed between fifteen and twenty weeks by measuring a chemical, called alpha fetal protein, in the mother's blood.

The Universal Carrier Screening Test

Genetic diseases can affect 3 to 4 percent of all children, but many of these conditions remain hidden in our DNA until a man and woman sharing the same grave genetic defect have a child. Now, modern science is enabling us to analyze the DNA extracted from a mother and father's saliva or blood, to see if they carry the gene mutations that lead to serious genetic diseases. (Testing for just one genetic disease today can cost from several hundred to several thousand dollars, and many conditions are so rare, testing for them does not make sense unless you know that you are in a high-risk group.) Thanks to recent advances in genetic sequencing technology, comprehensive carrier screening is now available. A nonprofit organization called the Beyond Batten Disease Foundation is working in partnership with the National Center for Genome Resources to create a low-cost universal carrier screening test for 400 of the most devastating genetic diseases. It's the first time that you can be tested for so many diseases at once at a cost of less than $500. Beginning in early 2010, the test will be available to potential parents through their healthcare providers. For more info about the test, please visit www.beyondbatten.org or call 1-877-6BATTEN.

- A comprehensive ultrasound evaluation in the second trimester, typically performed between eighteen and twenty weeks, evaluates growth, screens for birth defects, and looks for any physical markers suggestive of a chromosomal abnormality.

Diagnostic Tests

Diagnostic tests differ from screening tests in that they can provide a yes or no answer about certain genetic conditions. Diagnostic tests include:

- Chorionic villus sampling (also called CVS) in the first trimester, typically performed between ten and twelve weeks. (See page 54.) A small sample of cells, which contain the same genetic information as the baby, is removed from the developing placenta and analyzed to detect chromosomal problems.

- Amniocentesis is typically performed between sixteen and twenty weeks. About 2 tablespoons of amniotic fluid, containing some of the baby's cells, are removed. From these cells, a picture of the baby's chromosomes (also called a karyotype) can be made; this can rule out a number of genetic syndromes. Using the fluid from the amniocentesis, screening can also be performed for open neural tube defects.

Passenger Status: Fetal Development

At an airport, the passenger screening comes before the flight. In your pregnancy journey, screening actually happens before the pregnancy (ideally) or at the first visit and continues throughout the flight. Of course, much of that screening falls into your provider's hands (see above), but you too can be on alert for signs and signals that your passenger is uncomfortable. (In this case, you, the pilot, also have to assume the role of flight attendant to help your passenger get what he or she needs.) These are some checks you can perform to make sure that things are progressing the way they should be:

- In the middle of the second trimester, you'll become aware of your baby's movement patterns. This serves as a powerful tool to determine whether he's contented or if the environment of the womb may be uncomfortable. Your doc or midwife will provide guidelines for calling her if you perceive any significant change in your baby's movement.
- When your baby is growing normally and maintaining the right amount of amniotic fluid, you'll notice that you need to wear larger jeans. If this is not happening, call your provider. She will monitor the size of your belly at visits, but between visits, you're in charge. To measure the size of the baby yourself, see page 101.

- Monitor yourself for leaks or discharges. If you start to leak urinelike fluid through your vagina and you are not near your due date, you should call your OB. If it is tinged with blood, it may be a signal that your body is preparing to go into labor. If you detect an unusual odor, or if the fluid is bloody and heavy, call your provider immediately; you may be advised to have someone drive you to the hospital to get it checked out.

Safe Landing: Labor and Delivery

The approach to your final destination can be the most nerve-racking experience of the entire trip. Whether you're giving birth in a hospital, your home, or a tub of warm water, your first time can be a tough one—emotionally and physically—mainly because it's all a big unknown. We suggest you review our labor and delivery game on page 224 to get a picture of all the possible situations that can come up. In the meantime, use this checklist to do as much as you can to prepare for the big event.

- Develop a flexible birthing plan. While we admire any pregnant woman who comes up with a birthing plan describing in detail how she wants her delivery to go, we know from experience that you need to be somewhat flexible, because life is unpredictable. The best approach: Pick a birthing team that shares your values and philosophies. (See how to choose a provider on page 335.) In collaboration with your doc or midwife, you can then decide what kind of overall birth you want to have; for instance, a home birth with only calming words for pain management versus an elective C-section with lots of pain management—you get the idea.
- Tour the facilities where you're going to have the baby. The more you can familiarize yourself with the whos, whats, and wheres, the more comfortable and relaxed you'll be during delivery—and that plays a huge role in how your experience goes.
- Decide who is going to be in the delivery room with you for the birth.

- Have your bag packed and ready to go. (See complete list on page 249.) There's nothing worse than scrambling to find your fuzzy slippers when contractions are coming fast and furious. Enlist your significant other to make sure that the bag gets there at approximately the same time you do and before junior does. Don't forget to include some nonessential items (like photos of your family) too.

- Know your pain management options well before you actually need to employ one of them. (See our list on page 230.)

- Discuss options for banking cord blood. We support this practice (see page 246), but you'll need to make the decision well before delivery, so that the delivery team can take care of it at the time of the birth.

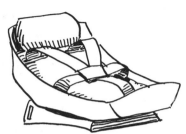

- Have your safety-approved car seat ready to go (more on page 345). No seat, no child coming home.

Taxi to Gate: Postpartum Issues

Once you've landed safely and the ten fingers and ten toes have all been accounted for, the real journey begins. In the first part of your parenthood journey—say, taxiing from the runway to the gate, or the first month or so after delivery—there are a number of issues you'll need to focus on to give the best care to your child, as well as to yourself.

See more details on postpartum issues in chapter 10.

- Decide whether or not to breast-feed. We enthusiastically support breast-feeding for all babies, though we recognize there are reasons why a mom may choose not to. The health benefits of breast-feeding for both you and your baby are enormous. If you're having trouble, you don't have to give up; you'll find some solutions for common problems on page 252, and there are lactation consultants at the hospital to help you. If you are destined for formula, ensure that it contains DHA to help your baby's brain.

- One of the great challenges you'll have early on is dealing with sleeping and feeding issues. Although you will need to wake up to feed your baby frequently at first, you can immediately take steps to help him distinguish night from day. Most important, you want to teach your child to soothe himself to go to sleep, so that he doesn't learn to rely on rocking or binkies or other crutches that will just make sleeping a bigger challenge as he gets older. (For more advice on sleeping, see page 261.)

- Use the chart on page 266 to keep your eyes on potential health problems that can occur in the month after delivery. There's never harm in calling your doctor if you're unsure of something or something doesn't feel quite right. A mother's instinct can be one of a physician's most powerful diagnostic tools.

- Don't neglect yourself. While you're certainly focusing the vast majority of your attention on your newborn, you don't want to put yourself at the back of the line. That means you need to keep an eye on potential medical problems that can affect new moms (see page 269) and monitor your own mental and physical health.

12

Your Pregnancy Toolbox

Essential Strategies for Improving
the Health of You and Your Child

No matter what kind of work we do, we all need special tools to help us do our jobs better. A plumber's toolbox contains wrenches, a chef's toolbox includes knives and measuring cups, and a teacher's toolbox may feature flash cards, microscopes, and gallons of glue. A pregnant woman also has her own special set of tools: specifically, knowledge, motivation, and action. Throughout this book, we've given you a lot to think about and act upon when it comes to figuring how your and your baby's bodies work together. Here we're going to add to your toolbox and give you a few more guidelines that can help you improve your chances of having the healthiest and safest pregnancy possible.

YOU TOOL 1

EXERCISE

We all know that pregnancy is not the time to be thinking about running ultramarathons, flattening your belly, or training for the Iditarod. But that doesn't mean that you should throw out exercise altogether. In fact, it's more important than ever, as you strengthen your body to handle the rigors of pregnancy, labor, and motherhood.

The aim is to stay fit and flexible. It's not about trying to get faster or lift more weight, it's about knowing that slow and steady wins the race. After all, pregnancy is a marathon, not a sprint, and anything you can do to build your endurance and improve your blood flow will help you make it to the twenty-sixth mile.

Here you'll find three exercise programs: one whole-body workout for during pregnancy, one short program to prepare for specific labor and delivery positions, and one to start immediately after giving birth. Please see the box on page 332 for precautions about starting any exercise program while pregnant or postpartum.

Workouts designed and written by Tracy Hafen and Joel Harper
(www.fitpackdvd.com).

PREGNANCY WORKOUT

Start with one-pound handheld weights, or no weights if you haven't exercised previously, and gradually increase the weight when the entire workout seems easy to accomplish. Increase the resistance by one-pound increments if possible, and don't increase more than once per week or use weights over five pounds. Whenever you have weights in your hands, keep your hands in sight, and always breathe. Perform two or three days a week and not on consecutive days.

Estimated time: less than thirty minutes depending on how much you want to do. See www.realage.com, doctoroz.com, and fitpackdvd.com to order a DVD that includes workouts for each trimester and another for right after delivery.

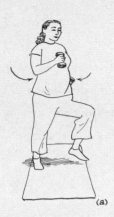

1. Marching Mom

(warms up your entire body)

Walk in place with lifted knees for thirty seconds. Swing your arms with your elbows at right angles. Keep your shoulders relaxed, down away from your ears. Remember to keeps your hands in sight. Take nice, deep breaths. Use your knees and ankles as cushions, and think floating, not pounding.

2. Rocky Mom

(warms up shoulders and arms, and increases muscular endurance)

Stand with your feet shoulder-width apart, knees barely bent, and hands at the sides of your waist, palms up. Start with your left arm and punch straight out in front of your chest, rotating your arm as you do, so that your palm faces down at the end of the punch. Alternate arms and punch twenty times with each arm. You can use furniture for balance; sometimes your center of balance may feel off. (*Advanced: Simultaneously kick your heel up toward your buttocks, using the same leg as arm.*)

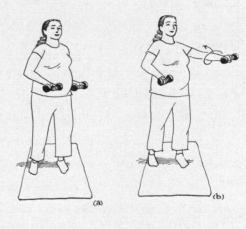

3. Overhead Punch

(warms up legs, shoulders, and arms; also helps with balance and muscular endurance)

While in a semilunge with your left foot forward and holding your left hand weight up by your left shoulder, elbow pointing down, punch straight up with your right hand. If you want to work more with balance, come up and down on your back toe as you punch up. Be slow and deliberate; no bouncing or flinging. Do ten times with each arm and then switch so your right leg is forward and repeat.

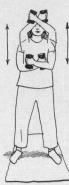

4. Car Seat Carry

(conditions biceps and shoulders)

Stand with your feet shoulder-width apart and your knees barely bent. Cross your arms at your wrists in an *X* in front of you, like a shield, with palms facing you. Lift and lower your arms in unison ten times. Then switch the front arm to the back and repeat with ten more times. Use furniture for balance if necessary. (*Advanced: Balance on your toes.*)

5. Lullaby Baby

(conditions arms and shoulders, and adds core stability and balance)

Stand with your feet shoulder-width apart and your knees barely bent. Cross your arms at your wrists in an *X* in front of you, like a shield, with palms facing you. Swing and lift your arms to your upper left side, then down in front of your belly, and then to your upper right side. Go back and forth ten times, then switch arms for

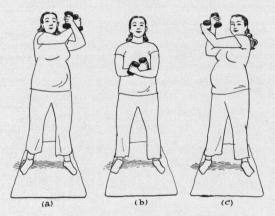

(a)   (b)   (c)

ten more. (*Advanced: To work balance, straighten the leg opposite the side you are coming up on; resist arching your back and keep a neutral spine.*)

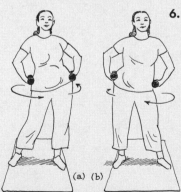

(a) (b)

6. Baby-Go-Round

(relaxes hips and back)

With feet shoulder-width apart and weighted hands on your waist, rotate your hips in a circular motion five times in each direction. Concentrate on elongating your spine and pulling the top of your head away from your tailbone as far as you can.

7. Car Seat Reaches

(works core, back, and arms)

While in a left-foot-forward lunge with arms out in front of you at shoulder height, put your left palm up and right palm down six inches above. Reach out shoulder height at a diagonal to your left, the front, and then right and front ten times. Switch so that your right leg is forward and your right palm is up and left palm is down; do ten more. (*Advanced: Lunge down with each reach and come up between reaches.*)

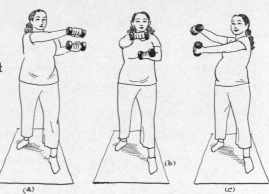

(a) (b) (c)

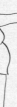

(a) (b)

8. Swing

(strengthens upper body and mobilizes shoulders)

Stand with your feet slightly apart and your knees soft, with arms by your sides. Hold in your tummy and raise your left arm to the front and your right arm to the back, palms facing each other. Stop just below shoulder height. Don't swing your arms; control the movement. Lower your arms to the starting position and bring your left arm to the back and your right arm to the front. Repeat twenty times, switching arms each time. Keep your hips facing forward.

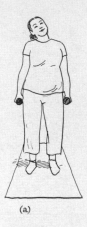 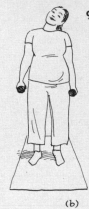

(a) (b)

9. Listening for Baby

(helps relieve neck and shoulder tension)

With your feet directly below your knees and continuing to hold your hand weights relaxed down at your side, inhale. As you exhale, slowly tilt your head to the right until you feel a stretch in your neck. Hold for two deep breaths. Slowly bring your head to the center, then tilt your head to the left. Hold while you breathe deeply two times. Repeat.

10. Crib Time

(strengthens back and arms)

Stand in a partial lunge with your left foot in front. Lean forward slightly at your hips. Rotate your torso barely to the left, so that your right shoulder is a little in front of the left, and let your arms hang straight down from your shoulders, with the palms facing each other. Use a rowing motion to pull your elbows up and back, lifting the weights to the sides of your rib cage ten times. Repeat with the right leg in front and the left shoulder forward. Keep the natural arch in your lower back throughout the exercise. (*Advanced: Do a full lunge as you lower the weights and come up as you row back; make sure that your front knee always stays above your ankle and does not move forward past your big toe.*)

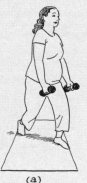 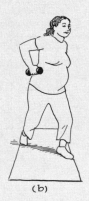

(a) (b)

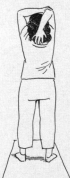

11. Back Scratch

(stretches upper back and triceps)

Without weights, grab your right elbow above your head with your left hand and slowly walk your right hand down your back. When you feel the stretch, hold for three deep breaths. Relax your shoulders down away from your ears. Repeat on the other side.

12. Supermom

(strengthens shoulders, butt, back of upper leg, and back; improves balance)

With feet together and hands at your sides, lift your left foot off the ground. Once you have your balance, lift your right arm up in front of you to shoulder height and simultaneously extend your left leg behind you, keeping your toes two to six inches from the floor. Bring your arm and leg back to the starting position between repetitions. Do ten and then switch sides. Think length rather than height as you reach. *(Advanced: Lift both arms simultaneously and keep your back foot lifted between repetitions.)*

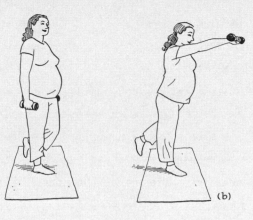

(a)　　　　　　　(b)

13. Pelvic Tilt

(lengthens the lower back and strengthens abs)

Stand comfortably with weighted arms relaxed down at your sides. Slowly tilt your pelvis back (tuck your hips under) by contracting your lower abdominals to lift your pubic bone up toward your navel as your lower back flattens and lengthens. Visualize your hips as the rim of a fishbowl; you want to spill water out the back only. Do five times.

14. Up the Stairs

(strengthens lower body and conditions arms and shoulders)

Rest the weights on opposite upper arms with your elbows up in front of you like a genie. Step back with your right foot into a mini left lunge and then lift your right knee up in front of you fifteen times. Switch sides and do fifteen more. Make sure that your back foot points directly forward on the mini lunge. Keep your upper body still and erect throughout the exercise. (*Advanced: Take a deeper lunge and straighten the lifted leg in front of you with the foot a few inches off the floor.*)

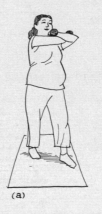
(a)

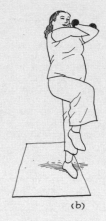
(b)

15. Two Things at Once

(stretches shoulders and upper back)

Stand with your feet shoulder-width apart, knees slightly bent. Reach both of your arms to the left at shoulder height while looking over your right shoulder. Hold the stretch and take three deep breaths. Moving slowly, reverse sides, reaching to the right while looking over your left shoulder. Repeat once. Keep your shoulders relaxed and down, and for variety during the pose, twist your hands in unison.

16. Soccer Mom

(strengthens legs, hips, and buttocks)

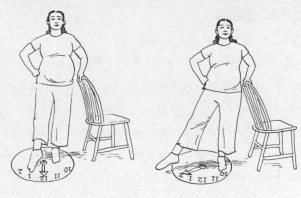

Hold on to a chair for balance. Lift your right leg forward, toe pointed, until it's high enough to give you a little challenge. Pause. Then bring your right leg back to the starting position with your foot flexed and then lift it at a two o'clock angle with the toe pointed. Pause. Repeat ten times and then switch legs. Try to keep your leg straight and lift only as high as you can without tucking your pelvis under or feeling discomfort in or near your hips. Keep the natural arch in your lower back at all times.

17. Seated Curtsy

(stretches hip muscles)

Sit in a sturdy chair and lift your left leg up, placing your left ankle on top of your right knee. Maintaining a straight spine, rest your left hand on your left knee. Take your right hand and gently pull up your left foot as if you wanted to look at the bottom of your foot. If you don't feel any stretch in this position, gently press your left knee down and think of a string pulling your lower back gently toward your calf. Take four deep meditational breaths, then switch sides and repeat with your right leg up. If you are not feeling the stretch, place your elbow on your up knee and lean farther forward; resist arching your back.

18. Twin Scoop

(conditions biceps and shoulders)

While seated and with your elbows slightly back and chest lifted, curl your arms up (palms facing each other). Do fifteen times. Then turn your palms up, extend your elbows away from your hips, and curl fifteen times. Then bring your arms in front of you so that your upper arms are parallel to the floor and curl for another fifteen. Finish with alternating side to forward, side, forward, and so on, fifteen times. Keep your back neutral and abs engaged. If you need support, rest your sacrum (the bottom of your spine) and upper back against the back of the chair. Keep your heels directly below your knees.

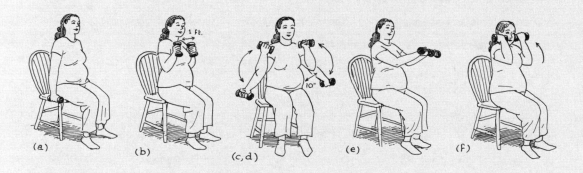

(a)   (b)   (c,d)   (e)   (f)

19. Ladybug Reach

(lengthens chest, neck, and arm muscles)

While standing, place your fingers on your shoulders and raise your elbows to your sides, shoulder height. As you inhale, reach out with one arm, making an arc with your hand. Follow the moving hand with your gaze. Focus on opening your chest. Exhale and bring your fingers back to the top of your shoulder. Alternate sides, five times each arm.

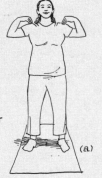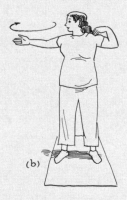

(a)   (b)

20. Pie Out of the Oven

(strengthens lower and upper body)

Stand, using a chair for support if needed, with your feet a little wider than shoulder-width apart and your legs turned out with your toes pointing slightly outward. Place your hands at your hip bones, palms facing up. Squat, taking your hips slightly back and down toward the floor and keeping your knees pointing in the same direction as your toes. As you squat, reach your arms forward from your hips and

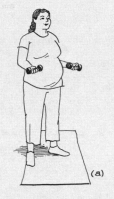 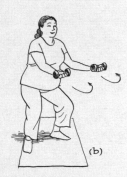

circle them upward and back in as you press yourself up, as if you were taking a pie out of the oven. Do fifteen times. After the last one, hold the squat position with weights on your hips for ten counts and do five Kegels (see page 216), squeezing the muscles you use to control your urine flow. Hold for two counts each. Maintain normal breathing. (*Advanced: Do biceps curls while in the hold.*)

21. Pedicure Reach

(stretches hamstring and calf muscles)

While sitting on the floor with your legs straight out in front of you, place your left leg with bent knee on top of your right straight leg and relax it there. While maintaining a straight spine, lean forward and reach your hands out in front of you at shoulder height. Take notice of your right foot and imagine that the sole of your foot is flush against a board. Pull the toes of your bottom foot straight back toward your knee. Take three deep breaths and switch sides.

22. Kicking Toys

(strengthens obliques and legs)

Lie down on your left side and rest your head
on your left hand or upper arm with your
hips flexed and your knees bent at a
45-degree angle so that your heels are

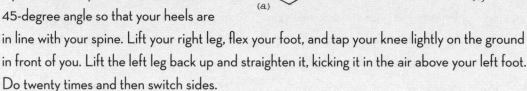

(a)　　　　　　　　　　　　(b)

in line with your spine. Lift your right leg, flex your foot, and tap your knee lightly on the ground
in front of you. Lift the left leg back up and straighten it, kicking it in the air above your left foot.
Do twenty times and then switch sides.

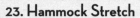

23. Hammock Stretch

(stretches hip muscles and hamstrings)

Sit on the floor with your hands behind you and your palms down,
fingers pointing backward, and elbows slightly bent. Place your
feet flat on the floor roughly two feet from your tailbone. Cross
your right leg on top of your left leg so that your right ankle is just above
your knee. Sit up straight. Focus on pressing your lower back toward your calf.
If you want a deeper stretch, gently press your right knee away from you. Hold for five seconds
and then switch sides.

24. Seesaw Abs

(strengthens core muscles)

While sitting on the ground with your legs bent
90 degrees and your feet on the floor, place
your hands behind your thighs for support.
Slowly lean back to activate your
abdominal muscles, and use them to
gently pull your belly button in. Hold the

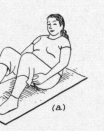
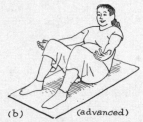

(a)　　　　　(b)　　　　(advanced)

position for five counts; do it five times. (*Advanced: Instead of using your arms for support,
extend your arms out to your sides.*)

25. Ballet Mom

(stretches muscles along trunk)

While seated with your legs in a V shape, place your left hand on the floor at your side and reach your right arm straight up over your head, leaning your upper body to the left while reaching up and over to the left with your right arm. Focus on reaching up more than over, so that both sides of your trunk stay elongated. Hold for two breaths and switch sides. Do two times.

26. Child's Pose

(stretches and releases your lower back and spine)

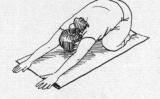

Kneel with your knees shoulder-width apart. Drop your hips toward your heels, placing your belly between your thighs and relaxing your head to the floor. Make sure that you do not rest your weight on your forehead and neck. You should avoid this pose if you have knee problems. Hold this pose for twenty seconds to two minutes. Perform Kegels during the pose.

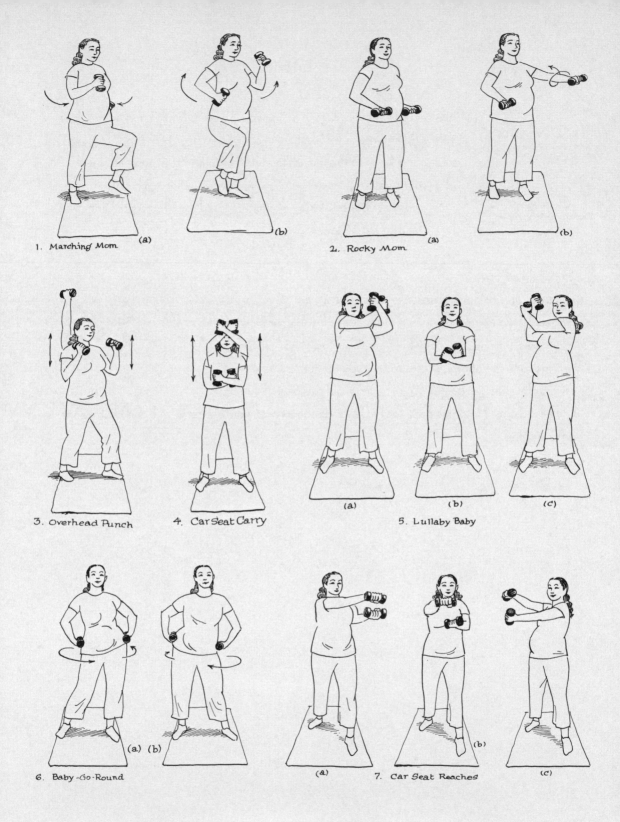

1. Marching Mom (a)

(b)

2. Rocky Mom (a)

(b)

3. Overhead Punch

4. Car Seat Carry

5. Lullaby Baby

(a)   (b)   (c)

6. Baby-Go-Round (a) (b)

7. Car Seat Reaches

(A)   (b)   (c)

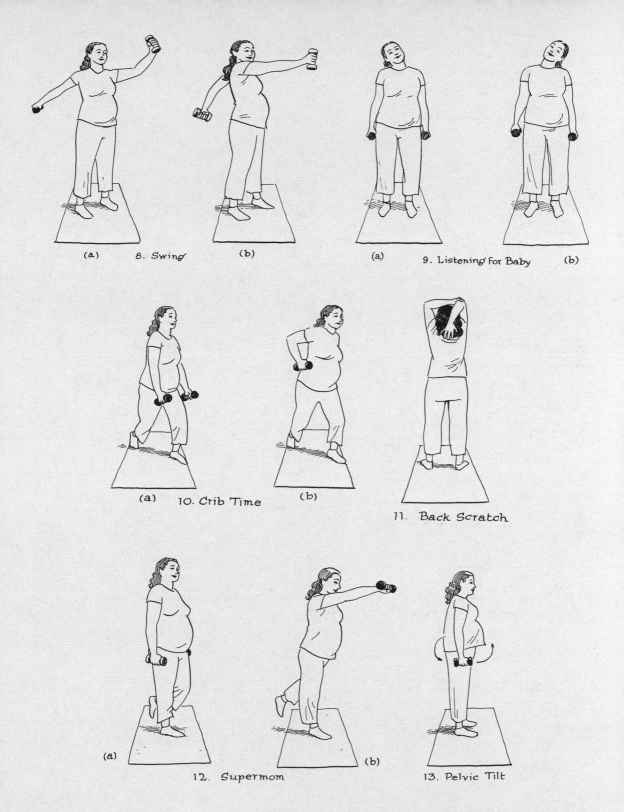

(a)   8. Swing   (b)   (a)   9. Listening for Baby   (b)

(a)   10. Crib Time   (b)   11. Back Scratch

(a)   12. Supermom   (b)   13. Pelvic Tilt

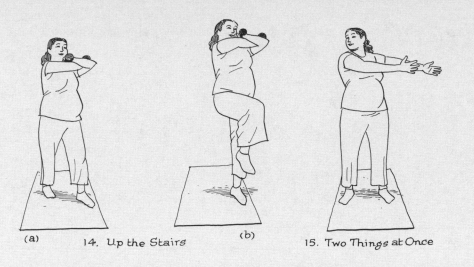

(a)   14. Up the Stairs   (b)   15. Two Things at Once

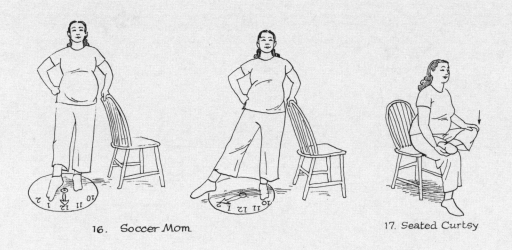

16.   Soccer Mom   17. Seated Curtsy

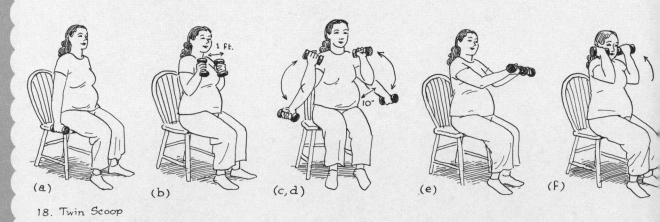

(a)   (b)   (c, d)   (e)   (f)

18. Twin Scoop

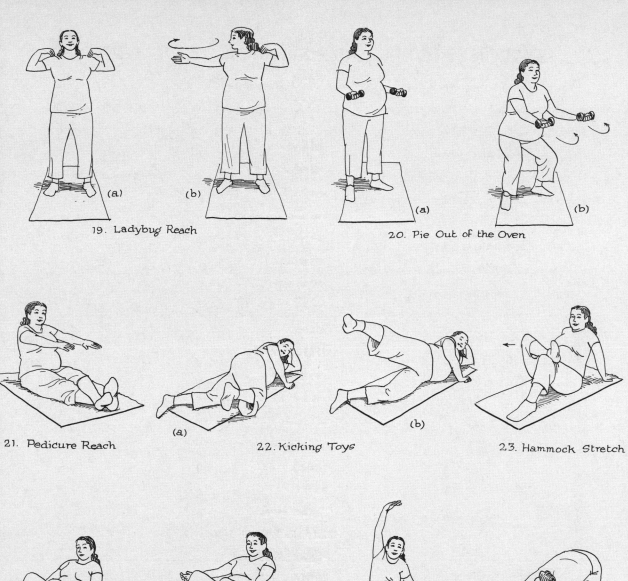

19. Ladybug Reach

20. Pie Out of the Oven

21. Pedicure Reach

22. Kicking Toys

23. Hammock Stretch

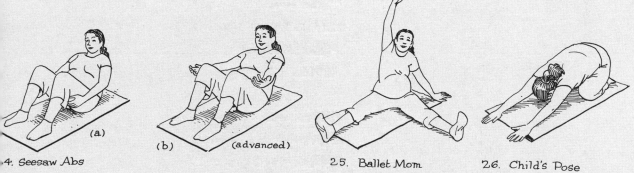

4. Seesaw Abs

25. Ballet Mom

26. Child's Pose

EXERCISES TO PREPARE FOR LABOR AND DELIVERY

Perform these three days a week during pregnancy. Many women find themselves trying several positions during labor and during the pushing phase. Some positions may feel more comfortable at certain points during labor or pushing, and other positions may seem better during other periods. You may also simply get fatigued using the same position for what could be hours. So it's smart to prepare your body for several labor and delivery positions. The following exercises will do that.

Estimated time: less than ten minutes.

1. Supported Squats

With feet shoulder-width apart and toes pointed forward or slightly out, clasp a very sturdy banister or rail at about chest height. Using your arms to support some of your weight, squat down as low as feels comfortable to your lower back and knees. Hold your lowest comfortable position for up to five seconds and come back up. Keep your focus forward. Try to work toward twenty repetitions.

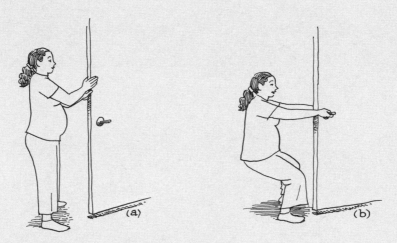

This exercise is particularly useful if you plan on using squatting or hanging rope positions for the end stage of labor or for delivery. You will gain the flexibility necessary to reach this position and the strength and muscular endurance needed to maintain it.

2. Delivery Circles

Comfortably lie on three firm pillows, one under your lower and two stacked under your upper back so that your entire back and head are at an upward angle. Make sure one of the pillows

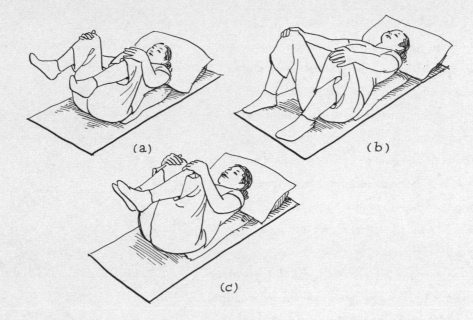

(a)

(b)

(c)

is under your right hip (and tilts you toward the left) to elevate the uterus off the inferior vena cava, since pressure on it can decrease the return of blood to the heart and decrease blood flow to the uterus. Place your hands below your knees, pull your knees up toward your chest, open them to the sides, and circle them down and around ten times. Then reverse the direction, taking the knees away from the chest, down and out to the sides, and around and up toward the chest again. Repeat ten times. Inhale on one circle and exhale on the next. Relax your face and mentally scan your body for tension, releasing it as you continue the circles.

This exercise stretches the lower back, opens the hips, and prepares your body for the most widely used (though not necessarily the most widely advocated) birthing position: on your back. You can increase the intensity and utility of this exercise by lifting up your head and tucking your chin slightly toward your chest. This engages the abdominals and neck muscles.

3. Rocking Table

If you need assistance, stack pillows under your abdomen for support during the exercise. It won't decrease its effectiveness.

(a) While on all fours (hands and knees), with your hands directly underneath your shoulders and your knees under your hips, slowly rock forward while inhaling and back while exhaling. Keep your spine in a neutral position. Do this ten times, keeping your elbows slightly bent.

(b) Then, while maintaining a neutral spine, shift your hips side to side ten times, not "wagging" your tail but shifting your body weight from side to side—especially your lower body weight. Keep the top of your head down so there is a straight line to your tailbone.

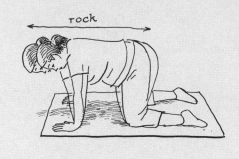

(c) Next do ten pelvic tilts with a relaxed neck, curling your tailbone under (pubic bone toward your navel). Return to neutral spine between each repetition. This is a relatively small movement involving the hips, pelvis, and lower back.

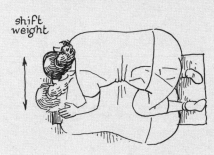

(d) Remaining on all fours, exhale and slowly lower your tailbone toward your heels, maintaining a neutral spine. Hold down for one deep inhale and exhale (roughly three seconds). On the next inhale, come back up to the starting position. Do ten times. You may need to open your knees out to the side some to accommodate your abdomen. Use pillow support as needed.

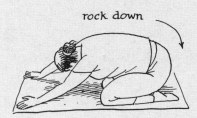

(e) Finally, still on all fours, come down to your elbows and put your hands into prayer position. Slowly rock forward while inhaling and back while exhaling. Keep your spine in a neutral position and your neck relaxed. Do this ten times.

These exercises prepare you for a variety of kneeling positions. Kneeling positions are particularly helpful during labor, especially if you have a posterior baby or extreme back pain with contractions.

4. Side-Lying Lifts

(a) Lie on your left side with your head resting on your left arm. Bend both legs about 90 degrees at the hip and knee, so that your knees are straight out in front of your hips. You can tuck a pillow between your knees and under your abdomen if necessary. (c) With your right hand resting on your right thigh, lift up your right leg, still bent, slightly higher than your shoulder and extend it straight down so that it is in line with your body, not out in front of you. Repeat twenty times. (b) Do the exercise again, only this time, grab the back of your thigh with your right hand and use the strength of your arm to help lift your leg. Repeat twenty times. Breathe normally throughout the exercise.

(d) Continue lying on your left side, with your legs and hips now bent at a 45-degree angle. Slowly place your right hand behind your head and (e) simultaneously lift up your right leg and elbow several inches so that you are doing a side crunch. Focus on gently pulling in your lower abdomen. Do twenty times. Continue regular breathing. Repeat the exercises lying on your right side.

This exercise prepares you for the side-lying labor and delivery position, which will usually be on your left side. If you have an epidural, you may need to use your arm to help support your lifted leg, or the nurses will attach a support bar to the bed for you to use in this position, which is why we've included the second exercise in part b.

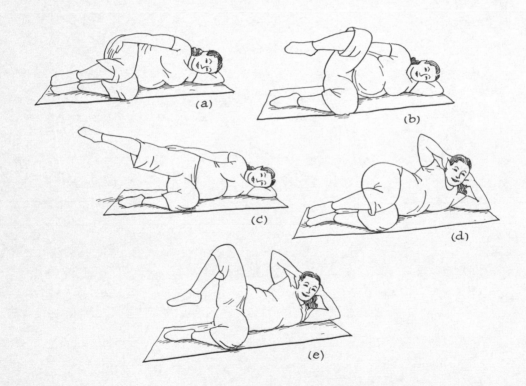

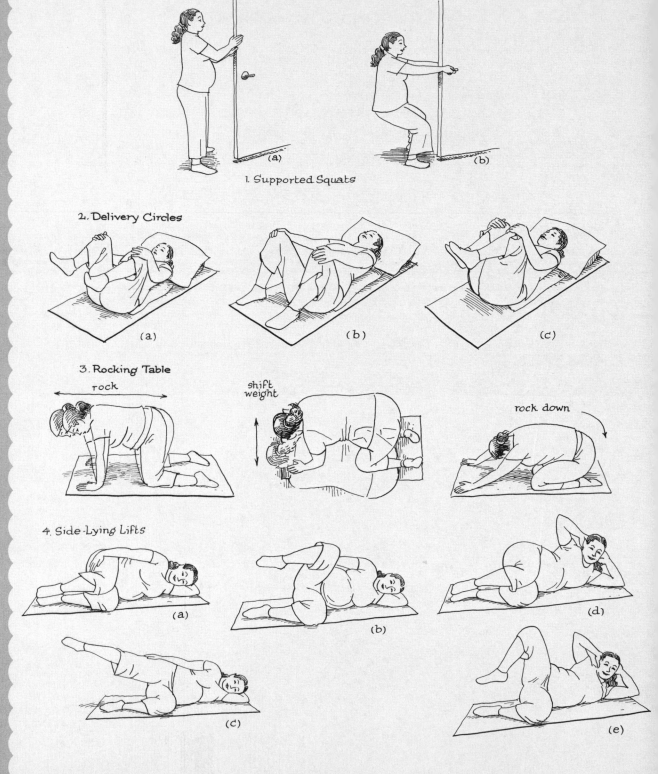

1. Supported Squats

2. Delivery Circles

(a)   (b)   (c)

3. Rocking Table

rock   shift weight   rock down

4. Side-Lying Lifts

(a)   (b)   (d)

(c)   (e)

POSTPREGNANCY WORKOUT

Although you may not be able to resume a full workout schedule for a few weeks after giving birth, with your doctor's permission you can begin certain exercises as soon as the day after delivery if you've had a vaginal delivery with no complications. Starting some exercises right away will not only help you recover more quickly and get your shape back sooner, it will also help you feel more in control at a time when that sense may be in short supply.

If you've had a C-section, your doctor will likely recommend a much longer waiting period before you are cleared to begin them.

Start with walking and Kegel exercises (tightening the muscles that control urine flow), as well as light stretching. This program focuses on tightening your core: primarily your abdominal muscles and the ones in your lower back. The reason? When you're pregnant, your abdominal muscles stretch to accommodate the growing fetus. That decreases back stability, due to the stretching of the muscles and magnified by the hormones that are causing your ligaments and cartilage to relax. And it also leads to diastasis recti, when the rectus muscles that run lengthwise down your abdomen pull apart because of the large uterus distending the belly wall. See the figure on page 279.

How do you know if you have a separation? Lie on your back with your knees bent and feet flat on the floor. Pull up your shirt, so that you can see your abdomen. Slowly curl your head and shoulders up off the floor. If you see a ridge or a bulge form down the center of your abdomen, you have a separation. You can also place a couple of fingers lengthwise along the center of your abdomen near your navel. Just barely lift your head and shoulders, and feel for

Do Your Kegels!

It's always a good time to do your Kegel exercises—that is, contracting and relaxing the muscles that help control urine flow. The slower, the better. Do them before you're pregnant, while you're pregnant, after you're pregnant. You'll keep the entire area strong and tight, which will enhance your pregnancy and delivery experience, as well as your sex life. See page 216 for more details.

Exercise Guidelines

First check with your doctor to make sure it's okay to exercise.

- Maintain a regular breathing pattern throughout all exercises. Don't hold your breath or strain.
- Wear a bra that provides good support but doesn't push against your breasts.
- After you've had your baby, nurse him just before exercise if possible. It will make you more comfortable during workouts.
- Drink plenty of water throughout the day, but especially when you're exercising. By the time you feel thirsty, you're already dehydrated.
- Exercise at a moderate intensity: a perceived exertion of 5 to 7 on a 10-point scale. If you become so out of breath that you cannot maintain normal conversation, or if you feel yourself overheating, stop. Once you've regained your breath and cooled down, resume at a more modest intensity.
- Avoid exercising on an empty stomach, but try to finish eating one to two hours before exercising.
- Avoid erratic, bouncy, or jerky movements while pregnant.
- Don't exercise on your back after the first trimester. Elevate your right hip by placing a pillow under it when doing exercises on your back.
- If you have any of these symptoms during exercise, stop and call your doctor: vaginal bleeding or spotting, unusual shortness of breath, visual disturbance, sudden headache, chest pain, unusual pelvic pain, racing heartbeat, amniotic fluid leakage, uterine contractions lasting longer than 30 seconds, preterm labor, or an unusual change in fetal movement patterns.

a dip or crevice running lengthwise down the center of your abdomen. If one, two, or three of your fingers can fit widthwise in this gap, you probably have a mild to significant separation. This can lead to lots of back pain over time.

These exercises will help tighten your core and eliminate the separation. Ultimately, this can be your lifelong program for strengthening and maintaining your entire core area. (Note:

If you have diastasis recti, do not do crunches, sit-ups, or heavy lifting, which can aggravate a separation.)

- Pull-ins: Keep the natural arch of your lower back and draw your navel in toward your spine. You can do this standing, sitting, or lying down. Start by doing twenty or so a couple of times a day, beginning the day after you have the baby, and work up to doing fifty to one hundred of them twice a day.

- Leg Slides Against the Floor: Lie on your back with your knees bent and feet flat on the floor. Find your neutral spine position, with your lower back just slightly off the floor. While keeping your back completely still, slowly slide one foot out along the floor until the leg is straight and pull it back in again. The arch in your spine should remain constant. Once you can do twenty repetitions with each leg while maintaining a stable spine and without detecting any ridge or bulge in your abdomen, you can move on to our next exercise. You may liberally use pillows to support the area under the knees to help keep the lower back as close to the floor as possible, not arching the spine beyond its natural arch.

- Leg Slides with One Leg Lifted: Assume the same position as above. Lift one foot off the floor with the knee still bent. Extend the leg out as you did before, but this time keep your foot a few inches above the floor. Do twenty repetitions on each side while keeping a neutral spine. Once you can do the twenty repetitions while maintaining a neutral spine and flat abdomen, you can move on to the next exercise.

- Single Leg Floor Touch: From the same starting position, lift one leg off the floor, keeping the knee bent. Now lift up the other leg to meet that leg. Keeping one leg still and both knees bent, slowly lower one leg toward the floor until your foot touches the floor, and bring it back up. Once you can do twenty repetitions on each side with a stable, neutral spine move to the next exercise.

- Leg Slides with Both Legs Lifted: This exercise is just like the second exercise, except that your stationary, bent leg is also lifted off the floor. So you'll begin with both legs bent and lifted off the floor. Extend one leg out, keeping it a few inches above the floor, and bring it back in, the whole time maintaining a neutral spine and a level abdomen. When you can do twenty repetitions on each side with no signs of abdominal separation, move on to the next exercise.

- Double Leg Floor Touch: This is like the single leg floor touch, except that you lower both bent legs together until your feet touch the floor, and then bring them back up to the starting position. This exercise series is effective for strengthening your abdominal muscles and helping you get a sense for maintaining neutral spine.
- Lean-Backs: Stand with your feet about hip-width apart and your arms extended straight out in front of you. Keeping a neutral spine and your torso motionless, hinge at the knees to lean back slightly. Your body should create a straight line from your head to your knees. Engage your abdominal muscles to keep your back from arching. Do this with a wall within six inches of your back so that you will not accidentally fall, or have a significant other spot for you.

YOU TOOL 2

CHOOSING YOUR CARE

You have almost as many options for pregnancy-related caregivers and pediatricians as you do at a Chinese restaurant. While the choice of a provider is a heck of a lot more important than the choice between lo mein and kung pao, the principle is the same: YOU are making a choice based on YOUR values (or tastes). Above all, the most important thing is to seek out someone who shares your priorities on pregnancy and child care; you want a relationship built on trust and support, not second-guessing. That may mean you want to go with an ob/gyn, or you may prefer a midwife if you're at low risk of encountering pregnancy-related complications. Instead of pushing your desires on a provider, find one who already shares your philosophy. After all, if you really like Chinese food, it doesn't make any sense to ask an Italian chef to cook up moo goo gai pan.

CHOOSING AN OB/GYN

One of the best ways to find an ob/gyn is to talk, talk, talk. Ask friends, ask neighbors, ask the woman standing in line behind you at the grocery store, and ask the pros—such as your internist— for recommendations. You can even call the delivery floor of a hospital and ask nurses and anesthesiologists for their recommendations. Many are more than happy to give them. Once you've narrowed down your choices, make appointments with at least two docs (yes, we said at least two) and ask them questions that are important to you. Many times, you're not looking for a right or wrong answer, you simply want to follow your gut and find someone whose goals and philosophies match yours.

Issues to Consider When Choosing an OB/GYN

- Is the doc board certified? See *YOU: The Smart Patient* for details about how to find out.
- If you have health insurance, does your health insurance cover this doctor's charges and the charges at the hospital with which he or she is affiliated?
- Ask her philosophy on birth. You'll gain valuable insights about her approach.
- Ask how much choice you and your partner will have along the way. People tend to have better experiences when they're encouraged to participate in the process.
- Convenience—you'll be going for appointments at least once a month.
- What is the reputation of the hospital with which the doctor is affiliated and how convenient is its location? You may need to get there in a hurry.
- Is the doc a solo practitioner or part of a group? Are midwives available?
- If solo, who covers when the doctor is away? Will you have a chance to meet the other partners?
- If in a group, will you always be seen by your personal doc, or will you rotate through doctors at each appointment? (We actually don't mind this, as you may deliver with one of the others, who may be on call when you go into labor.) Who will be present for the delivery?
- What is the doc's C-section rate? Under what circumstances does he or she call for a C-section?
- Is the doc's philosophy regarding episiotomy compatible with yours?
- What would the doctor do if you presented with a breech baby in labor?
- Is the doc's philosophy on pain management compatible with yours?
- What is the doc's policy on induction? Does she set a time limit on labor before inducing? How long past your due date will the doc permit you to go before inducing?
- Does the doctor have a policy on who may accompany you during prenatal visits and labor? Is the doc's feeling about doulas compatible with yours?
- If you have a complication, what is the doc's experience with cases such as yours? Would she refer you to a specialist?
- If you're considering a VBAC, what is the doctor's success rate with VBACs? (Ideally, it's between 60 percent and 80 percent.)

- If you're considering a water birth, is the doc's experience and philosophy with water birth compatible with yours, and will the hospital permit it?

CHOOSING A MIDWIFE

Midwives are an option for healthy moms with uncomplicated pregnancies; if complications develop, a midwife will refer you to an obstetrician. A woman may choose a midwife because she doesn't want to give birth in a hospital setting, because she prefers a less interventional approach to pregnancy, or because she wants her family to have greater participation in her pregnancy and birth process. Midwives tend to be more holistic and believe that women's bodies know how to give birth with minimal intervention.

Midwives may be solo practitioners or part of groups or "collectives" and usually are supervised by board-certified physicians who back them up in cases of emergencies. Some will provide prenatal care in your home. Those with offices tend to have larger appointment rooms to accommodate friends or family; provide a warmer, less clinical atmosphere; and give longer appointments than docs (averaging one hour versus twenty minutes). Midwives may provide extensive emotional and nutritional support often not provided directly by physicians.

If considering a midwife, you have two choices (in most states):

- Certified nurse-midwife (CNM): a registered nurse who has education and training in midwifery and is certified by the American College of Nurse-Midwives (ACNM) and also meets the standards of the North American Registry of Midwives (NARM). CNMs are internationally credentialed and may practice in hospitals or birthing centers, or attend home births. They are licensed to practice in all states and are licensed to prescribe medicine. All hospital midwives are CNMs, and many are in practice with obstetricians.
- Direct-entry midwife: These midwives are not licensed to practice in ten states and Washington, D.C. If you choose to use a midwife in one of these states and complications occur, you may end up in the emergency room, as your midwife will not be welcome at the hospital. Direct-entry midwives may be educated through self-study, apprenticeship, or at an independent midwifery school or college—not a nursing school. They practice

exclusively in nonhospital settings such as birthing centers and home births. There are four different types of direct-entry midwives:

- Certified midwife (CM)—same as a CNM but without nursing degree; meets qualifications of the ACNM
- Certified professional midwife (CPM)—meets qualifications of NARM
- Licensed midwife (LM)—licensed by state (not all states offer)
- Lay midwife—trained through self-study or apprenticeship; uncertified or unlicensed

Issues to Consider When Choosing a Midwife

- Is this midwife legally able to practice in your state? States have different requirements: licensure, certification, registration, permit.
- What is her education, training, experience, certification?
- Does she have hospital privileges?
- Are midwife care and this specific midwife collective covered by your insurance plan? Does your insurance cover transfer to a hospital?
- How long has this midwife been practicing? How many babies has she "caught"? (Midwives believe that mothers deliver babies themselves; midwives merely assist.)
- Who is the midwife's backup physician? Can you meet with him or her?
- If she is a solo practitioner, who covers when she is away? Can you meet her backup? What happens if two women are in labor at the same time?
- Will your midwife stay with you if you are transferred to a hospital?
- If she is part of a collective, will you meet the other midwives in the practice? Who will assist your delivery?
- If you are interested in a water birth, does she have experience with this?
- Are you in sync with her regarding the participation of family or friends?
- Under what circumstances does she recommend transfer to a hospital?
- What if you have a perineal tear or need an extensive episiotomy (done to expedite delivery) that needs to be sutured?
- At what point in your labor will she come to your home?
- Does she do postpartum visits after a hospital transfer?

CHOOSING A PEDIATRICIAN

This is a biggie. After all, here's the doc who's going to answer your questions about feeding, look at busted lips, and be there whenever things don't seem quite right. As with choosing an obstetrician or midwife, you want to find a pediatrician who shares your basic philosophy of health and child care. Some pediatricians are extremely aggressive and high-tech, wanting to intervene and treat any and every symptom. Others are less alarmist and have a more watch-and-wait approach. Some are open to complementary medicine; others are not. Some are willing to modify the American Academy of Pediatrics (AAP) vaccination schedule; others insist on following it to the letter. Keep your antennae up: If you feel rushed or that the doc is preoccupied during the interview, the same may be true during your visits. The most important thing is to connect with him or her on a personal level; after all, you're trusting this person to care for your most precious possession.

Here are some questions you might ask (both of yourself or, when appropriate, of the doc or office staff directly):

- Is the doc board certified?
- What is the doc's education, training, and experience? How long has he or she been in practice?
- Is the office convenient? In the first year, you'll be visiting the pediatrician fairly often—hopefully less so after that.
- What hospital(s) is the doc affiliated with?
- Does the doctor accept your insurance? Does his/her hospital(s)?
- Is the doc a solo practitioner? If so, who covers on evenings and weekends or when the doctor is away?
- Is the doctor part of a group? If so, will you visit your doctor exclusively, or will you see whoever is available (including, perhaps, a nurse practitioner)?
- Does the doc have early morning, evening, and/or weekend hours to accommodate working parents?
- Does the doc encourage email communication?
- How long can you expect to wait for a response when you email or phone with a question?

- How long is the response time for after-hours questions?
- Is the office clean and comfortable, and does it have a separate sick-child waiting area?
- Is the staff friendly?
- What is the doctor's attitude toward breast-feeding versus bottle feeding? Is it in sync with yours?
- How does the doc treat ear infections? This is a good litmus test for how interventionist he or she may be: Some dispense antibiotics liberally; others encourage that you watch and wait, as most ear infections resolve themselves within three days.
- Do you and the doctor share similar views about matters such as parenting issues (like cosleeping and circumcision)?
- Are the doctor's feelings about complementary medicine in sync with yours?
- Does the doc have a standard protocol for vaccinations? How flexible is he or she about the timing of vaccinations and the administration of optional vaccinations?
- Does the pediatrician's office have electronic medical records so that when Junior graduates from high school, his records are complete?

YOU TOOL 3
GUIDELINES FOR MEDICATIONS AND TOXINS

When you're pregnant and breast-feeding, it's not uncommon to obsess about every last thing that goes into your body and how it can affect your child—and that's a good thing (well, maybe not the obsessing part). One area that has parents-to-be more perplexed than an algebra-challenged ninth grader: medication. Some pregnant and nursing women don't want to take any medication because they fear it will have adverse effects as it crosses the placenta or enters their breast milk. But the reality is that pregnant and nursing moms can follow rational drug therapy to treat their own illnesses. If you need medication to make you healthier, the benefit most times outweighs the risk: Healthy mom equals healthy child. Below are some general guidelines when thinking about medications and toxins, as well as a specific list of common medications and their risk factors. See www.motherisk.org for more information. Remember that herbs are drugs too and should be treated accordingly. Just because something comes from a health food store and not a pharmacy doesn't necessarily mean it's benign.

GENERAL GUIDELINES

- Small amounts of alcohol consumed before you found out you were pregnant will not cause your baby to have fetal alcohol syndrome. If you're planning to conceive, quit several weeks before you begin trying to get pregnant. If you are a problem drinker or cannot quit drinking in pregnancy, seek help immediately.
- Quit smoking before you conceive. If you're pregnant and still smoking, stop pronto! If you can't do it on your own, seek professional help. Programs exist to help pregnant mothers stop smoking. See www.realage.com and www.doctoroz.com for our plan.

- Do not self-prescribe in pregnancy.
- Consult with your doctor about whether you should consider tapering off any medications that you might be taking for chronic conditions such as depression, asthma, diabetes, and so on. Do not stop cold turkey.
- If a medication you are taking is contraindicated for pregnancy, talk with your prescribing doctor about switching to an equivalent that is safe. In most cases, you have options.
- In general, older drugs may have more information on their safety for the fetus than newer, stronger drugs. This is because we have longer experience using them, even though formal studies may not have been conducted.
- If you need a medication for a medical condition, take the appropriate dose.
- Very few medications have proven to be unsafe to the unborn baby.
- Very few drugs are incompatible with breast-feeding.
- In late pregnancy, you may need more of a medication, because your size is larger and your body metabolizes some medications faster.
- For most herbal products, there is no safety data for your baby during pregnancy, so take extra precautions to read about and ask your doc about herbal remedies. You can find our recommendations throughout the book.
- If your occupation involves exposure to chemicals, find out what chemicals are involved and seek advice as to their fetal safety. Ditto for hobbies. And get manicures and color your hair only in well-ventilated salons.
- A lot of people will try to scare you about what is safe or not in pregnancy, and a lot of internet sites contain very poor information. Find out the facts. See www.drugsafetysite.com.

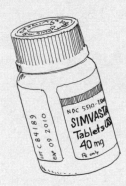

MEDICATION GUIDELINES

While most medications appear to be safe, you still need to consider these facts: About 2 to 3 percent of birth defects do seem to be linked to medications. Because there are so few data—few pregnant women would want to be in clinical trials testing the safety of medications during pregnancy—we do recommend that you try avoiding nonessential medications and exploring natural alternatives (a hot shower for nasal decongestion, for instance). That said, here are lists of medications that we would feel comfortable giving our wives and daughters during pregnancy, those we would have some reservations about, and those we would insist they avoid.

YES

These are generally considered safe during pregnancy (when given in appropriate doses and appropriate routes, especially if they have been used without adverse reaction prior to pregnancy).

Talk to your doctor before taking any medication or herbal remedy while pregnant.

- Allergy medications: chlorpheniramine (Chlor-Trimeton) and diphenhydramine (Benadryl)
- Asthma medications: budesonide (Pulmicort), Rhinocat
- Constipation relievers: docusate (Colace, Dulcolax), polyethylene (MiraLax), milk of magnesia, Metamucil, and Citrucel
- Cough medications: dextromethorphan (Robitussin DM)
- Diabetes medications: insulin and metformin (Glucophage)
- Diarrhea medications: loperamide (Imodium)
- Gas medications: simethicone (Gas-X, Mylicon)
- Heartburn medications: Tums
- Hemorrhoid medications: Tucks, Preparation H
- Hypothyroid treatments: levothyroxine (Synthroid)
- Infection medications: the antibiotics penicillin and erythromycin, which are used for many infections; nitrofurantoin (Macrobid), for urinary tract infections; cephalosporins such as cephalexin (Keflex) and cefazolin, used for a variety of infections; clindamycin (Cleocin), for lower GI infections; and metronidazole (Flagyl), used for urinary tract and other infections; the antifungal clotrimazole (Gyne-Lotrimin) for yeast infections; and the antiviral acyclovir (Zovirax), often used for herpes
- Insomnia medications: doxylamine (Unisom); Benadryl
- Nausea treatments: pyridoxine, metoclopramide (Reglan)
- Pain medications: acetaminophen (Tylenol)

(continued on next page)

MAYBE

Might have some risks associated

- Antidepressant medications: Antidepressants have FDA warnings, but the risks appear to be mild. There are rare complications for newborns with general classes of SSRIs, and one of them, paroxetine (Paxil), was once thought to cause birth defects, but studies haven't confirmed that problem.
- Diuretics/water pills
- Nasal congestion medications: pseudoephedrine (Sudafed), triprolidine (Actifed); avoid these in the first trimester.
- Pain medications with narcotics: not recommended for repetitive dosing.

NO

Don't take during pregnancy or while breast-feeding

- Accutane for acne. It has been associated with birth defects.
- Aspirin: In rare cases, baby aspirin may be recommended in the first trimester to moms who have had repeated miscarriages. Once past the first trimester, aspirin and drugs with similar action, such as the nonsteroidal anti-inflammatory drugs ibuprofen and naproxen, are not recommended as pain relievers, as they may cause a drop in prostaglandin levels, which causes a tube from the baby's heart to close off too early (a process that naturally happens after birth).
- Anxiety and insomnia medications: benzodiazepines like diazepam and midazolam.

Note: Check with your doc about medications for more specific conditions, like antiseizure medications and mood stabilizers. For herbal remedies, check www.americanpregnancy.org for the latest information on safety in pregnancy.

YOU TOOL 4

PREPARING YOUR HOME FOR BABY

Removing the disco ball from your spare bedroom isn't the only thing you need to do before you bring your baby home. Well before you deliver, it's a good idea to prepare for his or her arrival by readying his room (or area in your room) and making sure that you have all the key supplies you'll need—for him and for you. (This is a great job for your significant other.) If your baby will have his or her own room, paint in advance so that fumes have dissipated by the time baby comes home. While you're at it, cover all outlets, check smoke alarms, and be sure to remove all the cleaners and toxins from lower cabinets.

It's a good idea to register for the following items at a baby store, because you'll be getting lots of presents whether or not you have an official baby shower, and it's far better to receive things you need in the colors you prefer than some "creative" gifts that are totally not your taste and will require you to schlep from store to store returning them after the baby is born. Here's your checklist to make sure you've got everything in place before your baby comes home:

For baby:
- Infant car seat—and make sure you've practiced installing it!
- Crib, bassinet, or cosleeper (see "Crib Guidelines," below)
- Storage area for clothes and diapers
- Place to change the baby (changing table, padded foam form that attaches to any bureau top, changing pad if you plan to use the floor or bed)
- Large tote or diaper bag
- Diapers (Expect to use 350 disposables the first month; if using cloth, contact the delivery company, because you'll need 90 the first week; also buy 6 to 10 diaper wraps or plastic pants and 4 sets of diaper pins or "snappies.")

- Diaper pail or garbage can
- Alcohol-free wipes
- 10 to 12 extra cloth diapers for burping and other uses
- 5 to 10 T-shirts or onesies (kimono style easiest; avoid over-the-head)
- 3 to 5 pairs of booties/socks
- 1 or 2 knit hats
- 1 sun hat (if summer)
- 5 to 7 cotton sleepers or gowns
- 1 or 2 fleece sleepers, depending on season or temperature of room
- 1 bunting (if winter)
- 5 to 7 receiving blankets
- 1 or 2 thermal blankets
- 3 or 4 fitted crib sheets
- Waterproof mattress pad for crib
- 3 or 4 fitted sheets for pram, if using
- 3 to 5 soft washcloths
- 3 to 5 hooded towels
- Baby nail scissors or clippers
- Digital thermometer
- Baby brush and comb
- Mild soap
- Baby shampoo
- Vaseline
- Desitin or Balmex diaper rash medications
- Q-tips (not for ears!)
- Cotton balls
- Rubbing alcohol (for umbilical cord care)
- Mobile (high-contrast colors)
- Baby monitor
- Baby tub or large sponge to lay baby on in bathtub or kitchen sink
- If bottle feeding, bottles, nipples, bottle brush, formula
- Perfume- and dye-free laundry detergent

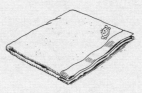

- Poly-Vi-Sol vitamin drops. We usually recommend 1 ml a day starting at age 2 months, but check with your doc. This vitamin preparation is important, as many infants become vitamin D deficient, as breast milk is somehow lacking in D.

Note: Wash all baby's clothes, sheets, and towels before use. There's no need to wash baby's things separately from your own or to use special baby detergent; the whole family can use perfume- and dye-free detergent. Avoid commercial fabric softeners and dryer sheets, as they contain harsh chemicals. If you must soften clothes, add either ¼ cup baking soda or ¼ cup white vinegar to the wash cycle. The vinegar will also take care of static cling. Seventh Generation and Ecover also make safe fabric softeners and static cling removers based on vegetable products and essential oils.

For you:
- If nursing, at least two cotton nursing bras, nursing pads, and one tube of udder cream or lanolin
- If pumping, either buy a portable pump (good for taking to work) or rent a hospital-grade one (stronger, but not easy to tote around), and buy glass storage bottles, and bottles, bottle brush, and nipples for baby
- Maxi pads (get overnights, the big ones)
- Tucks medicated pads
- K-Y Brand Jelly or Astroglide personal lubricant
- Witch hazel
- Plastic bags with ice (good for sore bottom and breasts)
- Waterproof mattress pad for your bed
- Ready-to-eat meals for freezer and pantry
- Easy-to-grab, healthful snacks
- Hands-free Bluetooth headset

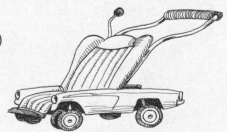

Other useful items to add to your wish list:
- Stroller (see "How to . . . Choose a Stroller," page 257)
- Sling or baby carrier (BabyBjörn, Snugli, and so on)

- Bouncy seat
- Battery-operated swing
- Gymini or similar colorful padded mat with suspended objects that baby can look at or kick while lying on his or her back
- Soft, colorful toys with varied textures and sounds but no removable parts (like button eyes)
- Rattles, rings, and toys that baby can grip
- Crib mirror
- Fabric books, board books
- CDs of nursery rhymes (or Mozart—your choice)
- A few days' worth of meals delivered to the house

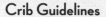

Crib Guidelines

- A firm, tight-fitting mattress, so baby can't get trapped
- No missing, loose, or broken screws or brackets
- No more than $2^3/8$ inches between crib slats, so baby's head and body cannot fit through the slats
- No corner posts over $1/16$ inch high, so clothing can't get caught
- No cutouts in the headboard or footboard, so head doesn't get stuck

YOU TOOL 5

POP'S PREGNANCY RECIPES

Many times during pregnancy, you're not going to feel like eating at all, much less grocery shopping and standing on your feet over a hot stove. So we've made this recipe toolbox especially for your partner. They're foods that are easy enough for him to make—with supervision, if needed—and easy on your stomach. Plus, they're tasty and healthy, and use many of the ingredients and nutrients that will satisfy your baby's nutritional needs. We've incorporated many recipes from Lifestyle 180, a program developed at the Cleveland Clinic to treat chronic diseases through lifestyle modification. The recipes all meet the following criteria:

- Saturated fat limited to fewer than 4 grams per serving of a main dish or 2 grams per serving of a side dish and desserts.
- No trans fats. (That's an easy one. Animals smell trans fat and know it's poison. They avoid it; so should we.)
- Sugars limited to fewer than 4 grams per serving of a main dish or dessert, or 2 grams per serving of a side dish.
- No added sugars or syrups.
- Only 100 percent whole grains.
- Sodium for the day should not exceed 1,500 milligrams (800 milligrams main, 480 side).

Also, when either you or your partner takes a trip to the grocery store, bring your magnifying glass and get ready to start reading. Forget what the front of the package says; that's usually just a marketing gimmick. Instead search the FDA nutrition label for the amount of saturated fat, sugars, and sodium. Then read the actual list of ingredients. We care about the first five: If there is any high-fructose corn syrup, added sugars, white grains (be suspicious of *wheat* or *enriched* as opposed to *whole wheat* flour), saturated fat, or trans fat (anything partially hydrogenated), put it back on the shelf.

The Ultimate Pregnancy Smoothie
1 serving (1 cup)

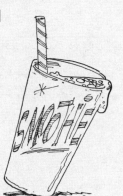

1 cup juice of your choice (papaya or mango nectar base is smoother and
    less acidic; less thick juices are preferable)

1 small banana or ³/₄ cup of your favorite berries

2 tablespoons whey protein

2 tablespoons flax, freshly ground (helps with constipation and provides
    omega-3s)

1 tablespoon hemp seed nut, hemp protein, or psyllium husk (for fiber)

1 tablespoon Salba or chia seeds (provide omega-3, calcium,
    magnesium, and protein)

1 tablespoon wheat germ (for B vitamins)

3 200-milligram fish oil capsules (break and use oil)

Combine all ingredients in a blender container. Cover; blend 30 seconds. Add ice cubes to change thickness or temperature if desired.

WHAT'S IN IT FOR YOU AND YOUR BABY

Calories: 274 Total fat: 9 g Aging (saturated and trans) fats: 1 g Healthy fats: 8 g Omega-3 fats: 2.6 g

EPA and DHA: 600 mg Fiber: 7 g Carbohydrates: 38 g Sugars: 24 g Protein: 11 g Sodium: 19 mg

Potassium: 277 mg Calcium: 122 mg Magnesium: 33 mg Selenium: 1 mcg

PREGNANCY SANDWICHES AND MAINS

Grilled Portobello Sandwich
1 serving

1 teaspoon olive oil

1 large portobello mushroom cap (outer skin and gills removed)

1 tablespoon soft goat cheese

1 slice whole grain bread, toasted

1 teaspoon bottled balsamic vinegar glaze

1 teaspoon minced fresh basil (optional)

Spread oil over both sides of mushroom cap. Grill over medium-high heat or cook in a nonstick skillet over medium heat 4 to 5 minutes per side or until tender. Spread goat cheese over toast. Slice mushroom cap; arrange over goat cheese. Drizzle glaze over mushroom. Garnish with basil if desired.

WHAT'S IN IT FOR YOU AND YOUR BABY

Calories: 190   Total fat: 10 g   Aging (saturated and trans) fats: 4 g   Healthy fats: 11 g   Omega-3 fats: 0 g

EPA and DHA: 0 g   Fiber: 3 g   Carbohydrates: 17 g   Sugars: 4 g   Protein: 9 g   Sodium: 190 mg

Potassium: 495 mg   Calcium: 76 mg   Magnesium: 25 mg   Selenium: 20 mcg

Bruschetta

1 serving

1 (6 inch) whole wheat baguette or bagel, split

1 ounce fresh mozzarella cheese or 1 slice (1 ounce) part-skim mozzarella cheese, thinly sliced

3 sundried tomatoes packed in oil, drained

¼ cup packed watercress or baby spinach

Lightly toast baguette if desired. Arrange cheese, tomatoes, and watercress over bottom of baguette; close sandwich.

WHAT'S IN IT FOR YOU AND YOUR BABY

Calories: 340 Total fat: 8 g Aging (saturated and trans) fats: 3 g Healthy fats: 9 g Omega-3 fats: 0 g

EPA and DHA: 0 g Fiber: 10 g Carbohydrates: 55 g Sugars: 9 g Protein: 28 g Sodium: 630 g

Potassium: 140 mg Calcium: 258 mg Magnesium: 7 mg Selenium: 0.27 mcg

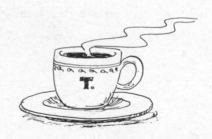

Smoked Salmon Sandwich

1 serving

¹⁄₄ cup (1 ounce) farmer cheese

1 slice whole wheat bread, toasted

¹⁄₈ teaspoon cayenne pepper

¹⁄₄ cup packed baby arugula

1¹⁄₂ ounces (2 thin slices) wild smoked salmon

Lemon wedge

Spread cheese over warm toast; top with cayenne pepper, arugula, and salmon. Serve with lemon wedge.

WHAT'S IN IT FOR YOU AND YOUR BABY

Calories: 320   Total fat: 11 g   Aging (saturated and trans) fats: 4.5 g   Healthy fats: 8 g   Omega-3 fats: 2 g

EPA and DHA: 2 g   Fiber: 1 g   Carbohydrates: 17 g   Sugars: 2 g   Protein: 37 g   Sodium: 250 mg

Potassium: 600 mg   Calcium: 263 mg   Magnesium: 55 mg   Selenium: 40 mcg

Lifestyle 180 Whole Wheat Penne Pasta
6 1½-cup servings

2 tablespoons extra-virgin olive oil

4 garlic cloves, thinly sliced

2 cups zucchini squash, diced

½ teaspoon salt

¼ teaspoon pepper

2 cups broccoli florets

12 ounces whole wheat penne

26 ounces basic tomato sauce

    or 1 jar (26 ounces) tomato-basil pasta sauce (no added sugar)

Bring a large saucepan of water to a boil. Heat oil in a large, deep skillet over medium heat. Add garlic; sauté over medium heat 1 minute. Add zucchini, salt, and pepper; sauté until tender, about 4 minutes. Stir in tomato sauce; bring to a simmer and turn off flame.

Lightly salt the boiling water; add broccoli florets and blanch for 3 minutes or until just tender. Remove broccoli with slotted spoon or strainer, drain well, and stir into tomato sauce mixture. Cook pasta in broccoli water according to package directions; drain and return to same pot. Add zucchini mixture; mix well. Heat if necessary.

Variation: For penne with meatballs, prepare Chia Sausage/Meatballs. (See recipe, page 355.) Stir 24 1-ounce meatballs into the tomato sauce along with the broccoli.

WHAT'S IN IT FOR YOU AND YOUR BABY

Calories: 159   Total fat: 6 g   Aging (saturated and Trans) fats: 0.5 g   Healthy fats: 5 g   Omega-3 fats: 0 g

EPA and DHA: 0 g   Fiber: 5 g   Carbohydrates: 23 g   Sugars: 6 g   Protein: 6 g   Sodium: 509 mg

Potassium: 191 mg   Calcium: 64 mg   Magnesium: 27 mg   Selenium: 14 mcg

Lifestyle 180 Chia Sausage/Meatballs
10 ½-cup servings (4 oz. serving size, or 3 small meatballs)

½ cup nonalcoholic red wine, vegetable juice cocktail, or vegetable broth

2 tablespoons chia seeds

¼ cup chopped fresh parsley

2 tablespoons minced garlic

1 tablespoon fennel seed

2 teaspoons seasoned salt

1 teaspoon crushed red pepper flakes

    (optional: use for hot sausage; omit for mild sausage)

½ teaspoon dried basil

¼ teaspoon dried oregano

¼ teaspoon freshly ground black pepper

¼ teaspoon dried thyme leaves

2 pounds ground turkey breast

In a medium bowl, combine wine and chia seeds; let stand 30 minutes to allow chia seeds to swell. Add remaining ingredients except turkey; mix well. Add turkey; mix until well blended. (At this point, mixture may be frozen in batches for future use.) Form into patties and cook in a nonstick skillet to internal temperature of 165 degrees F., or crumble into skillet; cook until no longer pink, stirring frequently. Use for pizza topping or stir into pasta sauce.

Variation: For turkey meatballs, add 2 egg whites and ½ cup fresh whole grain bread crumbs to turkey mixture. Form into 40 1-ounce (1-inch) meatballs. Place in 2 shallow baking pans coated with cooking spray. Bake at 375 degrees F. for 20 minutes or until meatballs are slightly browned and internal temperature reaches 165 degrees F.

WHAT'S IN IT FOR YOU AND YOUR BABY

Calories: 140   Total fat: 0 g   Aging (saturated and trans) fats: 0 g   Healthy fats: 2.5 g   Omega-3 fats: 0.5 g

EPA and DHA: 0 g   Fiber: 2 g   Carbohydrates: 3 g   Sugars: 0 g   Protein: 24 g   Sodium: 350 mg

Potassium: 33 mg   Calcium: 39 mg   Magnesium: 5.5 mg   Selenium: 0 mcg

Lifestyle 180 Quinoa Tabouli

7 ½-cup servings.

½ cup bulgur

⅓ cup cold water

⅓ cup fresh lemon juice

¼ cup extra-virgin olive oil, divided

1 cup cooked organic quinoa

1 cup diced tomato

1 cup cucumber, unpeeled, seeded, finely diced

½ cup fresh parsley, chopped

¼ cup chopped fresh mint leaves

¼ cup finely diced red onion

1 teaspoon minced garlic

½ teaspoon salt

½ teaspoon freshly ground black pepper

In a large bowl, combine bulgur, water, lemon juice, and 2 tablespoons of the olive oil; mix well. Let stand for 30 minutes or until most of liquid is absorbed. Stir in remaining 2 tablespoons olive oil and remaining ingredients; let stand 10 minutes to allow flavors to develop.

WHAT'S IN IT FOR YOU AND YOUR BABY

Calories: 122 Total fat: 8 g Aging (saturated and trans) fats: 1 g Healthy fats: 7 g Omega-3 fats: 0 g

EPA and DHA: 0 g Fiber: 2 g Carbohydrates: 11 g Sugars: 1 g Protein: 2 g Sodium: 165 mg

Potassium: 176 mg Calcium: 24 mg Magnesium: 29 mg Selenium: 1 mcg

Lifestyle 180 Pork Tenderloin with Szechwan Noodles and Broccoli
6 servings

Pork Tenderloin

3 tablespoons agave nectar

2 tablespoons rice wine vinegar

1 tablespoon balsamic vinegar

1 tablespoon reduced-sodium tamari sauce

1 teaspoon grated fresh gingerroot

1 teaspoon minced garlic

1 small (12-ounce) pork tenderloin

Combine all ingredients except tenderloin in a shallow dish and mix well. Then add tenderloin, turning to coat. Refrigerate at least 30 minutes or up to 4 hours. Meanwhile, prepare Szechwan Noodles and Broccoli. (See recipe on following page.)

Heat oven to 375 degrees F. Place tenderloin on rack on rimmed baking sheet. Pour marinade into a small saucepan; bring to a simmer. Cook until reduced to 3 tablespoons; cool 5 minutes. Coat tenderloin with half of mixture. Bake 15 minutes. Turn tenderloin over; brush remaining marinade reduction over tenderloin. Continue baking 15 minutes or until an instant-read thermometer inserted in the center of tenderloin reads 150 degrees.

Transfer to carving board; tent with foil and let stand 10 minutes. Cut crosswise into thin slices. Arrange Szechwan noodles and broccoli on four serving plates; top with tenderloin slices.

Lifestyle 180 Szechwan Noodles and Broccoli

8 ounces whole wheat spaghetti

2 tablespoons dark sesame oil

2 tablespoons reduced-sodium soy sauce

1 tablespoon balsamic vinegar

1 tablespoon agave nectar

1¹/₂ teaspoons hot chile dark sesame oil

¹/₂ teaspoon salt

¹/₂ teaspoon minced garlic

3 cups broccoli florets, steamed or simmered until crisp-tender

1 cup green onions, sliced

Cook spaghetti according to package directions. Meanwhile, in a large bowl, combine remaining ingredients except broccoli and green onions; mix well. Drain spaghetti and rinse to cool; add to bowl and toss well. Add broccoli and green onions; toss again.

WHAT'S IN IT FOR YOU AND YOUR BABY

Calories: 300   Total fat: 7 g   Aging (saturated and trans) fats: 1.5 g   Healthy fats: 1.2 g   Omega-3 fats: 0 g

EPA and DHA: 0 g   Fiber: 6 g   Carbohydrates: 38 g   Sugars: 8 g   Protein: 22 g   Sodium: 370 mg

Potassium: 499 mg   Calcium: 49 mg   Magnesium: 83 mg   Selenium: 50 mcg

Lifestyle 180 Fruited Pancake

Makes 4 servings (12 to 14 pancakes)

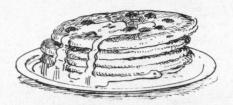

1⅓ cups whole wheat pastry flour

1 tablespoon baking powder

³/₄ teaspoon salt

½ teaspoon cinnamon

1 tablespoon ground chia seeds

1⅓ cups water

1 tablespoon pure vanilla extract

½ cup chopped, toasted walnuts

1 whole apple, coarsely grated

1 whole pear, coarsely grated

1 banana, halved lengthwise and thinly sliced crosswise

Agave nectar (optional)

In a large bowl, combine flour, baking powder, salt, and cinnamon; stir in chia seeds and mix well. Combine water and vanilla; add to the dry ingredients and mix well with a wire whisk. Stir nuts, apple, and pear gently into the batter; fold in banana. Mix well. (If batter seems very thick, depending on ripeness and juiciness of fruit, add 1 or 2 more tablespoons of water.)

Wipe a large nonstick skillet with a light film of vegetable oil and heat over medium heat until hot. Drop batter by ¼ cupfuls into hot skillet. Cook about 3 minutes or until bottoms are golden brown. Turn; continue cooking 1 to 2 minutes or until bottoms are golden brown. Transfer to warmed serving plates (may be kept warm in a 200-degree F. oven). Repeat with remaining batter.

WHAT'S IN IT FOR YOU AND YOUR BABY

Calories: 109   Total fat: 4 g   Aging (saturated and trans) fats: 1 g   Healthy fats: 3 g   Omega-3 fats: 0 g

EPA and DHA: 0 g   Fiber: 4 g   Carbohydrates: 18 g   Sugars: 4 g   Protein: 2 g   Sodium: 280 mg

Potassium: 88 mg   Calcium: 48 mg   Magnesium: 12 mg   Selenium: 0 mcg

Huevos Rancheros Burritos with Chipotle Chili Beans and Corn

4 servings

1 can (15 1/2 ounces) chili beans in spicy sauce, undrained

1 cup frozen whole kernel corn

1/4 cup salsa, preferably chipotle

3 large egg whites

2 large eggs

2 tablespoons reduced-fat sour cream

Cooking spray

4 large (10-inch) whole wheat flour tortillas

1/4 cup chopped cilantro

In a medium saucepan, combine beans, corn, and salsa. Bring to a boil over high heat; reduce heat and simmer uncovered 5 minutes. Beat together egg whites, eggs, and sour cream. Heat a large nonstick skillet over medium-high heat until hot. Coat with cooking spray. Add egg mixture; cook, stirring occasionally, until eggs are set. Break into chunks and stir into bean mixture.

Stack tortillas on a clean kitchen towel. Sprinkle a few drops of water over the top tortilla. Fold tortillas up in the towel; heat in microwave oven until warm, 20 to 30 seconds. (Do not overwarm, or the tortillas will be tough.) Place tortillas on serving plates. Divide egg mixture over tortillas; top with cilantro. Fold sides of tortillas in over filling; roll up, burrito fashion.

WHAT'S IN IT FOR YOU AND YOUR BABY

Calories: 333 Total fat: 7 g Aging (saturated and trans) fats: 2 g Healthy fats: 5 g Omega-3 fats: 0 g

EPA and DHA: 0 g Fiber: 8 g Carbohydrates: 46 g Sugars: 4 g Protein: 16 g Sodium: 734 mg

Potassium: 104 mg Calcium: 46 mg Magnesium: 3 mg Selenium: 6 mcg

Lifestyle 180 Chilled Avocado Asparagus Soup

5 1-cup servings

1½ cups packed fresh spinach leaves (2 ounces)

2 ripe avocados, peeled and pitted

2 cups cold water

2 cups fresh chopped or thinly sliced asparagus, woody bottoms removed

2 tablespoons fresh lemon juice

4 teaspoons reduced-sodium soy sauce

2 teaspoons chopped green onion

1 teaspoon minced garlic

¼ teaspoon chopped thyme

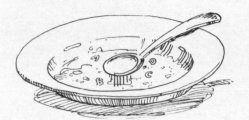

1½ teaspoons chopped fresh tarragon

½ teaspoon salt

Freshly ground pepper to taste

Pinch cayenne pepper

Olive oil, to taste (optional)

Combine spinach, avocado, water, asparagus, lemon juice, soy sauce, green onion, garlic, thyme, and tarragon in a blender. Cover; blend at high speed to a smooth puree, about 1 minute. Push mixture though a fine strainer set over a bowl. Season with salt, pepper, and cayenne pepper. Cover; chill at least 1 hour or until cold. Swirl in optional olive oil just before serving if desired.

WHAT'S IN IT FOR YOU AND YOUR BABY

Calories: 136   Total fat: 11 g   Aging (saturated and trans) fats: 1.5 g   Healthy fats: 9 g   Omega-3 fats: 0 g

EPA and DHA: 0 g   Fiber: 6 g   Carbohydrates: 10 g   Sugars: 2 g   Protein: 3 g   Sodium: 450 mg

Potassium: 525 mg   Calcium: 41 mg   Magnesium: 38 mg   Selenium: 2 mcg

Lifestyle 180 Roasted Sweet Potatoes
8 ½-cup servings

1½ tablespoons extra-virgin olive oil

2 teaspoons minced garlic

2 teaspoons ground cumin

1 teaspoon salt

½ teaspoon pepper

2 pounds sweet potatoes, scrubbed, cut into 1-inch chunks

Heat oven to 375 degrees F. Combine oil, garlic, cumin, salt, and pepper in a large bowl. Add sweet potatoes; toss until well coated. Place in a single layer in a 15 x 10-inch jelly roll pan. Bake 25 to 30 minutes or until tender.

WHAT'S IN IT FOR YOU AND YOUR BABY

Calories: 120 Total fat: 3 g Aging (saturated and trans) fats: 0 g Healthy fats: 2 g Omega-3 fats: 0 g

EPA and DHA: 0 g Fiber: 4 Carbohydrates: 23 g Sugars:: 5 g Protein: 2 g Sodium: 340 mg

Potassium: 372 mg Calcium: 38 mg Magnesium: 28 mg Selenium: 0 mcg

CALMING TEAS

- Cardamom cinnamon: Cardamom cinnamon tea bag (Republic of Tea is great and has no caffeine) with ¼ teaspoon of agave with splash of milk (cow or soy).
- Ginger (especially for morning sickness): Slice gingerroot into half-inch sections, simmer in 4 cups of water for 20 minutes, and add teaspoon agave and wedge of lemon.

FOLIC ACID BOOSTERS

- Hot grapefruit: Slice one grapefruit in half and place under broiler for 2 minutes, or until warm but not hot. Drizzle with 1 tablespoon honey, and crack fresh pepper and sea salt over the surface to taste.

Spinach Salad
2 1½-cup servings

2 cups packed baby spinach leaves

1 hard-cooked egg, peeled and chopped

¼ cup sunflower seeds

1 tablespoon orange juice

2 teaspoons extra-virgin olive oil

1½ teaspoons red wine vinegar

⅛ teaspoon salt

⅛ teaspoon black pepper, freshly ground

Combine spinach, egg, and sunflower seeds in a medium bowl. Combine remaining ingredients in a small bowl; mix well. Add to spinach mixture; toss well.

WHAT'S IN IT FOR YOU AND YOUR BABY

Calories: 250 Total fat: 17 g Aging (saturated and trans) fats: 2.5 g Healthy fats: 14.5 g Omega-3 fats: 0 g

EPA and DHA: 0 g Fiber: 6 g Carbohydrates: 12 g Sugars: 2 g Protein: 13 g Sodium: 440 mg

Potassium: 1,308 mg Calcium: 250 mg Magnesium: 183 mg Selenium: 8 mcg

Lifestyle 180 Chia Pumpkin Muffins
14 muffins

1½ cups whole wheat pastry flour

1 tablespoon chia seeds, ground

2 teaspoons baking soda

2 teaspoons cinnamon

½ teaspoon nutmeg

½ teaspoon salt

1 can (15 ounces) pumpkin, pureed

¼ cup canola oil

2 tablespoons agave nectar

¼ cup water or sugar-free apple juice

1 tablespoon pure vanilla extract

¾ cup walnuts, chopped

1 cup apple, coarsely grated, peeled, firm pack

Heat oven to 350 degrees F. Combine first six ingredients in a large bowl; mix well. In a separate bowl, combine pumpkin, oil, agave nectar, water, and vanilla; mix well. Add this mixture to dry ingredients, stirring just until dry ingredients are combined. Fold in walnuts and apple. Spoon batter into muffin tins lined with paper cups until almost full. Bake 30 to 33 minutes or until wooden pick inserted in center comes out clean. Transfer to a wire cooling rack; cool at least 10 minutes. Serve warm or at room temperature.

WHAT'S IN IT FOR YOU AND YOUR BABY

Calories: 150   Total fat: 9 g   Aging (saturated and trans) fats: 1 g   Healthy fats: 8 g   Omega-3 fats: 1 g
EPA and DHA: 0 g   Fiber: 3 g   Carbohydrates: 16 g   Sugars: 4 g   Protein: 3 g   Sodium: 265 mg
Potassium: 152 mg   Calcium: 29 mg   Magnesium: 36 mg   Selenium: 10 mcg

Lifestyle 180 Quinoa and Fruit Pudding
½-cup servings

1 cup organic quinoa

2 cups boiling water

½ cup cherries, dried

½ cup cranberries, dried

½ cup unsweetened apple juice

2 ripe medium bananas

1 teaspoon pure vanilla extract

1 teaspoon orange rind, grated

½ teaspoon cinnamon

Rinse quinoa in cold water; drain and add to boiling water. Reduce heat to low; simmer 7 minutes. Add cherries and cranberries; simmer until liquid is absorbed, 5 to 7 minutes.

Meanwhile, combine remaining ingredients in blender or food processor and puree until smooth. Combine pureed mixture with quinoa; mix well. Place in serving bowls; refrigerate until firm, at least 1 hour.

WHAT'S IN IT FOR YOU AND YOUR BABY

Calories: 130   Total fat: 1 g   Aging (saturated and trans) fats: 0 g   Healthy fats: 1 g   Omega-3 fats: 0 g

EPA and DHA: 0 g   Fiber: 3 g   Carbohydrates: 28 g   Sugars: 11 g   Protein: 3 g   Sodium: 0 mg

Potassium: 197 mg   Calcium: 16 mg   Magnesium: 41 mg   Selenium: 2 mcg

Lifestyle 180 Apple Pear Jicama Waldorf Salad
10 ½-cup servings

1 apple, unpeeled, diced

1 pear, unpeeled, diced

1 cup diced peeled jicama

1 cup seedless red grapes

3 tablespoons raisins

3 tablespoons sliced almonds

3 tablespoons chopped walnuts

3 tablespoons unsalted sunflower seeds

⅓ cup dressing of choice (see page 369) or Vegenaise nondairy dressing

Combine all ingredients except dressing in a large bowl. Stir in dressing and, if desired, agave nectar. Serve immediately or cover and chill up to 4 hours before serving.

WHAT'S IN IT FOR YOU AND YOUR BABY

Calories: 130   Total fat: 8 g   Aging (saturated and trans) fats: 1 g   Healthy fats: 5 g   Omega-3 fats: 0 g

EPA and DHA: 0 g   Fiber: 2 g   Carbohydrates: 13 g   Sugars: 8 g   Protein: 2 g   Sodium: 45 mg

Potassium: 150 mg   Calcium: 15 mg   Magnesium: 15.5 mg   Selenium: 2 mcg

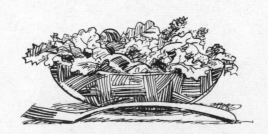

Lifestyle 180 Vegetable Frittata

2 servings

7 large egg whites

1 whole egg

1 tablespoon canola oil

1/2 cup sliced crimini or shiitake mushrooms

1/2 cup diced sweet onion

1/2 cup diced red bell pepper

1/2 cup diced zucchini squash

1 teaspoon turmeric powder

1/4 teaspoon salt

1/4 teaspoon pepper

Combine egg whites and whole egg; whisk well. Heat oil in a 10-inch nonstick skillet over medium heat until hot. Add mushrooms; sauté until golden brown, about 3 minutes. Add onion, pepper, zucchini, turmeric, salt, and pepper; sauté until vegetables are tender, about 5 minutes. Add beaten eggs evenly around vegetables and begin to gently fold in sides inward from rim of pan where the eggs begin to cook while tilting the pan in direction of the fold to allow the loose uncooked eggs to fill that area and cook. Continually doing this around pan will very quickly cook your eggs and begin to create the frittata. At this point you can finish cooking the top of the eggs by putting the pan under a preheated broiler or in a preheated 350 F. oven until eggs are done.

WHAT'S IN IT FOR YOU AND YOUR BABY

Calories: 196   Total fat: 11 g   Aging (saturated and trans) fats: 1 g   Healthy fats: 10 g   Omega-3 fats: 1 g

EPA and DHA: 0 g   Fiber: 2 g   Carbohydrates: 10 g   Sugars: 51 g   Protein: 16 g   Sodium: 503 mg

Potassium: 529 mg   Calcium: 41 mg   Magnesium: 31 mg   Selenium: 33 mcg

Lifestyle 180 Vegetable and Country Dijon Potato Salad

14 ½-cup servings

1½ pounds red potatoes, scrubbed, cut into ¾-inch chunks

1 pound green beans, cut into 1-inch pieces

¼ cup Dijon mustard

2 tablespoons white wine vinegar

1½ tablespoons extra-virgin olive oil

1 tablespoon chopped parsley

1½ teaspoons fresh lemon juice

½ teaspoon minced garlic

½ teaspoon salt

⅛ teaspoon pepper

½ cup finely chopped red bell pepper

½ cup finely chopped red onion

Cook beans and potatoes separately until tender, drain well, and set aside to cool. Meanwhile, in a very large bowl, combine mustard, vinegar, oil, parsley, lemon juice, agave nectar, garlic, salt, and pepper; mix well. Drain potatoes and green beans well; transfer hot vegetables to bowl and toss with dressing. Stir in bell pepper and red onion; toss again. Serve at room temperature or chilled.

WHAT'S IN IT FOR YOU AND YOUR BABY

Calories: 70   Total fat: 1.5 g   Aging (saturated and trans) fats: 0 g   Healthy fats: 2 g   Omega-3 fats: 0 g

EPA and DHA: 0 g   Fiber: 2 g   Carbohydrates: 11 g   Sugars: 2 g   Protein: 2 g   Sodium: 190 mg

Potassium: 244 mg   Calcium: 14 mg   Magnesium: 12 mg   Selenium: 0 mcg

LIFESTYLE 180 SALAD DRESSINGS

For all: Combine all ingredients in a small bowl; whisk well. Cover and refrigerate up to 1 week.

Asian Dressing
Makes ½ cup (8 servings)

4 tablespoons rice vinegar or champagne vinegar

1 teaspoon agave nectar

1 tablespoon dark sesame oil

2 teaspoons reduced-sodium soy sauce

1 tablespoon extra-virgin olive oil

1 teaspoon garlic, minced

½ teaspoon gingerroot, minced

WHAT'S IN IT FOR YOU AND YOUR BABY
Calories: 36

Rice Vinegar Dressing
Makes 1 cup (16 servings)

½ cup rice wine vinegar

⅓ cup extra-virgin olive oil

2 tablespoons agave nectar

1 tablespoon chopped fresh parsley

1 teaspoon minced garlic

½ teaspoon salt

½ teaspoon freshly ground black pepper

WHAT'S IN IT FOR YOU AND YOUR BABY
Calories: 35

Olive Oil and Lemon Dressing

Makes 1 cup (16 servings)

¾ cup extra-virgin olive oil

¼ cup fresh lemon juice

2 teaspoons minced garlic

¼ teaspoon salt

¼ teaspoon freshly ground black pepper

WHAT'S IN IT FOR YOU AND YOUR BABY

Calories: 98

YOU TOOL 6

JUST FOR DAD

Congratulations, pop! We're not going to celebrate with a cigar, but we will celebrate with a pat on the back, a shake of the hand, and a good old-fashioned Honey-Do list. Fact is, you can help out the mom-to-be in innumerable ways during her pregnancy. Think of yourself as part coach, part friend, part maintenance man, and, most of all, full partner.

Believe it or not, there is a very real thing called daddy brain: Expectant dads go through hormonal and brain changes that roughly parallel those of their pregnant mates; it's why there are such phenomena as sympathy weight gain and sympathy pregnancy. Prolactin increases 20 percent in dads in the weeks before the baby's birth, and the stress hormone cortisol doubles in dads during pregnancy. Even testosterone dips after the baby arrives, allowing the male brain to let down its ultramale guard and be receptive to bonding.

While men have little control over the physical course of their partners' pregnancies, they do harbor a lot of emotions about pregnancy and fatherhood and thus need to be involved and invested. Here are three areas in which you can really make a difference. Remember, the first step to being a great father is being a great father-to-be.

Logistical

- Ready the room. Painting's your job (no fumes for her). Also, get the crib and any other new furniture ready to go. Over the next few years, you're going to become a master assembler of cribs, strollers, and toys.
- Take charge of childproofing. Cover electrical outlets, move cleaning supplies, and so on. It may seem like ages until your baby will be crawling and exploring, but—trust us—it'll be here before you know it. Get this task out of the way now so that you don't have to worry about it later.

- Work on finances and budgeting. Price food, diapers, and clothes, and come up with a reasonable expense budget. Take the lead on making suggestions for how you're going to manage finances. If you think finances are tight now, just wait. Some people estimate that expenses associated with newborns are about $250 to $850 (not to mention upfront costs) per month; toddlers about $200 to $800 a month.
- If you haven't done so already, draw up a will, health proxies, and (if applicable) trusts, and make sure your life and disability insurance policies are all in place.
- See Tool 5 a few pages back? All yours, buddy.
- Add chores. You will win major fatherhood points—and improve the overall mood of mom-to-be—if you help with the cleaning, laundry, gardening . . . you get the picture. Remember, anything and everything you do around the house, baby related or not, will help ease her stress.
- Make the food runs. Even if it is four o'clock in the morning. Even if it involves black olives, bananas, and trout fins.
- Pack the hospital bag (see page 249), and help to assemble everything you need before the baby's arrival. (See page 345.)
- After the birth, ask how you can help with nursing (not literally, big boy). She's going to be exhausted, but she also needs to feed the child every three hours or so. Even if she's breast-feeding, you can help by getting up and bringing the baby to her in bed. Don't shove the whole responsibility off on her. Little savings in energy will have big benefits.

Emotional

- Talk, talk, talk, listen, listen, listen. Your conversations about the Red Sox, politics, and pop culture may have to take a backseat to morning sickness, ultrasounds, and in-law fury. Engage in those conversations. She needs them.
- While we're all for you being in good health, now's not the time to announce that you're overweight or going on a six-hundred-push-ups-a-day workout plan. As she's feeling angst about changes in her body that she can't control, you risk hurting her more by focusing too much attention on your physique during this time. By all means, keep eating healthfully

(men with pregnant partners do tend to gain weight as well), but no strutting and flexing, thank you very much.

- In the same spirit, watch what you're watching. If you linger over commercials with minimally clothed models, for example, the not-so-subtle message is that you're enjoying another woman's body during a time when your partner may or may not be feeling so good about hers. Sorry, *Maxim*, subscription canceled.

- We know you know that her body is changing in many ways, but we recommend that you pay close attention to the information in chapter 8 (not just chapter 7). She's going through a lot, and your understanding of those physical changes will be very much appreciated.

- Turn the other cheek. She's going to have mood swings—many, perhaps. So don't be surprised if she's yelling at you one minute and kissing you the next. And while it's fine to have disagreements, of course, remember that her hormones are making her do and say things she might not normally do or say.

- Remind yourself that you're no longer number one. It's easy to know that this is coming, but you may feel different once it's obvious that you will take a backseat. It may feel like a blow to your ego, but tell yourself that it's really a boost for your family.

- With everyone (read: in-laws) offering advice, try to keep it in perspective. They're not trying to tell you that you're doing a bad job—though it sure may seem that way. They have good intentions, so take a deep breath and relax when mum corrects the way you screw the nipples onto the bottles.

- Show your support in little ways: Give up your glass of wine, since she does too. Go to as many prenatal appointments as you can. Be an active participant in the birthing classes.

- Know her wishes regarding labor and delivery so you can act as her advocate.

Physical

- See our recommendations for increasing sensuality in your relationship on page 184. For her, closeness may not be about the sex, though some women do have an increased sex drive during pregnancy.

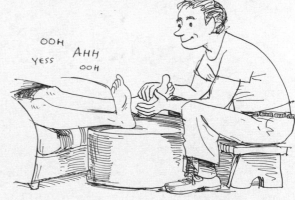

But she does appreciate the physical gestures that can have emotional implications: the hugs, the kisses, the hand holds. Initiate them. Often.

- See the most comfortable positions for sex on page 185. If she does want to be intimate, you want to make sure that she's as comfortable as possible.

- You've got two hands, right? Use them. On her back, on her neck, on her shoulders, on her feet. Rub, caress, knead. All the extra weight she's carrying means that she's holding a lot of tension. You can help her release it.

- During labor, have a couple of tennis balls ready to go. You can roll them over sore spots to help relax her muscles and ease the pain.

APPENDIX 1

The YOU Prepregnancy Plan

If you're one of those people who crank out to-do lists as fast as Starbucks cranks out lattes, then you may be on top of the game: You're reading about pregnancy before you're actually pregnant. Good for you. Smart thinking. That's why we developed this prepregnancy checklist—to give the blueprint for things you can do beforehand. (Remember that 50 percent of pregnancies are not planned, so it is important to take a healthy approach to prepregnancy planning.) If you're a woman of childbearing age and not using birth control, you should follow these steps to better your chances of a healthy pregnancy.

Clean Up Your Act (if it's rated R)
- Stop smoking.
- Stop drinking alcohol.
- Stop using recreational drugs.
- Avoid secondhand smoke.
- Floss every day.

Get in Shape

- Begin a regular exercise program.
- Attain a healthful weight (body mass index between 20 and 25 kg/m^2; see BMI description on page 68) and a waist size less than or equal to half your height. For the average five-foot-five-inch woman, that would come to around 32.5 inches at the belly button—with you sucking in like Scarlett O'Hara.
- Practice a stress reduction technique such as meditation, yoga, stretching, or walking.

Monitor Your Intake

- Take a daily prenatal vitamin that contains 400 mcg of folic acid.
- Limit caffeine to 200 mg a day.
- Avoid all trans fats.
- Choose organic low-fat meat, nonfat dairy products, and produce whenever possible.
- Avoid fish high in mercury (tuna, shark, tile, sword).
- Increase your intake of DHA with supplements or fatty fish to at least 200 to 300 mg daily; enjoy soy products, whole grains, and flaxseeds; increase your omega-3 intake by consuming walnuts, avocados, and canola oil.
- Avoid sushi, undercooked meat, soft cheeses (brie, gorgonzola), and unpasteurized cheeses and milk.
- Use acetaminophen (Tylenol) instead of ibuprofen (Advil, Motrin), naproxen (Aleve), or aspirin.

Minimize Your Exposure

- If you have not been exposed to toxoplasmosis, wear gloves when gardening or changing cat litter; afterward, thoroughly wash your hands.
- If painting, use latex paint and avoid spray paints and paint thinners.
- Avoid chemicals such as bisphenol-A (in plastic water bottles; look for the number 2 or 4 inside the triangle on the bottom of the bottle, but not 3, 6, 7, 8, or 9; 1 is acceptable but not reusable), phthalates (in composite dental

How Do You Know If You're Pregnant?

Some women can just "tell" if they're pregnant. Maybe they have a gut feeling, or maybe their bodies just feel a little bit different: Their breasts may feel more tender, or they may have immediate aversions to or cravings for food. The only way to confirm pregnancy is through the identification of the hormone hCG in either blood or urine. The blood test is done in the doc's office, of course, and the urine test can be done at home. But hCG doesn't show up in blood until about ten to fourteen days after conception, and a standard urine pregnancy test may not even show as positive for up to four weeks after conception. So it's possible you won't know for sure until at least after you've missed a period. If you just can't wait, highly sensitive home urine tests can give results between seven and ten days after ovulation—potentially before you've missed a period. Both standard and high-sensitivity urine tests are highly accurate. For home tests, use the first morning's urine (the concentration of hCG is higher), and wait five to ten minutes for results.

fillings; also released when plastic is microwaved), fluorotelomers (in linings of microwave popcorn bags, as well as stain-resistant carpets and furniture), and PCBs (polychlorinated biphenyls, which are organic compounds in fish caught from polluted waterways).

- Avoid pesticides.
- Avoid heavy metals such as mercury and lead.
- Avoid occupational or hobby exposure to organic solvents, such as toluene, xylene, benzene, tetrachloroethylene, ethylene oxide, acetone, and formaldehyde.
- Avoid exposure to anesthetic gases.
- Avoid exposure to excess radiation (X-rays, frequent long-haul flights) and radon.

If You're Diabetic

- Get your blood sugar under control a minimum of twenty-one days before conception; aim for a hemoglobin A1C of 6.4 percent or less.

- Follow a low-glycemic-index diet, including plenty of complex carbohydrates.

Select and See an OB/GYN or Midwife

- Update your immunizations, particularly chicken pox, measles, mumps, rubella, and influenza (seasonally).
- Discuss having genetic testing done before you try to conceive, especially if you are of Ashkenazi Jewish or Mediterranean ancestry or have a genetic disease with sickle-cell anemia trait.
- Review your personal and family history of diseases, especially diabetes, heart disease, asthma, high blood pressure, kidney disease, epilepsy, thyroid disease, phenylketonuria (PKU), thalassemia, iron deficiency anemia, and sickle-cell anemia.
- Review your reproductive history, including fertility issues, multiple miscarriages, an abnormally shaped uterus, endometriosis, sexually transmitted diseases, tubal problems, and polycystic ovary syndrome (PCOS).
- Have a blood test to determine your blood type and screen for toxoplasmosis, syphilis, HIV, and group B streptococcus.

See Your Dentist

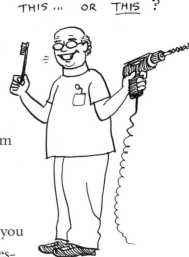

THIS ... OR THIS ?

- Get your teeth cleaned.
- Have all necessary dental work done, including fillings and treatment for gum disease.
- Be sure to drink fluoridated water or use a fluoridated oral rinse in addition to brushing at least twice a day with fluoridated toothpaste to prevent cavities and gum disease while you're pregnant.

See Your Other Docs

- Discuss continuing, stopping, or changing medications you may be on to treat other conditions, such as antidepres-

The Second Time Around

Once you've experienced pregnancy and childbirth, you're much better prepared to deal with potential complications the next time around. If you ran into any of the following problems during your first pregnancy, your chances of experiencing them again increase significantly. In most cases, preventive measures can be taken early on to minimize their impact on you and your baby, so be sure to talk with your OB before trying to get pregnant again.

- Antiphospholipid syndrome
- Rh disease
- Gestational diabetes
- Placental problems (like previa and abruption)
- Incompetent cervix
- Preeclampsia
- Cesarean section
- Congenital birth defects

An interesting note: If you've already had a pregnancy affected by a birth defect of the brain or spinal cord, ask your health care provider how much folic acid you need. Studies have shown that taking a larger dose of folic acid daily can reduce the risk of having another affected pregnancy. The recommended dose, of 4 milligrams (4,000 micrograms) per day, should be taken at least one month before pregnancy and throughout the first trimester.

sants, antihypertensives, diuretics, steroids, pain medication, and antiseizure medications.
- Discuss management of autoimmune disorders; examples include lupus and multiple sclerosis (MS).

APPENDIX 2

Fertility Issues

From a purely evolutionary perspective, you'd think that your body would make it fairly easy to get pregnant and keep the developing fetus safe and sound for forty weeks. After all, that's what ensures that the species and gene pools continue. But not so. About 15 percent of couples have trouble conceiving, increasing with age, and it can be a slippery slope even after conception occurs: About one-third of all conceptions fail. That figure includes ones in which women don't even know they're pregnant.

So pregnancy may be even more of a miracle than you think. If you're experiencing fertility problems, there are several things you can do to increase your odds. First, it's important to gain a little perspective about the things that are preventing your body from being able to conceive or to carry a child to term.

Fertility isn't just about the ability to get the sperm and egg to do the biological do-si-do; fertility is about having the ability to maintain fetal development past twelve weeks and to avoid some of the problems that cause miscarriage. A miscarriage essentially occurs when there's a hemorrhage in a layer of tissue in the uterus. The bleeding causes tissues next to the ovum to break down (see figure opposite), which

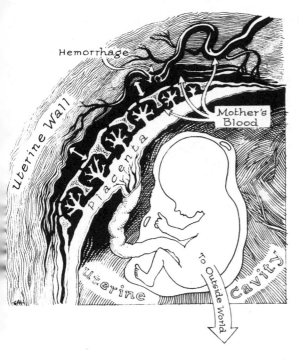

Hemorrhage

Uterine Wall

Placenta

Mother's Blood

Uterine Cavity

To Outside World

stimulates uterine contractions—contractions that result in the fertilized egg detaching from the uterine lining and thus being expelled by the mother. The blood hemorrhaging in the delicate space between mom and baby blocks nutrients and starves the child. Often, women aren't even aware that a pregnancy and miscarriage has occurred.

About 80 percent of miscarriages (also called spontaneous abortions) occur during the first twelve weeks of pregnancy, and half of those are caused by chromosomal abnormalities that are incompatible with a live birth. The risk of miscarriage increases with the number of previous births as well as with maternal and paternal age: A quarter of miscarriages happen in women older than forty. In the vast majority of cases, there's absolutely nothing you can do to prevent a miscarriage. What you can do is take certain steps to optimize your fertility and to provide the best possible environment for your fetus after you have conceived.

Before we give you our advice, it's important to know some important fertility facts and figures:

- You have about a 35 percent chance of getting pregnant within the first month of actively trying.
- If everything is working correctly, you have a 90 percent chance of conceiving within the first year of trying (and about 80 percent after six months). So our advice is that if you've been casually trying to get pregnant for six months without success, get serious about it over the next six months. After that, it's not a bad idea to see a fertility specialist to help you identify potential causes of infertility.

To figure out your best window of opportunity for conceiving, use this formula:

1. Record the length of your menstrual cycle from the first day of a your period to the day before your next period for several months, then take the average.
2. Subtract 14 from that number.
3. Each month, the best time to conceive is that number of days after the start of your period. Let's say that your period comes every 23 days. Subtract 14 from 23, which equals 9. So the 9th day after your period begins is the best day to make love if the goal is to get pregnant.

But you should get a head start, since sperm can live for three to five days in a woman's cervical mucus. You can also use your basal body temperature to pinpoint ovulation; more on that in a moment.

Common Causes of Infertility

Numbers may be all well and good, you say, but it's frustrating just the same if you have trouble conceiving. Because it is such a delicate process (see chapter 1), it shouldn't be a surprise that so many things can cause infertility. In fact, if we tried to explain all the causes of infertility here, you'd likely have enough time to get your yet-to-be-conceived child off to State U. before we finished. While advanced age is one of the major causes, here are a few others that affect fertility:

Stress

You hear stories all the time. As soon as a seemingly infertile couple decide to stop trying and go the adoption route, *bam,* the woman becomes pregnant. There's a reason for this: namely, the stress of trying so hard has stopped. Research shows that women who are emotionally expressive about fertility treatments have a harder time getting pregnant than those who are better able to deal with the stress of infertility internally.

This applies to men too. Stress seems to affect both sperm quality and quantity, making it more difficult to conceive. Historically, when we faced stress in our environment—a famine, for instance—our ancestors were in no position to make babies. In the male, increased levels of the stress hormone cortisol seem to inhibit production of normal semen. In the female, increased cortisol influences the other stress hormones coming from the ovaries and adds a supersonic drumroll to a delicate symphony. The resulting cacophony makes pregnancy very difficult. And contrary to popular wisdom, you *can* be too thin; to your body, that's also a form of stress. If you have a BMI of less than 20 Kg/m², you may increase your chances of getting pregnant by gaining five to ten pounds, not by Twinkies, please.

Polycystic Ovarian Syndrome (PCOS)

This hormonal condition affecting the ovaries is often accompanied by such features as facial hair, a stocky build, increased abdominal obesity, elevated lousy (LDL) cholesterol, increased triglycerides, increased inflammation, and increased blood pressure. The condition alters a woman's hormonal makeup, impeding ovulation and the formation of tissues needed for implantation of the egg. Metformin, a diabetes drug, has been used to help treat PCOS, as polycystic ovarian syndrome is a relative of metabolic syndrome and its close cousin, diabetes. An infertility drug called clomiphene (Clomid) is often used to help women with PCOS ovulate more consistently.

Tubal Factors

Typically, the blastocyst (the egg-sperm union) implants in the endometrial lining of the uterine cavity. But in ectopic pregnancies, which occur in about 2 percent of pregnancies, implantation takes place somewhere in the Fallopian tube—either near the ovary, in the middle, or where the tube inserts into the uterus. Nearly one-third of fertility issues are caused by tubal problems, such as a blockage or malfunction that prevents sperm from getting to the egg. Tubal damage—caused by surgery, pelvic infections, or the presence of an IUD, among other factors—can cause ectopic pregnancies. Even smoking and douching can cause the blastocyst to implant in the tube instead of the womb. If you've had pelvic infections or a prior ectopic pregnancy, the risk of experiencing another is about 15 percent. Nonwhite women have a higher risk, as do older women.

Signs of an ectopic pregnancy include abdominal pain, increased blood pressure, vaginal bleeding, or feeling a mass in your pelvic region. If your Fallopian tube ruptures, it's a life-threatening emergency that can cause your death. So if you have any question, see your obstetrician immediately. Docs can detect an ectopic pregnancy by evaluating hormone levels from a blood specimen and by ultrasound. If caught early, it can sometimes be treated with medication. Surgery can fix some tubal problems by tying down these delicate organs, which look like Venus flytraps.

Here are some tips to follow if you want to improve your fertility:

Time It. When's the ideal time during your cycle to have sex? (Anytime! he says.) If you're trying to increase your chances of conception, your best opportunity is one to two days before ovulation. To maximize sperm quantity and quality, have sex every two or three days starting five days before ovulation—because sperm can live for at least forty-eight hours in the vagina, you'll be covered. The challenge is that the actual day of ovulation can change from cycle to cycle. So what are the clues?

Cervical fluid: A change in cervical fluid can indicate that you are close to your peak ovulation day. Fertile fluid is stretchy and slippery; otherwise, it's more creamy and lotionlike. Just separate your vaginal lips and use a tissue or your finger to check the fluid at the opening, down near your perineum. Slowly open your fingers to see if it stretches to about the length of half a banana. If it does, it means you are getting ready to ovulate. Timing intercourse every other day for five days around this time should give you a good chance.

Waking temperature: While your waking temperature is lower before ovulation (97 to 97.7 degrees F.), it rises after ovulation (97.8). The elevation typically happens a day after ovulation because of the hormone progesterone, which induces heat. You can get a sense of when you're ovulating by taking your

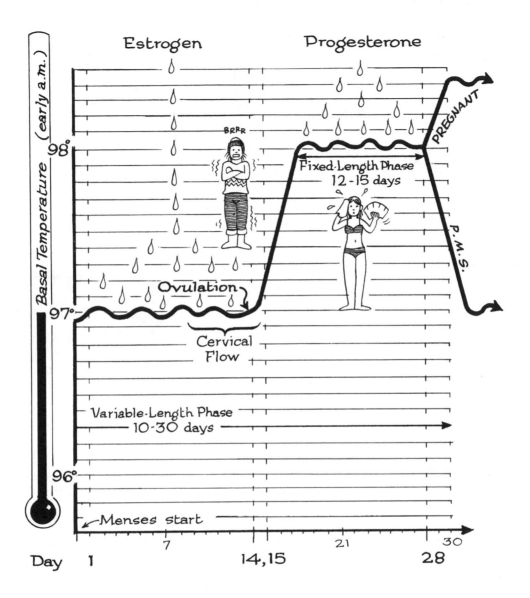

temperature first thing after waking, then plotting the numbers to a tenth of a degree. Ovulation has occurred when you see a more dramatic shift than the day-to-day fluctuations that happen during the rest of your cycle. That will give you an idea of which day in your cycle typically is your ovulation day.

Watch the Trans Fats. One of the best ways to increase fertility is to keep your lousy LDL cholesterol and your waist size low. Reducing the trans fats in your diet will help on both fronts. Research shows that the more trans fats in a woman's diet, the greater the risk of miscarrying. That's especially true when trans fats make up more than 5 percent of your daily calories. Eating too many simple carbs, as well as inadequate amounts of iron and protein, can also negatively affect fertility.

Don't Lubricate. We like admonishing you with a series of don'ts about as much as we like fried fish platters. One don't we can't avoid: sexual lubricants. While they can be helpful (and pleasing) in many circumstances, they actually can slow down sperm. And in the race of capture-the-egg, that can cost you the game.

Wait a Little: What's the best sex position for fertilization? Missionary? Reverse cowgirl? Something involving a leather ottoman? While the data are inconclusive that any sex position is better than another, it does seem that your odds go up with the missionary position and with the woman remaining on her back for fifteen minutes after the man ejaculates, which increases the chance that the sperm will make it upstream.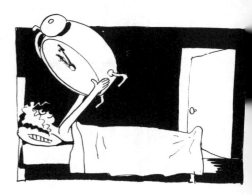

Don't Overdo It: If you exercise as if it's your job, you might be hindering your fertility. Vigorous exercise prevents ovulation. You will know by the irregularity of your menstrual cycles. Ask your doctor how you can modify your exercise plan to restore your normal pattern. No ovulation means nobody's going to be putting any cribs together anytime soon. While it's obviously important to stay healthy and exercise, in general we don't think you should run more than ten miles per week (or the equivalent in other forms of exercise). Because every woman's baseline fitness level is different and every pregnancy is different, it's impossible to know for sure how much is too much for your body and baby.

Male Factors

Obstacles to fertility in men include a low sperm count, poor semen quality, or immature or abnormally shaped sperm. Such demons as smoking, excessive use of alcohol and drugs, and obesity (as well as some nutritional deficiencies) can also be the triggers. Some other interesting notes:

- Mounting evidence suggests that male infertility may be added to the growing list of adult diseases that originate in the fetus. Researchers studying the epigenetics of DNA found that sperm DNA from men with abnormal sperm or low sperm counts contained high levels of methylation—one of the ways that the body regulates gene expression. That methylated DNA becomes half of the fetus's genome, a perfect example of how the epigenetic effects we talked about in chapter 1 can be passed on from one generation to the next.

- While some men who have been treated for testicular cancer may experience temporary infertility, a small minority of survivors are unable to father a child. The flip side is that men who experience infertility have a slightly increased chance of contracting testicular cancer later in life, so they should be diligent about performing regular testicular self-examination. Ask your doc to show you how.

- In addition to being the most prominent fat in the brain, the omega-3 fatty acid DHA is also abundant in sperm cells. Several laboratory experiments have found that DHA may improve sperm concentration. The jury is still out on the exact relationship between DHA and male fertility, but there seem to be some indications that DHA may produce faster, healthier sperm.

Tips for Dad-to-Be

It takes about ninety days for sperm to be manufactured and to mature, so, ideally, you should watch what you eat, drink, smoke, and expose your sperm manufacturing system to for three months prior to conception. For optimum fertility, sperm prefer a temperature slightly lower than the rest of your body. To keep your sperm delivery system working, it's also important to keep blood flowing to the area. For maximum potency, note the following dos and don'ts:

Do

- Eat your fruits and veggies, grains, beans, soy, nuts, oats, foods with flavonols (like broccoli, radishes, onions, tomatoes, and leeks), as well as other foods high in polyphenols (think bright-colored fruits and veggies), vitamins C and E, zinc, selenium, and omega-3s (salmon, trout, walnuts, chia, avocados, canola oil, and flaxseeds).
- Wear boxers, not briefs (lower temp in these).
- Avoid exposure to organic solvents, heavy metals, synthetic polymers, pesticides, PCBs, and ionizing radiation.
- Keep well hydrated while working out.
- Get a physical and discuss your personal and family medical history, including birth defects, sexually transmitted diseases, difficulty or pain with erection, ejaculation, or urination, and any medications you may be taking that could adversely affect your fertility. Among the possible culprits: antihypertensives, diuretics, antidepressants, antiseizure medications, antihistamines, antibiotics, chemotherapy, immunosuppressive drugs.

Don't

- Smoke.
- Drink excessively (more than two alcoholic drinks a day).
- Use recreational drugs.
- Take anabolic steroids.
- Eat fatty cuts of beef, dark-meat turkey, or fish containing mercury (bottom feeders).
- Use oil-based paints, spray paints, or paint thinners (and do use a fan).
- Work with your laptop on your lap.
- Lounge in the hot tub, steam room, or sauna; doing so can raise the temperature of sperm and kill them.
- Spend a lot of time wearing an athletic cup or jockstrap.
- Cycle if you experience numbness or tingling in the genital area or sexual dysfunction.

APPENDIX 3

Vaccinations

One of the most highly charged conflicts in the parenting world revolves around an issue that comes up just moments after your baby is born: to vaccinate or not to vaccinate?

Before we detail the issue, two important points: First, we are not going to adamantly tell you what to do one way or the other, since even the authorship team has varying opinions on the subject. What we hope is that you will explore both the pros and cons about vaccines (which we outline here), even do additional research, and make a thoughtful decision about what makes sense to you. Second, we want to make clear that this whole debate has nothing to do with which side loves their children more. People on both sides, even if they vehemently disagree, are passionately trying to protect their children's health.

In a nutshell, here's the conflict: There are surely enough data to show that vaccines do save lives and protect against illness. The size of that benefit may be debatable, but we consider it vast and significant. There are also safety concerns, as with any medication, in that there are not—and never can be—enough data to guarantee the safety of vaccines in any given individual, especially as they interact with other vaccines, drugs, foods, and that person's specific environment.

So what are we left with? In one corner, we have a group of people who examine the data and believe the advice of the majority of pediatricians and the government. They conclude that vaccines are much more likely to benefit their children than harm them and are helpful to the long-term health not only of children but of the population at large. They cite data showing that immunizations prevent many infant deaths every year and studies concluding that nonimmunized children experience more disease events that are categorized as "side effects of vaccine" (such as epilepsy, delayed development, and impaired communication) than occur in immunized children. Some individuals blame vaccines as the cause of epilepsy, delayed development, or impaired communication; as it turns out these problems arise in close approximation to vaccine administration—but close approximation does not indicate cause and effect. Since more unimmunized children have these problems than immunized children, blaming the vaccines should not be justified. In the other corner, we have those who believe that vaccines are detrimental to the long-term health of their children, that no studies effectively demonstrate a vaccine's safety, and that the full range of serious consequences caused by vaccines is being minimized and ignored.

The great news is that there is some common ground: Both sides acknowledge that the debate has forced vaccines to become safer, and that's a good thing. Beyond that, your decision may ultimately come down to (1) what kind of person you are at heart (trusting of the medical profession or skeptical of it), (2) how tolerant you are of risk, and (3) your family medical history. One thing is clear: not vaccinating your child increases her risks of getting one of the vaccine-preventable diseases.

To help you make an informed choice, we questioned over one hundred experts in the field. Here's a summary of some of the major arguments for and against vaccination:

The Issue	Are vaccines safe and effective?
Support Vaccines	Vaccines decrease mortality. They prevent 20,500 infant deaths a year in the United States (compared to the prevaccine era) and other disorders such as brain dysfunction, paralysis, and even cancer in children and adults. By reducing the prevalence of these infections in the population through vaccination, we can reduce the risk to those not able to be vaccinated or for whom vaccines may not work (those with immune deficiencies, those who are receiving treatments that hinder immunization, those who are too young). If immunization rates were to decrease, the risk of infection would increase for all children, and especially for the most vulnerable members of society. There's no doubt that vaccination can cause some injuries. For example, we believe polio vaccine, which prevents polio in 1 in 245 immunized, causes polio in 1 in 1 million to 2 million back when the vaccine was made from a live weakened virus. The rate is zero reported cases for the inactivated vaccine currently used in the U.S. and Scandinavia. Measles vaccine causes about 4 cases of serious brain dysfunction a year in the United States (and prevents 2,000 to 4,000 such brain dysfunctions and several hundred deaths from the actual disease), and the rotavirus vaccine caused intussusception—a serious condition often requiring surgery or a radiologic procedure—in 1 of every 10,000 to 14,000 kids immunized. This spurred development of a new vaccine; that new vaccine does not appear to be associated with intussusception risk. Moreover, it prevents hospitalization for diarrhea in about 1 in 200 kids. (The "Vaccine Injury Table" of the National Vaccine Injury Compensation Program lists side effects that have been acknowledged by the government.)
Against Vaccines	Large studies such as those in Europe that show no adverse effects from vaccines in more than 2.5 million kids are epidemiological, meaning that they show patterns in the population rather than biological cause and effect in the individual. Large studies ignore the significant number of stories by parents who have witnessed sudden declines in the health of their children after vaccination.
The YOU Docs' Take	Safe does not mean without risk. It means benefit greater than risk for the general population. Vaccines save lives and prevent disease, but all seventeen childhood vaccines combined may carry serious risks for anywhere from 1 child in 2,000 to 1 child in 10,000. The chance that childhood vaccines benefit the typical child are at least twenty times greater than the chance of serious injury.

(*continued on next page*)

The Issue	Do vaccines cause autism?
Support Vaccines	Large-scale epidemiologic studies in a number of countries, including Finland, the Netherlands, the United Kingdom, Japan, and the United States, clearly demonstrate that vaccines are not responsible for the epidemic of autism. Vaccines might trigger autism in a small number of genetically primed individuals who most probably would have developed autism even if they hadn't received the vaccine.
Against Vaccines	The stories of parents describing the transformation of their previously healthy children into children with autism spectrum disorder soon after and in immediate relationship to vaccination are too strong and too common to avoid the conclusion that vaccines can cause autism.
The YOU Docs' Take	Vaccination is not the cause of the autism epidemic, but it might trigger autism in genetically susceptible children. We cannot currently identify such vulnerable children prior to vaccination. As genetic triggers become better known, and as testing becomes safer, less expensive, and more available, we may be able to identify all individuals at risk for vaccine-triggered diseases and avoid vaccinating them. For all who choose vaccination, make sure that your child is in good health, is hydrated with water before getting the shot, and is not receiving antibiotics. If your child or a close family member is sick, schedule his vaccines for another time. Treat any postvaccine fever and irritability aggressively, hydrate with water or sports drinks, and proceed according to your pediatrician's instructions.
The Issue	Are vaccines even necessary?
Support Vaccines	If we had vaccines for more pathogens, we could decrease the incidence of more diseases—for example, vaccines against Alzheimer's disease, AIDS, and bacterial infections such as MRSA, a potentially fatal staph bug that is alarmingly resistant to antibiotics.
Against Vaccines	There are hundreds of pathogens for which there are no vaccines, and the CDC makes very good recommendations for staying healthy while being exposed to those pathogens (disease-causing agents, such as viruses and bacteria). The same recommendations should hold true for those diseases for which we have vaccines.

The YOU Docs' Take	Our grandparents and their parents didn't get vaccinated, and a number of us didn't get many of the current vaccines. We missed seven days or so of school for chicken pox (varicella), and some of us will suffer shingles when that virus resurfaces in us later in life. Our caregivers suffered with us and stayed home from work too. We weren't allowed to play outside, go to the movies, or go to camp in the summer until the polio vaccine was deployed. One in a thousand of our parents' generation who got measles developed brain dysfunction. German measles led to deafness, blindness, and brain dysfunction if infection was contracted in utero, and more kids died in previous eras due to vaccine-preventable diseases. Vaccination has promoted a better quality of life and has allowed more of us to survive and have children of our own. We're for 'em.
The Issue	**What are we exposing our kids to?**
Against Vaccines	If children receive the entire panel, they get 32 vaccinations (17 vaccines, but some are given more than once to achieve complete protection) over six years and are injected with 113 vaccine antigens. That's a lot of unnecessary chemicals to put into a child's body and three times as many as was recommended two decades ago. This is also more than many European countries recommend.
Support Vaccines	Kids and even adults are exposed to many more than 113 new antigens every hour in a new environment such as a zoo or museum. Plus, the smallpox vaccine alone contained 203 antigens. The great news? By wiping out smallpox through mass vaccinations in the past, no one currently gets those 203 antigens.
The YOU Docs' Take	The safety of vaccines and vaccine additives has improved, and we are more comfortable with their safety based on scientific study and years of experience. Of course, more can always be done to improve the quality of vaccines, and the current debate is pushing that research forward.
The Issue	**How important are vaccines in a global and unpredictable world?**
Support Vaccines	Vaccines are necessary because we live in a world—and travel in a world—where we come into unexpected contact with people who have been exposed to disease or may be asymptomatic carriers.
Against Vaccines	Those who are not especially high-risk do not need to be exposed to vaccines.

(continued on next page)

The Issue	How important are vaccines in a global and unpredictable world? (*cont.*)
The YOU Docs' Take	If you can identify your child as low-risk for certain diseases (see bottom box on page 400)—and this is not easy unless you and your child do not and will not have much contact with the outside world—you can be more flexible in terms of timing vaccines. For example, if you, your partner, and your child's caregivers are not carriers of hepatitis B, we recommend waiting to give this vaccination until two months of age or later. Do note that varying from the recommended schedule places the burden of record keeping on you, but if you're up to the task, it may be safer for Junior.
The Issue	Can we wipe out diseases with vaccines?
Support Vaccines	Through vaccines, we can achieve herd immunity, making diseases so uncommon in the environment that some are eventually eradicated (and we no longer need the vaccine). The best example is the global elimination of smallpox. We were very close to eliminating polio until a few countries declined immunization for several years, allowing it to resurface in their populations and then spread to others. Until those outbreaks can be eliminated, polio vaccination is still a necessity.
Against Vaccines	Modern medical advances such as sanitation systems and personal hygiene have also played a major role in wiping out diseases, and children do not need to be vaccinated for diseases that they're at little risk of contracting or suffering life-threatening complications from.
The YOU Docs' Take	We love the smallpox story but think it is unlikely to be repeated for many diseases. We hope we are wrong. We urge you to protect your child according to the current standards set by the American Academy of Pediatrics, which has considerable flexibility, and we urge you to discuss this issue with your pediatrician before delivery.
The Issue	Should we use vaccines to protect others?
Support Vaccines	Vaccinating children helps protect others who might be particularly vulnerable to these life-threatening diseases, such as grandparents, infant siblings, and people who suffer from disorders that compromise their defenses against disease or who are undergoing immune-suppressing therapies.
Against Vaccines	People who are vulnerable need to take preventive measures against contracting diseases. And disease risk has gone down substantially as many others are getting vaccinated. My child need not bear the responsibility for other people's health by being vaccinated.

The YOU Docs' Take	Herd immunity is a wonderful thing. If you're concerned about the health of the general population, your choice is clear; if you're concerned solely for the health of your child, your choice may be more difficult.
The Issue	**Who should make decisions about vaccination?**
Support Vaccines	The issues around research and ethics are too tough for those not scientifically trained to understand. Complicating the issue is the fact that the gold-standard studies are unethical: How could you carry out a double-blind study of a large group of children, randomly assigning half to be immunized and half not, and leave the second group of kids vulnerable to serious and often deadly diseases?
Against Vaccines	Individuals need to customize their own programs with willing physicians as advisers. The one-size-fits-all schedule is dangerous for too many kids.
The YOU Docs' Take	We think that you are smart enough to digest the arguments in this toolbox and make rational decisions for your children. Most readers will follow the official guidelines established by the American Academy of the Pediatrics, which offer the least chance of missing important vaccinations. Others will follow alternative schedules to reduce to the smallest degree possible the potential perceived complications. Since our society recognizes its responsibility to protect all children, laws and regulations may exclude unvaccinated children from public programs such as schools, day care, and camps.
The Issue	**Have the YOU docs presented the issue fairly?**
Support Vaccines	You could have done a better job. Giving equal space to those against vaccines makes it seem as though they have a valid argument. You try to be too nice, and maybe you guys don't understand the science well enough.
Against Vaccines	You guys seem to ignore the personal stories of parents whose children suffered real illness and injury right after vaccination. You do not tell the story of how the establishment is hiding data concerning side effects or misleading themselves about the robustness of weak studies.
The YOU Docs' Take	If both sides think that we are giving the other side too much credit, we've probably hit the sweet spot in this argument. But we also believe that we need a new way of presenting the information to help mothers and fathers discuss the options with well-meaning but busy pediatricians who are understandably frustrated addressing the same concerns dozens of times weekly. That's why we're applying a formulation called the Number Needed to Treat.

The Number Needed to Treat

To help you understand the risk-benefit relationship with regard to immunization, we calculated for each vaccine a number called the Number Needed to Treat—that is, how many kids have to be inoculated to save a life or prevent a case of that particular disease. (For more information on how we calculated these numbers, please see our explanation on www.realage.com and www.doctoroz.com.) The advantage of this number is that it gives you some perspective on how effective a vaccine can be.

Factoid: As of 2009, forty-eight states allowed parents to excuse their children from vaccination requirements on religious grounds, and nineteen of those states also allowed exemptions for parents with secular philosophical concerns. About 3 percent of U.S. children are excused from immunization by parents; in some areas, the rate is as high as 15 to 20 percent.

How to read it: The smaller the number, the better the figure. For example, when the number needed to treat is 2, that means that for every two vaccines given, you've prevented one death or disease. When the number is big, it's the opposite. For every, say, 5,000 vaccines given, you've prevented only one death or disease. If you're not comfortable with numbers and statistics (and even if you are), we strongly encourage you to copy this chart and discuss it with your pediatrician to help you understand the numbers as well as you can.

Because vaccination has made many of these diseases uncommon, you may not be familiar with the possible outcomes of contracting them. We encourage you to read our summary of the risks of each disease at the end of this toolbox.

The big things you can take away from these numbers:

In most cases, vaccines prevent high-impact ailments for which there is currently a low probability of contraction. It's up to you to decide where the balance point lies between risk and benefit, according to your own sensitivities. Remember, if there were a simple answer, we wouldn't even be having this debate.

It's important to focus on the Number Needed to Vaccinate to Prevent a Case, not only the Number Needed to Vaccinate to Prevent a Death, because infection often leads to hospitalization (and potentially a host of other exposures and lifelong complications), not to mention that infections put others around you at risk as well.

These numbers are calculated by comparing the number of cases of a disease before versus after vaccines were used. And they lead to a fundamental question: Is the risk of getting the infection great enough to warrant vaccination, or is it small enough that the risk of the vaccine isn't worth it? Only you can answer that, because we each have our own philosophical take on where to draw that line.

	Number Needed to Vaccinate to Prevent a Case	Number Needed to Vaccinate to Prevent a Death
Varicella	2	46,512
Rotavirus	2	104,167
Measles	8	9,091
Newborn influenza	13	50,000
Pertussis (whooping cough)	22	998
Mumps	26	102,564
Hepatitis A	39	33,613
Hepatitis B	75	21,053
Rubella	84	235,294
Smallpox	138	11,869
Strep pneumococcus	186	2,424
Diphtheria	200	2,195

(continued on next page)

	Number Needed to Vaccinate to Prevent a Case	Number Needed to Vaccinate to Prevent a Death
Haemophilus influenzae type b (Hib)	201	4,020
Polio	245	2,129
Influenza in pregnant women	952	63,492
Meningococcus (cerebrospinal meninococeal meningitis)	2,689	22,409
Tetanus	7,421	8,547

Your Vaccination Options

The bottom line is that you can educate yourself to make informed, conscious, and customized choices based on your family's beliefs and values. Essentially, you have three options.

The Option	Vaccinate according to U.S. government's and American Academy of Pediatrics' approved guidelines
Support This Approach	The American Academy of Pediatrics and the U.S. Centers for Disease Control and Prevention have assembled the most knowledgeable people in the world to come up with a schedule that makes the most sense for the public health. The schedule is based on the knowledge of diverse experts who are best able to synthesize what is known about human developmental biology, the epidemiology and clinical characteristics of the disease, and the characteristics of the particular vaccine.

Against This Approach	Many of these experts earn income by administering or researching vaccines or consulting with pharmaceutical manufacturers. While they are concerned about the health of the general public, few value your individual child's health as greatly as you do. And some recommendations are clearly designed for society in general even if you as an individual might not benefit. For example, the recommendation to immunize against hepatitis B at birth is illogical if you, your spouse, and your caregivers are all low-risk. But the advice is wise for the U.S. population as a whole, if you as an individual don't think that the parents at high-risk for hepatitis (like IV drug abusers) will bring their children back to the pediatrician in a timely fashion.
The YOU Docs' Take	The advantage of the standard plan is that it represents a broadly based scientific consensus on how to maximize protection of each child. In addition, most docs follow it, making it easier to avoid mistakes, especially if you're moving or switching pediatricians at any point. Combining injections saves money (since many insurers won't pay for alternative plans) and avoids traumatizing the child with multiple injections at every doctor's visit. The downside, some believe, is that some of the early vaccines (like hepatitis B at birth) are unnecessary for low-risk babies.
The Option	**Vaccinate according to a popular pediatrician's guidelines or your own plan**
Support This Approach	Spreading out vaccines reduces the insult to your child's immune system caused by administering multiple antigens and toxins at once. Delaying the vaccines allows the infant's immune system to develop so that she can cope more effectively. And when she has completed the schedule, she still gets all the protection offered by the standard approach.
Against This Approach	If you do follow an alternative program, you have to be diligent in your record keeping to help out the doc's office, since the staff there might not be used to the alternative schedule, and it's essential to complete each series for full immunity. Further, no study has been conducted to randomly allocate kids to an alternative schedule versus the standard schedule, so we do not know if it is as safe and as protective as the standard schedule. If you are going to use an alternative schedule, check with your insurance company to make sure that the vaccines are covered, as some companies cover only the traditional schedule. If you need to pay for the visits yourself, you may want to consider using the public health department services at a lower cost.

(continued on next page)

The Option	Vaccinate according to a popular pediatrician's guidelines or your own plan (cont.)
The YOU Docs' Take	Here, you'd still get the recommended vaccines, but they're spaced apart a little more, thus exposing your child to fewer foreign substances at once and spreading out that exposure over a longer period of time. The downside is that it means more doctor visits, more exposure to sick kids at those doctors' offices, more money, more periods of post-shot grumpiness, and greater risk of your child contracting a disease during infancy.

The Option	Not to vaccinate your child
Support This Approach	Some believe that all vaccines are unnecessary, especially for people with few risk factors. They also believe that some health benefits are achieved if a child overcomes an illness, such as less asthma and gains lifelong immunity. If you believe that health is an "inside-out" phenomenon—meaning that if you have a strong immune system, it will prevent you from getting sick—you may decide that you and your children can stay healthy without vaccines. When deciding whether or not to vaccinate, many parents may not know that vaccines are not always mandatory for entering the public school system. Every state has its own rules, but nineteen states have what is called a philosophical exemption, meaning that you have a very simple right to refuse. The other two types of exemptions, religious and medical, are beyond the scope of what we want to discuss here. But it's important for you to know that you don't always have to vaccinate simply to get your kids into school.
Against This Approach	You never know when your child might be exposed to certain diseases, whether through traveling on airplanes or public transportation, visiting foreign countries, going to day care or school, or being taken care of by a babysitter or relative who may be an unwitting carrier. Choosing not to vaccinate puts both your child and your community at risk via loss of herd immunity or protection, because the majority of individuals are not vaccinated/immunized. If this individual decision makes you or your child contagious, that can set up a larger outbreak of a significant or life-threatening infection.
The YOU Docs' Take	Children deserve our protection. All children are at risk from vaccine preventable disease. Some children are at higher risk. That includes children living in cities who take public transportation, whose parents work in health care, who travel (or whose parents travel), and who live in communities with immigrants. We also recommend immunization for kids who live around people at high risk for contracting diseases, such as grandparents and those whose immune systems may be compromised; those who spend time in settings with other children, such as in day care; and children caregivers who may be exposed through any of these means.

Vaccine Schedule Options

Below you'll find both the official AAP schedule and an alternate one. We include the alternate one because you may have heard of it, so it is here for you to review with your pediatrician. No matter what you decide, we do want to offer some basic guidelines and principles for vaccines and immunity.

- Pregnant women should avoid getting the influenza vaccine in their first trimester. After that, we consider that immunization safe enough, but you should talk to your doctor about it and always make sure that the vaccine is thimerosal free (single-dose vials are thimerosal free). We believe all pregnant women should seriously consider it, since they are at higher risk of severe or even fatal flu. If you choose not to get the flu shot, you can boost your immune system during the winter by taking 2,000 IU of vitamin D daily.

- If your child is at risk of contracting influenza either because you or his caregivers are or because he is exposed to crowds or in day care, he should receive his first flu vaccine at six months and then annually thereafter. One of the reasons you don't want your baby to catch the flu is that antiviral medications such as Tamiflu (oseltamivir) are either contraindicated due to side effects in those under one year of age or have not been tested for safety in that population.

Factoid: Oseltamivir (Tamiflu), zanamivir (Relenza), amantadine (Symmetrel), and rimantadine (Flumadine) are all Pregnancy Category C medications, indicating that no clinical studies have been conducted to assess the safety of these medications for pregnant women. In animal studies, both amantadine and rimantadine have been shown to cause miscarriage or birth defects when administered at substantially high doses. No adverse effects have been reported among women who received oseltamivir or zanamivir during pregnancy or among infants born to such women. Overall, antiviral drugs should be used during pregnancy only if the potential benefit justifies the potential risk to the embryo or fetus.

- We strongly support breast feeding, as it does offer some immunity to babies, but it is far from foolproof, especially since most mothers who breast-feed discontinue the practice by six months after delivery and breast feeding can be sporadic at times.
- The best ways to prime your child for successful immunization are to make sure that he has a good night's sleep (toddlers need twelve to fourteen hours of total sleep a night plus naps), is not showing symptoms of any illness, is well hydrated, and has had adequate amounts of vitamins A, C, and E for at least a week prior to being immunized. Breast milk provides these vitamins, but recommend you supplement with a baby multivitamin such as Tri-Vi-Sol or Poly-Vi-Sol—1 ml a day starting at age two months (see page 347).

Here are two user-friendly forms that you can use to help track either the standard vaccination schedule or a reasonable alternative devised by Dr. Bob Sears:

American Academy of Pediatrics Schedule

	Diphtheria Tetanus Acellular Pertussis (DTaP)	Rotavirus	Pneumococcal	Haemophilus influenzae type b	Polio	Measles Mumps Rubella (MMR)	Varicella	Hepatitis A	Hepatitis B
2 months	*	*	*	*	*				*
3 months									
4 months	*	*	*	*	*				*
5 months									
6 months	*	*	*	*					
7 months									
9 months									
12 months						*	*	*	

(continued on next page)

	Diphtheria Tetanus Acellular Pertussis (DTaP)	Rotavirus	Pneumococcal	Haemophilus influenzae type b	Polio	Measles Mumps Rubella (MMR)	Varicella	Hepatitis A	Hepatitis B
15 months	*		*	*	*				*
18 months								*	
2 years									
2½ years									
3 years									
3½ years									
5 years	*				*	*	*		

- Influenza: yearly beginning at 6 months.
- Meningococcal: given before age 11.
- The last dose of polio, MMR, varicella, and DTaP can be given anytime between 4 and 6 years.

Alternative Schedule by Dr. Bob Sears

	Diphtheria Tetanus Acellular Pertussis (DTaP)	Rotavirus	Pneumococcal	Haemophilus influenzae type b	Polio	Mumps	Measles	Rubella	Varicella	Hepatitis A	Hepatitis B
2 months	*	*									
3 months			*	*							
4 months	*	*									
5 months			*	*							
6 months	*	*									
7 months			*	*							
9 months					*						
12 months					*	*					

(continued on next page)

	Diphtheria Tetanus Acellular Pertussis (DTaP)	Rotavirus	Pneumococcal	Haemophilus influenzae type b	Polio	Mumps	Measless	Rubella	Varicella	Hepatitis A	Hepatitis B
15 months			*	*							
18 months	*							*			
2 years					*			*			
2½ years											*
3 years							*				
3½ years											*

Risk of Disease

Before making your decision, take a moment to read through the following information. We provide it not to scare you but to let you know the risks of contracting the various ailments against which pediatricians vaccinate.

- Diphtheria—attacks the throat and heart, can lead to heart failure and death. The infection is thought to respond to antibiotics. There are fewer than four cases a year in the United States (advocates would say, Thanks to vaccines).

- Pertussis (whooping cough)—causes severe coughing that makes it hard to breathe, eat, or drink; can lead to pneumonia, convulsions, brain damage, and death. Most serious for kids under three because secretions are thick and windpipes are tiny. Older children typically develop a cough and recover uneventfully.

- Tetanus (lockjaw)—can lead to severe muscle spasm and death. It's a serious infection but not typically deadly.

- Polio—can cause muscle paralysis; it paralyzes muscles used to breathe and swallow and can lead to death. Most with polio have mild symptoms, but a small percentage get paralysis or debilitating motor impairment.

- Measles—causes fever, rash, cough, runny nose, watery eyes; can lead to ear infections, pneumonia, brain swelling, and death. Individuals who are against vaccination add: If there is an outbreak of measles in your area, buy some Mycel vitamin A drops and give your child approximately 10,000 IU in juice for five days (or a single dose of 200,000 IU of vitamin A orally for children over one year of age, and 100,000 IU in a single dose for children six months to one year of age). If he contracts measles, it will likely be a mild case, and he will have lifetime immunity. Supporters of vaccination ask: Why play Russian roulette with your child's life? In a recent U.S. outbreak among unvaccinated children, several died, and several suffered permanent brain dysfunction.

- Mumps—causes fever, headache, painful swelling of salivary glands; can lead to meningitis and brain swelling. In very rare cases, mumps can cause testicles to swell, which can lead to infertility. Much more common: a parent's spending seven days with the child at home while she recovers.

- Rubella (German measles)—causes slight fever, rash, and swelling of glands in the neck; can cause brain swelling or bleeding. If a pregnant woman contracts rubella, it can cause miscarriage or put her baby at high risk for neurological problems that resemble autism or life-threatening birth defects involving loss of brain, hearing, cardiac, and endocrine function. If you were not immunized earlier in life, get immunized more than three months prior to pregnancy, or as soon as possible.

- *Haemophilus influenzae* type b—can cause meningitis, pneumonia, and epiglottitis (a severe throat infection that can lead to choking and death). This infection is less frequent in babies who are exclusively breast-fed, but it's an issue after six months, and especially when breast feeding wanes or stops.

- Hepatitis B—can cause infection of the liver that can lead to liver cancer and death. Unless you and your partner are high-risk, it doesn't need to be given at birth and can be delayed until two months; some argue that any time before age ten is also fine.

- Pneumococcal conjugate vaccine—protects against bacteria that commonly cause ear infections as well as potentially fatal illnesses such as meningitis and bacteremia (infection of the bloodstream). Those most at risk are those with predisposing factors, like certain upper respiratory tract infections and other conditions, many of which do not affect most healthy children.

- Meningococcal conjugate vaccine—prevents against four types of bacterial meningitis (infections and inflammation of the fluid and sacs around the brain and spinal cord) that can cause high fever, headache, stiff neck, confusion, brain damage, hearing loss or blindness, and death. While this infection is unquestioningly severe when it happens, it is sporadic.

- Rotavirus—causes severe acute gastroenteritis (vomiting and diarrhea) that can lead to hospitalization and death. By the time children are two years of age, the vast majority have had a rotavirus infection and are immune going forward.

- Hepatitis A—a liver disease that can cause mild flulike symptoms, jaundice, severe stomach pains, diarrhea, and in rare cases, death.

- Varicella (chickenpox)—a highly contagious, common disease that can cause low-grade fever, rash, complications including pneumonia and encephalitis, and in severe cases, death. Fetuses of women who contract varicella during the first two trimesters of their pregnancy can acquire congenital varicella syndrome; if a woman is infected between five days before giving birth and two days after, the baby will acquire the virus, which can be fatal. In addition to preventing chickenpox, the vaccine can also protect adults from contracting shingles, a very painful condition that affects more than 30 percent of unvaccinated adults.

- Influenza—a highly common and contagious disease that can cause fever, aches and pains, cough, congestion, and lead to pneumonia, and, in rare cases, death. The vast majority of cases are an inconvenience, not deadly. Out of 400,000 pregnant women in the United States who contract influenza each year, 400 die of it and an equal number are believed to have children with some significant abnormality because of it. Keeping the immune system strong with vitamin D during the winter, along with obsessive hand washing and great sleep, helps avoid the flu.

Vaccine Requirements by Schools, Day Cares, Head Start, and Camps

Highly recommended (required by virtually all school systems nationwide)	Recommended (sometimes required for school or day care—check your state)	Optional (not commonly required)
DTaP (the *a* means that it's a less reactive form of the pertussis vaccine) Polio MMR (or separate measles, mumps, and rubella) Hepatitis B (but does not need to be given at birth) Varicella Hib	Hepatitis A Meningococcal conjugate Pneumococcal conjugate especially important if you have depressed immunity (spleen removed), diabetes, asthma, or other heart or lung diseases	Rotavirus (unless your child is in day care, in which case it is highly recommended) Influenza (ditto for this one, and highly recommended for all children with asthma, congenital heart disease, and other risk factors—see page 412)

Our Recommendations on Specific Vaccines

- If you, your partner, or a caregiver is a carrier of hepatitis B, request the first dose of the vaccine at birth. In everybody else, we recommend waiting until two months of age. At this time, it can also be given as part of a combination vaccine.

- Hepatitis A is not common in the United States, but it is very common in other parts of the world. The Centers for Disease Control and Prevention has recommended this vaccine to all children ages one and older since 2006, in part because of increased travel and immigration, but also in an attempt to eliminate indigenous hepatitis A from the United States. If your school system does not require it, if you do not live in a high-risk community, if all who prepare food for your child wash well, and if you do not travel to countries with a high incidence, consider it optional.

- The rotavirus vaccine is a live oral vaccine, so one of the side effects is vomiting and diarrhea—exactly the symptoms it is supposed to protect against, but exponentially milder than the disease itself. A prior version of this vaccine was withdrawn from the market in 1999 because it was linked to a severe condition known as intussusception, a blockage or twisting of the intestine that may require surgery or a radiologic procedure and rarely can be fatal. The new vaccine is not associated with intussusception. We recommend that you definitely opt for this one if your child is in day care or other high-risk circumstances.

> Factoid: New research shows that a child's IQ can be lowered when the mother contracts the flu during pregnancy—perhaps another reason to consider a vaccine for yourself, especially if you're at high risk.

- Because influenza is so common and affects young children so severely (20,000 U.S. children under age five are hospitalized with complications of the flu each year), and because children under one year of age are not given antiviral therapy, the recommendation of yearly flu shots beginning at six months of age is not unreasonable. (Children age two and above can

What We Did

Some of the YOU authors explain what they did when it came to immunizations for their children:

Oz family immunization regimen: We gave no immunizations for six months, and most immunizations were given about a year after recommended, with the hope that the children's immune systems would mature. Yet at the same time we needed to complete the recommended immunizations before school started to avoid battles with the health department. We gave no immunizations that we were not legally obliged to administer in New Jersey, and none of the kids got hepatitis B when they were babies. On the positive side, we agreed with most of the recommended immunizations in New Jersey.

Lisa breast-fed all the kids, and none of the children was in day care, so we had two important risk factors on our side. We had no genetic fears except that I probably have borderline ADHD. We placed lots of emphasis on the child being healthy at the time of immunization, and we were careful about their diets, but we did administer vaccines in groups to reduce the children's fears and visits to the pediatrician.—Mehmet Oz, MD

Roizen family immunization regimen: We went with the standard (AAP and CDC) schedule of immunizations; hepatitis B vaccination did not exist at that time. Nancy breast-fed both children but returned to work as a pediatrician after three months. Since she saw sick kids and our kids shared a babysitter, we had all the high-risk factors for childhood diseases. We had no genetic fears except that I also probably have borderline ADHD. Other than making sure that the children observed normal sleep patterns and were well hydrated, we did nothing special prior to immunization. Our children received the vaccines in groups, as recommended, to reduce their fears and visits to the pediatrician.
—Michael Roizen, MD

See what other members of the authorship team did, on www.realage.com and www.doctoroz .com.

take the nasal spray as long as they don't have asthma and are not immuno-compromised.) Just make sure that the preparation is thimerosal free (from a single-dose package). Children at high risk for complications from the flu who should get vaccinated include those with asthma, immune suppression, chronic kidney disease, heart disease, HIV/AIDS, diabetes, sickle-cell anemia, long-term aspirin therapy, and any condition that can reduce lung function. If your child is in day care or a member of your household is elderly or at high risk for flu, we also recommend vaccination. If the flu vaccine is not required for school and you would like to opt out, take precautions to avoid transmission, including frequent hand washing, not sharing cups and utensils, learning how to sneeze and cough into a sleeve, and avoiding even small crowds during flu season.

Further Reading

Because this topic is so complicated and conflicted, we recommend that you explore it further. These are some of the resources that we found extremely helpful when thinking about the issue:

Saying No to Vaccines: A Resource Guide for All Ages, by Sherri Tenpenny

Vaccinated: One Man's Quest to Defeat the World's Deadliest Diseases and *Autism's False Prophets: Bad Science, Risky Medicine, and the Search for a Cure,* by Paul A. Offit

Vaccine Safety Manual for Concerned Families and Health Practitioners: Guide to Immunization Risks and Protection, by Neil Z. Miller

Do Vaccines Cause That?: A Guide for Evaluating Vaccine Safety Concerns, by Martin Myers and Diego Pineda

The Vaccine Book: Making the Right Decision for Your Child, by Robert W. Sears

Red Book: 2009 Report of the Committee on Infectious Disease, by American Academy of Pediatrics (www.aapredbook.aappublications.org)

APPENDIX 4

The Basics of Preemies and Multiple Births

There are many variations of the typical pregnancy scenario (many of which we've covered throughout the book), but we'd like to spend a little more time on two scenarios that are indeed quite common: premature birth and multiple births. While it's true that not all preemies are multiples, many multiples are preemies, and both situations present you with different things to consider during pregnancy and delivery. To help you prepare, let's review some of the basics.

Premature Labor

Technically, premature labor is defined as labor that starts before thirty-seven weeks (the time when a baby's lungs are fully matured). If labor happens before twenty-four weeks, it is virtually impossible for the baby to survive outside the womb, for many reasons. In any case, the thing to remember is that in any preterm situation, something is going on inside the womb that is not agreeing with the baby, and your body decides baby is safer outside than in.

Risk Factors

Women at risk are those who've had previous premature children, who have had cervical surgery, or who have had certain infections (like chlamydia). Abnormal placental location such as previa and/or premature separation of the placenta may all be reasons a woman may go into premature labor. The thought is that when the cervical membranes get infected, the subsequent immune response can trigger the whole contraction process.

What Happens

When a woman presents with preterm labor in the hospital, the care team will hydrate her and give her magnesium sulfate or other medications to slow down contractions or stop the labor. In true preterm labor, the cervix will continue to dilate and the baby will deliver, no matter how far along the pregnancy is. Docs try to slow down the labor process to buy enough time to give you corticosteroids, which help mature the baby's lungs. It takes between seven and ten days of steroids to get lungs mature before the thirty-seventh week.

After Delivery

Many babies delivered prematurely are almost ready to function on their own except for breathing, even if they need a little extra time for organ development. When the baby can't breathe on his own, the doctors will immediately take him to the neonatal nursery for oxygen. There you'll work with the team to figure out how best to feed and interact with your newborn. Many preemies are too small to suck, so if you want to breast-feed, you may have to pump and use a preemie nipple on a bottle. See our tip on kangaroo care on page 275.

What You Can Do

By following our guidelines throughout the book, you'll decrease your chances of having a premature delivery. Listen to your doc, and if something does not seem right, don't hesitate to call and at least get her opinion. Pay special attention to the things that can help most: Take DHA and folic acid, stop smoking, and make sure that you don't go to either extreme when it comes to weight (see page 69).

Multiples

Fraternal twins occur when two separate eggs are fertilized in the same cycle—often the result of ovarian stimulation or multiple embryo transfer during fertility treatment. Genetically, they're no more similar or different than any other siblings. Identical twins, which account for one-third of twin births, come about when a single fertilized egg subsequently splits in two. Identical twins share the same genes but are never truly identical because they may receive different amounts of nongenetic cellular material. In the womb, but even more after birth and throughout life, identical twins continue to differentiate because they are exposed to different environments, a phenomenon known as epigenetic drift.

Depending on when the embryo divides, identical twins can be completely separate, share a placenta, share a placenta and an amniotic sac, or be conjoined (Siamese). While the rate of identical twins is constant worldwide—one set per 250 births—the rate of fraternal twins is influenced by race, heredity, maternal age, number of prior births, and the use of fertility drugs.

Multiples have been on the increase since the advent of assisted reproductive technology, which accounts for 77 percent of multiple births. While multiples can be twice the fun (and work!) of singletons, they also double the risk of preeclampsia (maternal high blood pressure), postpartum hemorrhage, and, therefore, premature birth and maternal death, so you need to be monitored closely throughout your pregnancy.

Some other things to consider if you're carrying multiples:

In Utero Issues

Women carrying multiples typically have more prenatal visits than women carrying one child. Your doctor may also use ultrasounds to detect any issues that may arise. Some of the common issues with multiples:

- One child, to put it bluntly, can hog the placenta. That means the other child isn't getting the nutrients he needs and can suffer from growth restriction.
- Overcrowding compromises the cervix, putting you at risk of preterm labor.
- If one child is breech, that increases the rate of C-section.

Your Body

Women carrying multiples shouldn't double their weight. Aim for about a ten-pound increase above a singleton pregnancy (see page 68 for details). It's especially important to monitor your nutritional intake and make sure that you're getting enough protein. Since back pain is more common in women carrying multiples, pay close attention to your exercise routine after checking with your doctor to make sure it is okay (swimming is a good option), and be conscious of your posture throughout the day. Sometimes women report that a maternity belt helps relieve the low back pain associated with a larger abdomen throwing their center of balance off. You may also need to be on bed rest toward the end of pregnancy. Trust your doctor to help provide these guidelines.

The Vanishing Twin

If your doc tells you that you're carrying twins, triplets, or an entire baseball team before twelve weeks, don't be surprised if one or more embryos vanish at your next visit. In the first trimester, one or more embryos may disappear in one-third of twin pregnancies, half of triplet pregnancies, and two-thirds of quadruplet pregnancies. You can ensure that more survive if you have good prenatal care and see an OB who specializes in high-risk pregnancies.

Delivery

Because of the tight space in the uterus with multiples, it is not uncommon for at least one of the babies to be heading the wrong way, and this, along with other conditions that may necessitate a earlier delivery, can increase your likelihood of having a C-section. Twins can be delivered vaginally if their gestation period is longer than thirty-two weeks, if the baby closest to the cervix is larger than the other and his head is down, and if there's no sign of fetal distress, especially in the second twin.

APPENDIX 5

Postpartum Depression Scale

As you've read in chapters 8 and 10, postpartum depression is both common and frustrating for everyone involved. We've given you some guidelines for determining your level of the blues, but this official test, called the Edinburgh Postnatal Depression Scale (EPDS), will give you even more insight into whether you need professional help.

Please circle the answer that comes closest to how you have felt *in the past seven days*, not just how you feel today.

1. I have been able to laugh and see the funny side of things:

    As much as I always could
    Not quite so much now
    Definitely not so much now
    Not at all

2. I have looked forward to things:

    As much as I ever did
    Rather less than I used to
    Definitely less than I used to
    Hardly at all

3. I have been anxious or worried for no good reason:

    No, not at all
    Hardly ever
    Yes, sometimes
    Yes, very often

4. I have blamed myself unnecessarily when things went wrong:

    Yes, most of the time
    Yes, some of the time
    Not very often
    No, never

5. I have felt scared or panicky for no very good reason:

    Yes, quite a lot
    Yes, sometimes
    No, not much
    No, not at all

6. Things have been getting on top of me:

    Yes, most of the time I have not been able to cope at all
    Yes, sometimes I haven't been coping as well as usual
    No, most of the time I have coped quite well
    No, I have been coping as well as ever

7. I have been so unhappy that I have had difficulty sleeping:

    Yes, most of the time
    Yes, sometimes
    Not very often
    No, not at all

8. I have felt sad or miserable:

    Yes, most of the time
    Yes, quite often
    Not very often
    No, not at all

9. I have been so unhappy that I have been crying:

    Yes, most of the time
    Yes, quite often
    Only occasionally
    No, never

10. The thought of harming myself has occurred to me:

    Yes, quite often
    Sometimes
    Hardly ever
    Never

SCORING: Answers for the first three questions are scored on a scale of 0, 1, 2, and 3. Answers 4 to 10 are scored in descending order: 3, 2, 1, and 0. Add the scores of your answers together. If you scored above a 12, it's a sign that you probably need to have your depressive symptoms checked out.

APPENDIX 6

In Utero Growth Chart: Average Size

We don't want you to obsess over your baby's weight (or your own), but you do want to make sure that your baby's weight doesn't swing too far up or down (see chapter 4 for more details). This chart gives you the norms of a baby's size for each week of development.

Gestational age	Length (inches)	Weight (ounces, then pounds)
	(crown to rump)	
8 weeks	0.63	0.04 (ounces)
9 weeks	0.90	0.07
10 weeks	1.22	0.14
11 weeks	1.61	0.25
12 weeks	2.13	0.49
13 weeks	2.91	0.81

14 weeks	3.42	1.52
15 weeks	3.98	2.47
16 weeks	4.57	3.53
17 weeks	5.12	4.94
18 weeks	5.59	6.70
19 weeks	6.02	8.47
20 weeks	6.46	10.58
	(crown to heel)	
20 weeks	10.08	10.58
21 weeks	10.51	12.70
22 weeks	10.94	15.17
23 weeks	11.38	1.10 (pounds)
24 weeks	11.81	1.32
25 weeks	13.62	1.46
26 weeks	14.02	1.68
27 weeks	14.41	1.93
28 weeks	14.80	2.22
29 weeks	15.2	2.54
30 weeks	15.71	2.91
31 weeks	16.18	3.31

(continued on next page)

Gestational age	Length (inches)	Weight (ounces, then pounds)
32 weeks	16.69	3.75
33 weeks	17.20	4.23
34 weeks	17.72	4.73
35 weeks	18.19	5.25
36 weeks	18.66	5.78
37 weeks	19.13	6.30
38 weeks	19.61	6.80
39 weeks	19.96	7.25
40 weeks	20.16	7.63
41 weeks	20.35	7.93
42 weeks	20.28	8.12
43 weeks	20.20	8.19

Source: www.babycenter.com

ACKNOWLEDGMENTS

From the YOU Docs—Mike Roizen and Mehmet Oz

Some people spend their Sundays in church or watching football or eating big breakfasts. We do some of that, too (except the big breakfast part), but the YOU team also spends at least some of its Sunday on a weekly conference call that's part congressional hearing, part mud-wrestling match, and part *Saturday Night Live*. During that call, we discuss, debate, and brainstorm, and then we send each other off with our assignments for the week. A week later (and a whole lot of heavy lifting in between), we're back at it again—reviewing, critiquing, and even sneaking in a laugh or two. What you're reading now is the result of a truly group effort that works because of the diverse and dedicated minds on our team.

Clark Kent is no match for Ted Spiker as a writer or as a performer of superhuman tasks. Professor Spiker (he really is one in real life at the University of Florida) runs a tight ship. We never take on water, despite the perfect storms into which we routinely sail, and we always have ample intellectual provisions on our Sunday morning calls. His superhuman efforts result in accessible, enjoyable works that exalt our readers to take charge of their health destiny.

We are proud to have Gary Hallgren's acclaimed medical cartoons grace our pages, but even more honored to have Gary grace our lives. We enjoy watching him draw magical images that bring alive complex topics so all our readers can enjoy the childlike enthusiasm the YOU docs have for our work.

Like most mortals, we cannot always keep up with Craig Wynett's brilliant ability to connect seemingly disparate facts, but that is his genius and all our readers benefit from his brilliance. His overarching concepts light the pathways to knowledge in our books, and he designs and articulates these seamlessly with all the docs on each call. Craig transforms the YOU books with profound insights that form the foundation of the text and cause our Sunday morning conferences to break down in laughter, only to be resurrected as the insight shines through.

Master Ob-Gyn Dr. Margaret Mckenzie brings a sophisticated common sense to every project she engages, whether it's educating residents at the Cleveland Clinic or helping us share the essence of her specialty with our readers. We love the colorful spices she brought to the book-writing party. We really interrupted her life many times more than she planned as she became the constant partner in the process, and along with Linda, Lisa, Nancy, Tracy, Dr. Ellen Rome (who was working on another book with us, yet diverted to help keep us on track on this one), and many readers (over forty pregnant or recently pregnant women commented on each edition and each section or chapter of each edition) kept us understanding the better half's points of view. Her meticulous attention to detail improved the quality of the book.

Lisa Oz works tirelessly behind the scenes to ensure we don't take ourselves too seriously and always, always, always stay focused on the needs of the readers. Thank goodness that one of us married her. Nancy Roizen's honest and insightful editorial advice keeps us on our toes. Thank goodness that one of us married her.

Linda Kahn taught the doctors quite a bit about medicine as well as the mother's perspective on pregnancy. And that wasn't even her day job responsibility of helping to organize and edit our book. She continued to provide very profound criticisms of our work and help us revise the text into the wonderful final result. She reminds us that "no pain, no gain" applies to books as well. Without Linda, we would have a far inferior product.

Joel Harper teamed up with Tracy Hafen to craft the elegant YOU: Having a Baby Workouts for each trimester. Their tireless efforts resulted in a wonderful exercise video that will benefit many pregnant women. Dr. Art Markman understands human motivation as reflected in the brilliant stress quizzes he created. Besides being a pleasure to work with, he helped us combine decades of research into a succinct quiz that we hope will fascinate you.

Adam Snavely worked tirelessly to fact-check and research many of the questions created whenever scientists are researching a book. He was helped by Jeff Roizen and Lauren Karp, who labored hardily to root out answers to even the esoteric questions.

Finally, our agent Candice Fuhrman's innovative insights and tough commentary helped redirect our work to truly suit the needs of women having babies.

While the hours of conference calls, research and writing were often exhausting, this powerful group functioned seamlessly to resolve style and content conflicts.

We also want to thank the group at Free Press (Simon & Schuster) who so enthusiastically supported this material and has dedicated themselves to bringing our ideas to the world. Dominick Anfuso joins Martha Levin (with Carolyn Reidy) as captains of the wonderful ship at Free Press (Simon & Schuster). The top-notch crew of Jill Siegel, Carisa Hays, Suzanne Donahue, Mark Speer, Nancy Singer, Ruth Lee-Mui, Nancy Inglis, Alex Noya, and Leah Miller are always seeking solutions to our many needs and have committed themselves to making our books the best possible experience for our dedicated readers.

Most of the recipes came from the Lifestyle 180 team of master chef Jim Perko, nutritionist Kristin Kirkpatrick, and medical director Elizabeth Ricanati. These Lifestyle180 recipes are based on guidelines for YOU healthy foods, and were tested for enjoyment and capacity to be made by pregnant ladies and their significant others (who made the meals and washed the dishes).

We are indebted to our close partners at RealAge.com, including Val Weaver, Keith Roach, Carl Peck, Axel Goetz, Marty Munson and Meredith Wade, and of course cofounders Charlie Silver and the late Martin Rom, and former COO Rich Benci, who all planned to and did depart after Hearst acquired it. We appreciate the continued support of the former Discovery Health team, including Carol Tomko, Alon Orstein, Wayne Barbin, and John Whyte. And as always, thanks to Billy Campbell for being such an honorable lifelong friend. And we thank the great team at *Good Morning America* including Patty Neger and Diane Sawyer, who made waking up early to discuss health a lot of fun.

Thanks to all of our friends at *The Oprah Winfrey Show,* especially Jack Mori, Terry Goulder, Jill Van Lokeren, Candy Carter, Shari Salata, Lisa Erspamer, Chris Martin, Leslie Grisanti, Ann Lofgren, Jenn Horton, Harriet Seitler, Tim Bennett, Erik Logan, Doug Pattison, Lisa Halliday, and Don Halcombe. The Oprah radio team, including John St. Augustine, Lauren Kahn, Theresa Rodriguez, and Tracy Square, organized interviews with opinion leaders in pregnancy. Special thanks to Ms. Oprah Winfrey for pulling these great souls together into one remarkably cohesive team and for teaching us to always put the audience first.

Our books contain so broad a range of topics that we are compelled to ask advice from many world experts who selflessly share their insights in the true academic tradition. We list them all here without details of their contributions in order to save space for the actual book, but we deeply appreciate your dedication to your specialties and willingness to sacrifice your time in helping craft the most scientifically accurate book on aging possible. We thank Shari I. Lusskin for her contributions to the brain chapters and Lise Eliot for her help in the senses chapter, as well as Jennifer Ashton, Mary D'Alton, Sherri Tenpenny, Ivan Kronenfeld, Jon Lapook, Regina Brett, Paul Rosenberg, George Rodgers, Jennifer Ashton, John Ellis, Marsha Lowry, Dominique Campodonico, Michelle Narens, Alena Marie Kelly, Alan Cinchon, Iyaad Hasan, Jodi Hazen, Tiffani Mauldin-Frederick, Sarah Mohr, Suzanne Dixon, Nazallee O'Hearn, Amy Byram, Breck Thomas, Erinne Dyer, Erica Foreman, Megan Pruce-Ferington, Susan Parnell, Mitzi Reaugh, Manu Singh, Anna Robins, Jennifer Roizen, Susan Sonnenberg, Rachel Tangen, Rosaleind Wattell, Bethany Yu, Alfonse Gallizia, Brian Kolonick (who helped us greatly with the male Tool Box), and especially Drs. Dean Ornish, Mark Hyman, Elliott Philipson, Mark Rosen, Mark Batshaw, William Camann, Johanna Goldfarb, Paul Offit, Justin Lavin, Rocio Moran, Charis Eng, Sharon Malon for teaching us and reviewing our work.

From Mehmet Oz

Dr Oz thanks his colleagues in Surgery for their continued support, including Dr. Craig Smith, Dr. Yoshifuma Naka, Dr. Mike Argenziano, Dr. Henry Spotnitz, Dr. Allan Stewart, and Dr. Mat Williams. The physician assistants, especially Laura Altman and Tom Cosola, the nurses in the OR and floor, and our spectacular ICU team always care meticulously for my patients. My office staff, including Lidia Nieves, Michelle Washburn and Celia Taylor, kept me on time and on target as I combined a life of heart surgery with media. Our divisional administrator Diane Amato offered unique insights to books and life. Thanks to the dedicated staff at New York-Presbyterian Hospital, including Herb Pardes, Steve Corwin, Bob Kelly, David Feinberg, Bryan Dotson, Alicia Park, and Myrna Manners for their heart felt advice.

My parents, Mustafa and Suna Oz, taught me that the cream always rises to the top. My parents-in-law Gerald and Emily Jane Lemole led by example while raising all my brother—and sister-in-laws. Besides being our coauthor, the love of my life Lisa had four uneventful pregnancies with Daphne, Arabella, Zoe, and Oliver and always shows me how to life live right.

From Michael Roizen

Dr. Roizen wants to thank his administrative associates Qintene Graham and especially Beth Grubb, who made this work possible. And to thank many of the staff at the Cleveland Clinic and physicians elsewhere who answered numerous questions. Many of the Clinic's Wellness Institute staff and associates made scientific contributions and constructive criticisms, and allowed the time to complete this work. Cleveland Clinic CEO Toby Cosgrove has said that the Clinic will continue to be one of, if not the best, in illness care, and that wellness is what the clinic will do for every employee and person we touch. I am fortunate to work with such a talented and creative group who helped our thought processes as Nabil Gabriel, Dr. Beth Ricanati, Dr. Martin Harris, Dr. Brigette Duffy, Joe Hahn, David Strand, Scott McFarland, Cindy Hundorfean, Chris Ayers, Dennis Kenny, Paul Matsen, Bill Peacock, Cindy Moore, and many nutritionists and exercise physiologists, chef Jim Perko, Drs. Rich Lang, Tanya Edwards, Rene Seballos, Steve Nissen, Jim Young, David Bronson, Anthony Miniaci, Glen Copeland, and clinicians and leaders that span the gamut from inner city school teachers to executive coaches.

Our family was fully engaged—with Jeff as our MD, PhD research associate; and Jennifer and Nancy as critical readers, joined at times by the "enlarged family" of the Katzes, Unobskeys, Wattels, and Campodonicos. I also want to thank Sukie Miller, Diane Reverend, Eileen Sheil, Susan Petre, John Maudlin, Zack Wasserman, and others for encouraging and critiquing the concepts.

Having a great partner to ablate stress daily is clearly a magnificent way to help life and even writing be better—thank you, Nancy.

From Ted Spiker

I'm thankful that the worst side effect that my beautiful wife Liz experienced during her pregnancy with our twins was an outrageously itchy belly. Since the day that her water broke eleven years ago (in between clothing racks at the mall, six and a half weeks before her due date), my life has never been the same. Thank you to Liz, Alex, and Thad for being such a wonderful, fun, and inspiring family. I'm also appreciative of my entire family (Alex and Thad's grandparents, aunts, uncles, and cousins), friends, the whole YOU team, my colleagues and students at the University of Florida, and all the various magazine editors and writers I've worked with over the years.

From Craig Wynett

To my family: my wife Denise, sons Ryan and Jim, cat Abbey, and dogs Ned and George. Collectively you have given me plenty of baby-related experience to draw on. A few of these "experiences" we have advised readers to avoid at all cost; many more are truly worthy of emulation.

From Margaret McKenzie

For my parents Jean and John Mckenzie, who led the example of greatness. To God, Clairmonte, Claire, Mackenzie Cappelle, thanks for your love which sustains me. To all my patients who inspire me to be my best. For all my teachers and students who fueled my passion to share knowledge. To my coauthors of this book Craig, Linda, Mehmet, Mike, and Ted, thanks for your inspiration to share the whys of the miracle of new life.

From Linda G. Kahn

Thank you to the YOU team—Drs. Michael Roizen and Mehmet Oz, Craig Wynett, and Ted Spiker—for welcoming me on board. Who knew waking up at six a.m. on Sunday mornings could be so rewarding? Thanks, too, to Dr. Margaret McKenzie for generously answering all of the questions I'd been harboring since my own first pregnancy eleven years ago. To Candice Fuhrman, for her excellent matchmaking skills. To Jackie Skeris, Krista Abrahams, and Soo-Mi Yun for providing insightful feedback on the manuscript. To my husband, Rob, my parents, Patricia and Stephen Gross, and my sisters, Karen Fittinghoff and Diane Leifer, for their support. And last, but not least, to our children, Elliot, Eva, and Leda, for being *very* quiet while Mommy was working.

From Gary Hallgren

A shout-out to Cliff McKee, artist and teacher, Ferndale High School 1962. He said if I worked it right, my abilities could take me around the world. He was right, and if I still haven't made it to Asia, it's only because I always get distracted by Italy. The detour into the body with Drs. Oz and Roizen has been most pleasurable, exotic and informative, however. Congratulations, belatedly, to my sweet wife Michelle for doing what this book outlines so well and producing a fantastic human being . . . twenty-five years ago. I am referring to my beautiful, talented and supportive daughter, Annabel, who has canceled every doubt I ever had about parenthood.

INDEX

resiliency of, 7
self-education about, 8
shape of, 17, 69, 147, 170, 175–76
size of, 170
transformations of, 7
YOU Tips about, 184
See also specific body part
body mass index (BMI), 68, 69, 376, 383
bonding, 48, 130, 132, 133, 139, 142, 147, 184, 243, 271
bottle-feeding, 123, 340
"boutique" ultrasounds, 104
bowels, 237, 241, 248, 277.
See also constipation; diarrhea
Bradley method, 190
brain
baby's, 110–28
basic structure of, 114
biology of, 140–43
and body image, 176
"critical periods" for, 111–20
and crying babies, 266
damage to, 93
and depression, 137, 150–51, 161
development of, 6, 15, 93, 96, 98, 110–34, 161
and DHA, 141, 160, 307
and exercising with newborn, 277
and fat, 141, 161
father's, 371
feminization of, 288
and fever, 267
and gender, 120, 123
and glucose, 93
and hormones, 141, 142
and metabolism, 96, 141
mother's, 140–43
and neurons, 115, 116–18, 119, 122, 123, 129, 142, 147
and nutrition, 15, 34, 70, 72, 73, 78, 81, 288
and pain, 274
plasticity of, 115
and second pregnancy, 379
and seizures, 268
and sensory development, 121–34
size of, 141
and sleep, 137, 147, 148

and stress, 137, 140–43, 144, 145, 154
and strollers, 257
and toxins, 39
and vaccinations, 393, 408
vomiting center of, 76, 77
and YOU Prepregnancy Plan, 379
See also specific part of brain
brain stem, 121
Braxton Hicks contractions, 212, 227
breast-feeding
benefits of, 178, 252, 261, 307
and crying babies, 265–66
and delivery, 241
and dental work, 39
and DHA, 160
and dieting, 67
discussions during doctor's visits about, 300
and exercise, 332
Factoid about, 123
and fat, 67
in first month, 252–55, 257–61
and holding the baby, 254
and medications, 342, 344
and partner's responsibilities, 372
and pregnancy plan, 298, 307
and premature birth, 414
preparation for, 178
and preparing your home, 347
problems during, 255, 257
and selecting caregivers, 340
and sensory development, 123
and sex, 173, 174
and skin, 181
speed of, 253
support concerning, 298
tips for, 254–55, 257–61
and vaccinations, 401–2, 408, 411
web sites about, 298
and weight, 67, 276
See also breast milk; nipples
breast milk
content of, 252
dumping of, 260–61
and estrogen, 47
and mother's health, 270
and placenta formation, 49
pumping of, 252, 253, 258–59, 260–61, 270, 414

quality and quantity of, 253, 255, 258, 259, 260
storage of, 259
supply and demand for, 258
and taste, 127
and toxins, 38
and vaccinations, 402
vitamins in, 402
breasts
and body image, 176–79
and delivery, 246, 248
and determining pregnancy, 376
engorgement of, 252, 271
and exercise, 332
implants in, 259
leaking, 177, 179, 253, 259
massaging of, 253, 271
and mother's health, 271
pain in, 253, 271
pumping, 252, 253, 258–59, 260–61, 270, 414
reduction in, 259
sagging, 259
self-examination of, 187
and sex, 172
size of, 176–77, 195, 205–6, 252, 259, 271
sore, 177
stimulation of, 248
swollen, 271
unwashed, 123
weight of, 72
YOU Tips about, 186–87
See also breast-feeding; breast milk; nipples
breath/breathing
baby's first, 236–37
and brain development, 117
calling the doctor about, 267
and contractions and cramps, 212
deep, 62, 227
and delivery, 227, 230, 237, 241
and development/size of fetus, 105
and exercise, 332
Factoid about, 213
and milestones, 42
and mother's health, 270
and picking a birthing class, 190
and placenta, 47
and premature birth, 97, 414

men
  depression in, 272
  and fertility issues, 383, 386–88
  See also partners
meningitis, 394, 408
meningococcal conjugate, 398,
    404, 408, 409
menstruation, 195, 386
mental retardation, 245
mercury, 38, 39, 62, 80, 84, 288,
    376, 388
metabolism
  and brain, 96, 141
  and development of fetus,
    91–94, 98
  and energy, 91, 92, 93
  and epigenetics, 79
  and exercise, 108
  and fat, 91
  and formation of placenta, 49
  and hormones, 91
  and medications, 342
  and nutrients, 91
  and size of baby, 91–97
  and thyroid, 95
  See also blood sugar; glucose;
    insulin
metformin, 108, 383
methylates, 38, 292
methylation, 31, 35, 387
Micronase, 108
midbrain, 114
midwives, 191, 229, 282,
    299–303, 306, 336, 337–38
milestones, 40, 41–43
minerals, 79–81, 252, 291.
  See also specific mineral
miscarriages
  and age, 381
  causes of, 381
  and CVS, 54
  and DVT, 211
  and fertility issues, 380–81
  and genetics, 22, 26
  and nausea, 76
  and nutrients, 81
  overview about, 48
  prevention of, 381
  and Rh factor, 53
  risk of, 381
  and rubella, 407
  stillbirths as, 249
  and toxins, 39
  truth about, 48

and ultrasounds, 101
and YOU Prepregnancy Plan,
    378
mixed-handedness, 144
MMA (chemical), 177
molar pregnancy, 76
Montgomery's tubercles, 179
mood swings, 137, 147, 148,
    149–53, 172, 173, 182,
    271–73, 373.
  See also depression; postpartum
    depression
morning sickness, 14, 49, 75–79,
    80, 86–87, 216
mother
  brain of, 140–43
  competing needs of baby and,
    2
  essential nutrients for, 79–81
  health of, 50, 269–73, 308
mother-daughter stress, 156–57,
    296
motion sickness, 78
motor skills, 127, 130
mouth problems, 195–97. *See also*
    teeth
movement, fetal, 41, 91, 105, 106,
    114, 127–28, 149, 265, 302,
    305, 332
muchal translucency, 303
mugwort, 126
multiple births, 235, 241, 413,
    415–17
multiple sclerosis (MS), 379
mumps, 378, 397, 403, 404, 405,
    406, 407, 409
muscles, 108–9, 246, 293
musculoskeletal system, 7, 205–8,
    216–17
music, 133, 157, 209, 296
myelin sheath/myelination,
    118–20, 129

nails, 40, 42, 43, 177, 273
naming your child, 256, 274,
    297
naproxen, 344, 376
naps, 264, 295
narcotics, 232
National Center for Genome
    Resources, 304
National Domestic Violence
    Hotline, 186
nature-nuture issues, 2

nausea
  and brain biology, 142
  and development of fetus, 98
  and eating, 66, 75–79, 83,
    86–87
  and genetics, 76
  and hormones, 172
  medications for, 343
  and miscarriages, 76
  and nutrition, 14, 15, 75–79,
    286, 289–90
  and saliva, 70
  as side effect of pregnancy, 7
  and smell, 142, 160
  and teeth, 216
  and toxins, 76
navel rings, 253
nervous system, 80, 84
neural plate, 113, 114
neural tube, 112
neural tube defects, 54, 80, 114
neurological development, 132
neurons, 115, 116–20, 122, 123,
    129, 142, 147
neurotransmitters, 116
new-moms groups, 298
newborn influenza, 397
niacin, 187, 290
night feeding, 254, 262, 308
night sweats, 183, 273
nipple rings, 253
nipples, 172, 177, 178, 179, 241,
    246, 255, 257, 258, 266
nitric oxide, 100, 142, 172, 208
nitrous oxide, 232
nonstress test, 102, 104, 302–3
North American Registry of
    Midwives (NARM), 337
nose/nostrils, 41, 196, 203. *See
    also* smell
nuchal translucency test, 54
nurseries, readying of, 155, 296
nursing. *See* breast-feeding
nutrients/nutrition
  bad, 288–89
  basic goals for, 82
  and body image, 16
  and brain, 34, 70, 72, 73, 78, 81
  and breast-feeding, 67
  and carbohydrates, 107
  and crying babies, 265–66
  and delivery, 229, 248
  and development/size of fetus,
    98, 106

rotavirus, 397, 403, 405, 408, 409, 410
rubella, 300, 378, 390, 397, 403, 404, 405, 406, 407, 409

Salad Dressings (Lifestyle 180 recipes), 369–70
saliva, 70, 203, 304
salivating, 127
salt, 75, 211
Save the Blood, 244, 245, 307
scalp, massage of, 134, 181
schizophrenia, 78
sciatica, 206, 207
scopolamine patch, 70
screening tests, 303–4
Sears, Bob, 402, 405–6
seat belts, 217
Seated Curtsy (exercise), 317
second pregnancy, 379
second trimester
    doctor's visits during, 301–2
    and fetal development, 305
    pregnancy plan for, 296, 301–2, 304, 305
    prenatal tests in, 303, 304
Seesaw Abs (exercise), 320
seizures, 250, 268
selective serotonin reuptake inhibitors (SSRIs), 162, 344
selenium, 291, 388. *See also specific recipe*
semen, 383, 386. *See also* sperm
senses
    and biology of brain, 142
    development of, 121–28
    YOU Tips about, 129–32
    See also specific sense
serotonin, 151, 162, 198
sertraline, 162
serum screening test, 303
sex
    after birth, 174
    and brain development, 123
    and breast-feeding, 173
    contractions during, 212
    and delivery, 248
    and doctor's visits, 300, 301
    environment for, 158
    and estrogen, 172, 173, 174
    and exercise, 184
    and fertility issues, 384
    foreplay, 174

and hormones, 170–72, 173, 193
and men, 184–85
and nutrition, 288
oral, 174
and placenta previa, 52
positions for, 174, 185–86, 374, 386
postpartum, 173, 174
during pregnancy, 172–75
and premature birth, 173
and progesterone, 172
and relationship with partner, 173, 174–75, 184, 373
and sex drive, 10–11, 170, 172–75, 373
and side effects of pregnancy, 196
and stress, 185
YOU Tips about, 184–87
sexual abuse, 242
sexual lubricants, 174, 386
sexual orientation, 145
sexually transmitted diseases (STDs), 188, 274, 302, 378, 388
shingles, 393
siblings, 274–75, 297
sickle-cell anemia, 300, 378, 412
sickness
    and brain vomiting center, 76, 77
    and eating, 66, 75–79, 83, 86–87
    and exercise, 86
    and medications, 87
    severe, 78
    and smell, 86
    and stress, 87
    You Tips about, 86–87
    See also morning sickness; nausea
side-lying hold, 254
Side-Lying Lifts (exercise), 328–29
Single Leg Floor Touch (exercise), 333
sinusitis, 203
size, fetus/baby
    and big babies, 89–90, 94–97
    and blood sugar, 90, 93, 94–95, 96, 97
    and breech position, 235
    and delivery, 236, 240, 241, 248

and diabetes, 90, 94–97, 99
and genetics, 34
measuring, 100–101
and metabolism, 91–94
and milestones, 41, 42, 43
and too big babies, 89–90, 94–97
and underdevelopment of fetus, 89
in utero growth chart for, 420–22
See also development, baby; weight
skin
    and body image, 179–81
    color of, 246, 267
    dark spots on, 278–79
    and delivery, 245
    and estrogen, 172
    Factoid about, 187, 275
    and getting your body back, 278–79, 281
    and kangaroo care, 275
    lump under, 269
    and milestones, 41, 42
    and premature birth, 275
    and stretch marks, 179
    stretching of, 7
    thickness of, 303
    and when to call the doctor, 268, 269
    YOU Tips about, 184, 187–89
skin-to-skin contact, 132, 275
sleep
    benefits of, 147
    and brain, 137, 147, 148
    and circulatory system, 209
    and depression, 138
    and dreams, 148
    environment for, 158
    Factoid about, 140
    and feeding your baby, 258
    of fetus, 140
    in first month after delivery, 261–64, 272
    importance of, 147–49
    managing, 261–64
    and massage, 132
    and medications, 158, 343
    and milestones, 42
    and mother-baby sleeping together, 263–64
    and mother's health, 272
    and naps, 264

normal cycle for, 147–48
position for, 159
and pregnancy plan, 295, 297, 298, 308
and skin-to-skin contact, 275
and stress, 138, 147–49
and vaccinations, 402, 411
YOU Tips about, 158–60, 217
smallpox, 390, 393, 394, 397
smell
and biology of brain, 142
development of, 117, 122–23
Factoid about, 111, 117, 122
and gender, 117
and infections, 204
and milestones, 42
and mother's health, 270
and nausea, 76, 77, 78, 160
and pets, 276
and sickness, 86
and sleep, 263
of vagina, 270, 306
See also nose/nostrils
Smoked Salmon Sandwich (recipe), 353
smoking
and asthma, 197
and baby development, 38
and delivery, 229
and depression, 151
and development of fetus, 98
discussion with doctor about, 300
and feeding your baby, 261
and fertility issues, 383, 386, 387, 388
and formation and function of placenta, 50, 52, 60
guidelines about, 341
and premature birth, 415
and stress, 145
as toxin, 292
and YOU Prepregnancy Plan, 375
Soccer Mom (exercise), 317
sodium, 75, 349. See also specific recipe
sonograms, 301
sorbitol, 215
soy milk, 288
special care nursery, 137
sperm
and biology of pregnancy, 4–5, 23, 24–27

and fertility issues, 382, 383, 384, 386, 387, 388
quantity and quality of, 383, 384
shape of, 386
See also semen
spicy food, 122
spina bifida, 37, 54, 80, 112
Spinach Salad (recipe), 363
spinal cord, 112, 113, 114, 120, 121, 122, 379, 408
spinal epidural, 232
spitting up, 269
spleen, 56
spontaneous abortions. See miscarriages
sprains, 206
startle reflex, 128, 130
stature, 98, 383
stem cells, 245
stepping reflex, 128
sterile water, injections of, 230
steroids, 142, 151, 236, 388, 414
stillbirths, 211, 249
stimulation, 129–31, 246
stools
baby's, 266, 267, 278
mother's, 270, 277
streptococcus, 378, 397
streptomycin, 124, 126
stress
acute, 143–44
and ADHD, 118
and adrenaline, 144, 145, 151
and age, 26
about baby's health, 155
and biology of conception, 26
and body image, 176
and brain, 111, 137, 140–43, 144, 145, 154
and choosing caretakers, 131
chronic, 143–44, 154, 165
and cortisol, 144
and depression, 138, 150, 151
and development, 144
and doulas, 152
effects of, 138–39
and epinephrine, 145
and exercise, 157
Factoid about, 144, 145
of fathers, 371
and feeding your baby, 138, 257
and fertility, 382–83

and formation and function of placenta, 61–62
and genetics, 33
and goal of pregnancy, 8
healthy/positive, 138, 139
and hormones, 145, 165
and hot flashes, 183
and immune system, 61
knowledge about, 137–38, 146, 154, 155
during labor, 157
management of, 8–9, 62, 137–52, 154
managing, 62, 111, 137–52
and massage, 132
for men, 383
mother-daughter, 156–57
negative, 138
new-mommy, 155
nonspecific, 122
overview about, 137–40
and pregnancy plan, 283, 294–99
and premature birth, 61, 137, 144
prevention of, 294–99
prioritizing, 140
professional treatment for, 138
quiz about, 9
science of, 143–46
and sex, 185
and sexual orientation, 145
and sickness, 87
and sleep, 138, 147–49
and soft health issues, 170
and support, 156, 157
and surrogate worriers, 62
web sites about, 62
work, 155–56
and YOU Prepregnancy Plan, 376
YOU Tips about, 108, 154–57
stress test, contraction, 104
stretch marks, 179, 188–89
stretching, 109, 133, 211, 265, 331, 376
stripping the membrane, 240
stroke, 34, 38
strollers, 257, 347
sucking, 42, 116, 127, 128, 246, 253, 414
sudden infant death syndrome (SIDS), 252, 262

ABOUT THE AUTHORS

MICHAEL F. ROIZEN, M.D., is a *New York Times* #1 bestselling author and co-founder and originator of the very popular RealAge.com website. He is chief wellness officer and chair of the Wellness Institute of the Cleveland Clinic and the enforcer of *The Dr. Oz Show.*

MEHMET C. OZ, M.D., is also a *New York Times* #1 bestselling author and Emmy Award–winning host of *The Dr. Oz Show.* He is professor and vice chairman of surgery at New York Presbyterian-Columbia University and the director of the Heart Institute.

The following is an excerpt from the YOU docs' new book, *YOU: Raising Your Child: The Owner's Manual from First Breath to First Grade,* **available now.**

In this book, which covers child health and development from birth to about age five, you're going to learn about cutting-edge research and a variety of developmental approaches. Among all of us on the authorship team, we've had fourteen children, and two of us are pediatricians—including one who's a full-time developmental pediatrician. So we've spent much of our personal and professional lives thinking and caring about the very same issues as you. A lot has changed since the days of Dr. Benjamin Spock—in terms of how the world works, the challenges of parenting that your parents didn't face, and what we've discovered about how a child's mind and body develop. You'll learn that kids are like dolphins (both *ping* their needs to their parents). You'll learn that some of the best parenting lessons are taught by children (they subtly send messages about where their skills, talents, and desires lie).

You'll learn that kids actually learn *more* by doing *less* (cool brain section up ahead!).

You'll learn that children are like mirrors (their brains are, actually), reflecting behavior that you, their caregivers, and other influential people in their lives model.[*] And you'll learn that the most powerful messages you send your kids—from day one all the way up to day 6,574[†]—may involve absolutely no words at all.

We'll teach you about these amazing insights the best way we know how—through biology. Ultimately, all of these lessons do come down to biology, even the ones that you wouldn't necessarily think would, like behavior. After all, we've always believed that explaining "why" can make the "what to do" much, much easier.

Along the way, we're going to ask you to join in a game of pretend, as you assume a metaphorical role as river guide. See, the way we think about child development—and smart parenting—is to imagine a child's journey though life as a boat ride down a long, often unpredictable river. You, as the guide, help control the direction and speed, while your

---

[*] That's actually one of the reasons why children raised in the same family can be so different; not only do you change the way you parent with subsequent children, but also the environment changes as well.

[†] That's eighteen years (including four days for leap years). Add another day if the child is born in 2007, 2011, or 2015.

youngster sits back and takes in everything around him (including watching you, so that he can eventually learn to paddle or steer on his own). This analogy, we hope, will help you understand parenting on several levels:

- ⊃ **Consider the boat that is your child's genetics.** Everyone's is shaped a little bit differently, and that plays a role in how you can navigate the river, but it's hardly the only factor that determines the quality of your trip together.

- ⊃ **Your paddle really serves as your own behaviors, actions, and words.** It helps you steer the boat in terms of where you go and what your passenger sees. You can bring your boat to a standstill, you might crash into a rock and get stuck, you can choose which path (of many) the boat takes, you can go fast when needed and slow down when you need a break. You, for much of the time, are in control. But the biggest lesson of all when it comes to paddling is this: Sometimes you don't need to paddle at all to get where you want to go. In fact, there is such a thing as overpaddling—trying so hard to do right that you actually send your vessel in the wrong direction. Lots of times, you're better off going with the flow. Our mantra: Parent smart, not hard.

- ⊃ **The river represents the environment in which your child lives.** Sometimes there's rough water, and sometimes there's calm water. Sometimes you have a wide river with lots of choices of where to steer a boat and sometimes, in narrow sections, you just have to ride the rapids. The bottom line is that no matter how expert a guide you are, the environment has a bigger impact on you and your youngster's ride together than anything else. One of the great lessons we learn from traveling the river is that the easiest places to travel are the channels that are well worn and well traveled, and you'll encounter windows of opportunity in which to find those easy-to-navigate places. Your child will actually help direct you there.

- ⊃ **Your boat carries all the equipment you'll need.** You have maps to help you predict rough waters ahead ("I want to get a tattoo!" announces your daughter). And you have life vests too, in case you run into some trouble. Both of them come in the various support systems that you already have and will develop en route, including your partner, friends, extended family, doctors, and even the internet, books, and other resources that can help you navigate a river that many before you already have voyaged successfully.

- ⊃ **The destination?** Well, those are all the traits, skills, attitudes, emotions, and behaviors that make up the person your son or daughter eventually becomes. As you can guess by now, your child's destination depends greatly on which path you take, and how you lead the way—not by your words but by your actions. But a big lesson we'll be exploring is that what you want for your child might not be right for her, so it's important that you learn to read her signals and help her go where she naturally wants to go.

➲ **Your ultimate goal as guide is to teach your passenger enough about the river so that she can start to take the helm.** This handing-off process starts very early (think toilet training), and culminates when your passenger has attained all the skills necessary to be her own guide: how to make important decisions, how to be calm and confident in the face of adversity, and how to live a productive, satisfying, independent life. If all goes well, she'll be giving you a ride about two decades from now.

Since you're reading this, chances are that you've already embarked upon your river ride. Think of this book as one of your river maps, helping you plan the itinerary that you will lead you and your child to your desired destination. Two qualities make for exceptional river guides: experience and knowledge. While you may or may not have the experience of parenting, we believe that this book can help you with the second part of that equation. Throughout the book, you'll learn about science and strategies, you'll use the strategies, tools, and tips, and we'll cover all the big topics important to parents, including how to help your child sleep better, how to help your child maintain a healthy weight, how to best treat a fever, and hundreds and hundreds of others. Here's how the book works:

➲ In the first three chapters (as well as throughout the book), we'll concentrate on this whole notion of creating the optimum environment for raising your child—and the things that you can do to maximize your child's potential and happiness. It may seem as if we're dabbling in psychology, but what we're really teaching you is neurology: that is, the science of how the brain best learns and develops. This development relies on the stimuli (environment) that you provide and the healthy habits that you instill from your heart and from the start.

➲ After that, we're going to move into more of the hard-core health and medical concerns that parents have. What do you do if you have trouble breast feeding? Why is your child a picky eater? How do you treat allergies? What do you do if your child is sick? What is that bright red rash on your child's rear end? As doctors and as parents, we know that it's hard to keep the big picture in mind when day-to-day tribulations and health anxieties keep demanding your focus. Your book takes you through the most prevalent childhood health issues and tells you how to diagnose, treat, and prevent them.

○ We'll also provide practical guidance on some decisions and actions you'll have to make and take, such as picking a pediatrician, finding a day care program, child-proofing your home, and installing car seats (80 percent of them are installed in-correctly, so it's vital info).

○ In our signature YOU Tools section, we'll show you kid-friendly ways to keep your offspring in shape, we'll share simple, great-tasting recipes that your whole family will enjoy, and we'll summarize the various points of view about the hotly debated topic of vaccines. First-time parents will find our YOU Tool for newborns espe-cially helpful; there we'll offer info on diapering, feeding, sleeping, bathing, and all the other mysteries of caring for an infant.

○ Our YOU Plan gives an overview of critical developmental milestones you can expect (but not obsess over, please), as well as some tips and tricks that will make the various stages from birth to age five a little bit easier. Think of it as the pocket version of our detailed map—good for a quick glance when you're in a hurry or need a refresher.

○ In our appendix, we'll cover issues that may be important to some of you, such as multiple births, nontraditional families, and a handful of specialized health con-cerns such as autism and attention deficit/hyperactivity disorder, or ADHD.

We know, we know. So exciting, so titillating, so promising that you can't wait to jump right in and devour dozens of pages on the fine art of applying cream to a diaper rash or teaching manners (not to mention the much more big-picture topics.). But before you begin, we want to introduce you to a few high-altitude thoughts about parenting*—the recurrent themes that, while perhaps not front and center every day, should be on your radar screen as you undertake the greatest job in the world.

---

* Did you know that parenting seems to lower your blood pressure? One of the many benefits, for sure.

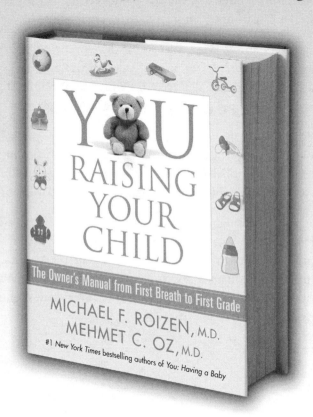
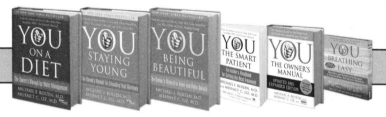